SURGERY
SURGICAL NURSING

Fourth Edition

Selwyn Taylor
DM, MCh, FRCS, Hon. FRCS (Ed), Hon. FCS (SA)

Dean Emeritus, Royal Postgraduate Medical School,
Hammersmith Hospital; lately Surgeon, King's College
Hospital and Belgrave Hospital for Children, London;
Honorary Consultant to the Royal Navy

Madeleine Birchall
SRN, RCNT

Clinical Teacher to the Theatre Course,
Brompton Hospital and Cromwell Hospital, London

HODDER AND STOUGHTON
LONDON SYDNEY AUCKLAND TORONTO

British Library Cataloguing in Publication Data

Taylor, Selwyn
　　Surgery and surgical nursing.—4th ed.—
　　(Modern nursing series)
　　1. Surgical nursing
　　I. Title　II. Birchall, Madeleine　III. Taylor,
　　Selwyn. Principles of surgery and surgical
　　nursing　IV. Series
　　610.73′677　　　　RD99

　　ISBN 0 340 33629 3

Fourth edition 1985

Typeset in 11/12 pt Bembo by
Macmillan India Ltd., Bangalore

Printed and bound in Great Britain
for Hodder and Stoughton Educational
a division of Hodder and Stoughton Ltd.,
Mill Road, Dunton Green, Sevenoaks, Kent,
by Richard Clay (The Chaucer Press) Ltd., Bungay, Suffolk

Editors' Foreword

This well established series of books reflects contemporary nursing and health care practice. It is used by a wide range of nursing, medical and ancillary professions and encompasses titles suitable for different levels of experience from those in training to those who have qualified.

Members of the nursing professions need to be highly informed and to keep critically abreast of demanding changes in attitudes and technology. The series therefore continues to grow with new titles being added to the list and existing titles being updated regularly. Its aim is to promote sound understanding by presenting essential facts clearly and concisely. We hope this will lead to nursing care of the highest standard.

Preface

In the last five years The Nursing Process has probably done more to improve the quality of nursing care and the patient's happiness than any other single factor. What a pity that it first arrived in the UK so heavily disguised in sociological jargon.

In plain English it draws attention to four basic tasks for the nurse in dealing with her patient:

1 To find out about the patient's daily life, habits and background.
2 With 1 in mind to draw up a plan of appropriate nursing care.
3 To put 2 into action with the collaboration of the staff.
4 To evaluate 3 continuously so as to speed the patient's recovery.

In brief, the accent is on nursing and not administration.

However, no nurse can begin to treat a patient's complaints without a broad knowledge of the pattern of disease and trauma, how the tissues respond and what agents are available to assist recovery. This short book sets out to describe these facts in a simple and compact form. The nurse must consult larger textbooks in the library when more information is required. In the new edition the surgical contributor has been joined by a nursing author and we believe this has produced a more balanced text. Much updating has been done, the chapters are regrouped and more space is devoted to pre-operative, theatre and postoperative care. This modestly priced volume is intended to fill the gap between the large and comprehensive work of more than one thousand pages and the short revision book which is used as a pocket reference guide. We have tried to make it interesting and readable, with line drawings rather than photographs for illustrations. For these we are particularly grateful to Jack Bridger Chalker. The aim throughout has been to keep the presentation as concise as possible without loss of clarity.

Selwyn Taylor
Madeleine Birchall

Contents

I

Inflammation, Ulceration and Gangrene

Inflammation

Inflammation is the reaction of the tissues to an injury such as trauma, infection, heat, cold, chemicals or electricity. Infection due to bacteria is, however, by far the commonest cause of inflammation.

Symptoms and signs

The Romans, who knew all about inflammation, summed up the signs and symptoms in four neat little words. They are

rubor,   *calor*,   *tumor* and *dolor*

Rubor is the redness which is seen in the skin overlying an area of inflammation. It is due to the fact that at first there is an increased blood supply to the particular part. Later, when the circulation to the overlying skin becomes slowed, the stagnant blood gives it a purplish colour. This is usually an indication that pus has formed.

Calor or heat is always felt over an area of inflammation, especially when the condition is acute. This is due to the increased flow of blood through the tissues.

Tumor means swelling and is due to the exudation of fluid into the tissues. Later, a swelling may be due to the formation of pus and is called an abscess.

Dolor or pain is always felt where there is inflammation. When inflammation is acute, then the pain is usually of a throbbing nature; if less acute, it may be a dull ache or merely a feeling of discomfort.

The general signs and symptoms of inflammation are the result of the body's attempt to deal with the injury or infection. There is a rise of temperature, which may be minimal when the inflammation is slight or may reach very high levels when the infection is acute or develops suddenly. The pulse rate is raised because the heart has more work to do, pumping a larger amount of blood to the affected area. In addition, the increased action of the heart is an endeavour to rid the body of toxic products.

When the inflammation is severe, there are signs of toxaemia; this means that toxic substances resulting from the breakdown of tissues and bacteria are absorbed by the blood stream. The patient complains of the following symptoms: malaise or a feeling of being unwell, lack of appetite, headache and frequently a feeling of mental depression. When such a toxic patient is examined, it is noted that the skin is hot and dry and the tongue is furred. The urine is excreted in small amounts and is dark in colour because it is concentrated. The patient is dehydrated and is usually constipated.

Pathology

The word pathology, which is derived from the Greek (*pathos*, meaning disease, and *logos*, science of), describes the study of changes which occur in the tissues and the reasons why they take place. When inflammation is present, the reaction of the tissues to an injury which does not destroy them takes the following course.

In the first place the blood vessels supplying the area dilate and more blood, with its component red and white cells, flows to the infected part. This provides additional oxygen, antibodies and other chemical defence substances together with white cells. The increased blood supply produces warmth and redness in the affected area. The blood vessels not only become dilated, but under certain circumstances the finer ones, called capillaries, allow cells to pass through their walls into the surrounding tissues. At the same time some of the fluid part of the blood (serum) also passes out and accumulates in the tissues causing the swelling which is so typically seen in an inflamed area. The white cells, which pass out into the tissues, attempt to destroy and mop up the bacteria. In so doing, many of them die and this collection of dead white cells, tissue fluid and bacteria constitutes pus. The pressure which is exerted by the increase of fluid in the tissues and the presence of pus stimulates the nerve endings to the part and causes pain. When the increased blood flow, or *hyperaemia* as it is called, is severe, the pulsation of the blood vessels may be transmitted to the nerve endings; this explains the throbbing pain which is felt in an infected finger.

Pathology, or the science of disease, becomes daily a more complicated affair and has been divided up by the various specialists who contribute to it. There is the histopathologist, who describes the changes which he sees in pieces of tissues removed from the body, suitably stained and put under the microscope. He is also responsible for the postmortem examination of patients who die from disease or injury. In addition there is the clinical pathologist, who studies the changes occurring in the living patient. He can tell us what deviations from normal take place in the bloodstream, in the urine and so on. There are many other specialized pathologists such as bacteriologists, virologists, immunologists, haematologists and chemical pathologists.

Laboratory tests

White blood cells. The changes in the blood which take place in inflammation are important. The number of white blood cells in 1 cubic millimetre of blood from a normal person is 5000 to 10 000. When inflammation occurs, levels of 15 000 to 50 000 may be obtained. The condition in which there is an increase in the number of circulating white cells is called a *leucocytosis*. It is made up largely of an increase in the *polymorphonuclear leucocytes*; these are the multilobed nucleated white cells which are chiefly responsible for the *phagocytosis* or mopping-up of foreign material. In an overwhelming and possibly fatal infection the white cell count may fall (*leucopenia*), or the polymorphs may disappear (*agranulocytosis*) due to depression of the function of the bone marrow where they are manufactured, by bacterial or chemical toxins. When inflammation occurs deep to the surface of the body, there may be no outward sign of rubor, calor, tumor or dolor, but there will be the general signs and symptoms of toxaemia and the increase in the white cell count will usually give a very good indication of the presence of inflammation.

ESR. There is another test which, while being in no way specific for inflammation, is very useful. It is called the erythrocyte—or red cell—sedimentation rate, usually written ESR or BSR. This is measured by taking a small quantity of a patient's blood, diluting it with a citrate solution so that it does not clot and standing it up in a vertical tube (Fig. 1.2). When inflammation is present, it is found

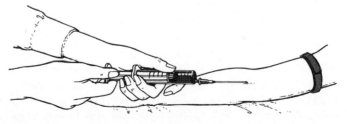

Fig. 1.1 Venepuncture.

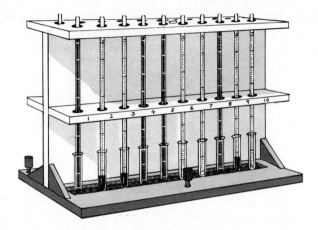

Fig. 1.2 Rack of tubes for determining the blood sedimentation rate, ESR.

that the rate at which the red cells settle to the bottom of the tube is increased. The ESR or BSR is also increased in other conditions so that this test is not diagnostic, but it is a useful one where it is necessary to follow the course of a chronic disease such as rheumatoid arthritis.

End results of inflammation

Inflammation terminates in one of three ways:

1 *Resolution* is what happens when the tissues are not destroyed, return completely to normal and are not affected by pus formation or fibrosis.

2 *Suppuration* or pus formation indicates that there has been death of part of the tissues. This dead tissue, together with the white cells from the bloodstream and bacteria, constitutes pus. A collection of pus is called an *abscess*, and since pus is fluid its presence may be detected when near the surface by the sign of fluctuation. When an abscess distends, the overlying skin becomes purplish in colour, and if it bursts through the surrounding tissues it exposes an infected raw area called an *ulcer*. If tissue in the neighbourhood of an abscess is pressed upon and loses its blood supply it dies and this is called *gangrene*. The dead tissue which comes away from an infected area is called a *slough*. In the case of bone, this process is called *necrosis* and the dead portion is called a *sequestrum*.

3 *Fibrosis.* When cells are destroyed by an inflammatory process, repair takes place by means of fibrous tissue. A scar consists of fibrous tissue and when this overgrows and is heaped up it is described as keloid.

Complications of inflammation

The course which inflammation takes depends largely on two factors, the first is the type of injury to which the tissues are subjected and the second is the resistance which they have to this injury. For example, if a small area on one finger is burnt, the inflammation is likely to be strictly localized. If, however, the area becomes infected with pathogenic bacteria, then the inflammation is likely to spread beyond the tissue actually destroyed. If the type of infecting organism is a staphylococcus, there will probably be a circumscribed abscess containing thick yellow pus. If, on the other hand, the infecting organism is a streptococcus, then it is possible that the area of inflammation will spread much more widely beyond the local injury. A knowledge of the way in which inflammation spreads is important.

Cellulitis. When inflammation spreads widely through the tissues the condition is called cellulitis, because all the cells are involved in the same process. Clinically it is likely to show as a red, tender, brawny affection of the tissues, but without actual pus formation. The type of organism often determines the pattern of inflammation. For example, the streptococcus manufactures enzymes which facilitate the spread of infection widely through the tissues while staphylococci tend to remain localized, producing an abscess containing thick yellow pus.

Lymphangitis. When the inflammatory process spreads by means of the lymphatic channels, it is called lymphangitis. This is seen, for example, when a patient with a severe whitlow on a finger shows a fine red line running up towards the wrist and elbow. These red streaks overlie the lymphatic channels which have become involved by the inflammation.

Adenitis. When the lymph carries the products of inflammation to the regional lymph nodes, the latter become tender and enlarged; this condition is referred to as lymphadenitis. For example, a patient with a whitlow may have tender enlarged axillary lymph nodes which are readily palpable in the armpit.

Bacteraemia. If the resistance of the tissues to the local inflammatory process is not good the infection may spread into the bloodstream. The presence of bacteria in the bloodstream is called bacteraemia and is a serious complication. These bacteria can be detected by the pathologist if he takes some of the blood and cultures it in a nutrient medium such as broth, in an incubator.

Septicaemia. If the organisms which have entered the bloodstream are so virulent that they are able to multiply in the blood, the condition is described as septicaemia. With such a complication the patient will be dangerously ill with a high swinging temperature. Septicaemia indicates that the individual has very poor immunity i.e., resistance to that particular strain of organism.

Pyaemia. When an abscess is present in the body and erodes the wall of a blood vessel, small particles of pus may enter the bloodstream and this is described as pyaemia. These fragments of septic material may lodge in any part of the circulation, but are most likely to be filtered off in the lungs, liver, kidney and brain. If there is not good local resistance in the tissues an abscess will form where the particles of pus are arrested.

Opportunist infection. Rarely, when the body's normal resistance has been diminished by long illness and the administration of many antibiotics, an organism of low virulence, such as the fungus *Aspergillus*, will multiply in the lungs and other tissues and may cause death.

Chronic inflammation

Chronic inflammation is the result of a long-continued mild stimulus which provokes a marked proliferation of the tissues. Chronicity may be the end-result of acute inflammation when some structures develop considerable local resistance, as in osteomyelitis and empyema, or it may be the result of low-grade inflammation from the outset. There are three main groups of conditions causing chronic inflammation:

1   Specific granulomatous infections, of which tuberculosis, syphilis, actinomycosis and leprosy are important.
2   Infection by organisms whose virulence has been diminished by antibiotics, especially when they have been given in inadequate doses.

3 Foreign bodies such as non-absorbable sutures of thread and silk, or particles of silica, which used to be a constituent of glove powder.

Treatment and nursing care

The treatment of inflammation is both general and local: general, in order to improve the patient's general condition and thus his immunity to the inflammatory process; local, in order to speed up recovery from the local inflammatory process and keep it as strictly confined as possible.

General treatment. It is necessary for the patient to rest in bed so that the body's energy may be mobilized to fight the invader. The surroundings should be cheerful, there should be plenty of fresh air without draughts and the patient should be kept warm. Each individual needs help and encouragement to adjust to illness. Reassurance, together with a simple explanation of the process of inflammation, will help the invalid along the road to recovery.

Diet. When the temperature is high and the patient toxic, solid food is usually refused. Under such conditions the digestive powers are severely impaired and a simple fluid diet is indicated. Fresh fruit drinks with glucose provide calories, are refreshing and contain vitamin C. Meat extracts and soups are a source of water and provide some protein, vitamin B and fat. Flavoured milk drinks have all the essential nutrients. Tea and coffee are usually appreciated.

The diet in convalescence should contain well-balanced proportions of the essential food constituents: protein, carbohydrates, fat, mineral salts, vitamins and water, and should usually be of sufficiently high calorific value to supply the bodily needs. The ideal ratio of protein, carbohydrate and fat is of the order of 2 : 2 : 1. It is important that an adequate amount of protein is included as this is necessary for the repair of damaged tissues. Protein may be given in the form of milk, eggs, cheese, fish, poultry, meat and the ubiquitous soya bean. An adequate amount of fibre should also be included since it helps the patient to have a regular bowel motion. Vegetables, salads and fruit together with brown bread are ready sources of fibre. Some patients are used to taking bran with their breakfast cereal.

Intravenous alimentation. When the patient cannot obtain nourishment by mouth or nasogastric tube, it is given intravenously (IV). Indeed if the patient can take nothing orally it is possible to provide complete replacement by an IV infusion. In addition to the saline which is then necessary, sterile containers of glucose solution provide the carbohydrate, amino acids the nitrogen, and it is possible, though not always desirable, to given an emulsified preparation of fat. There are commercial packs which contain a balanced mixture together with sodium, potassium and other essential salts and vitamins. Forced intravenous feeding or hyperalimentation can be of crucial value in patients greatly debilitated by extensive burns or loss from intestinal stomas.

Serving of meals. It is the nurse's responsibility to encourage the patient to take nourishment. Meal times should not be viewed as a chore to be accomplished with haste. No two patients are the same and so an individual approach to preparation of the patient and presentation of the meal is important. Attention to comfort is essential. Toilet facilities should be offered before mealtimes. If the patient is to remain in bed, arrangement of the pillows for comfort and support is necessary. If the patient is able to sit out of bed, this may be preferable.

The way in which meals are served may do much to tempt the patient's appetite. The tray should be clean and set with everything which may be required. Well-planned meals, offering variety, colour and interest, and served attractively will help to promote appetite. The food should be served in small amounts with the offer of more if desired. Hot food should be served hot on hot plates; cold meals on cold plates. The patient should not be rushed through his meal: separate courses should be offered one at a time.

Advice and help from one of the hospital's dieticians in the planning of a patient's meals can be invaluable, and essential for those patients who have special dietary requirements or preferences. Some hospitals have introduced a daily menu to help the patients select their meals in advance; a system which promotes the individual approach to patients whilst also helping to prevent wastage.

Fluid balance. Water is an important constituent of all body tissues; when there is pyrexia, body metabolism is increased and an extra intake of water is essential. It may also help in the excretion of waste products. In health and under ordinary atmospheric conditions, about 800 ml (approximately 30 fluid ounces) of water are lost in the expired air and from the skin daily. The volume of urine passed in twenty-four hours is about 1500 ml (approximately 50 fluid ounces). In order to replace the amount of water lost and provide the daily requirements, about 2.5 to 3 litres (4 to 5 pints) are required. When there is fever an increased amount is lost from the skin and 3 to 3.5 litres (5 to 6 pints) of water should then be taken. Water forms a large part of food, and if the patient is not taking a normal diet a fluid–balance chart may be required to show whether sufficient water is being taken, whether it is drunk or has to be augmented by intravenous infusion.

General hygiene. Attention to personal cleanliness, with particular care of the skin, is of paramount importance in the bed-ridden patient and does much to raise morale. With the increase in sweating, the risk of pressure areas becoming sore is high. A daily blanket bath will be necessary. In some instances where there is a very high temperature and rigor, sponging of the skin and a change of bed linen and bed clothing will be required more often.

Frequent change of the patient's position and use of pressure-relieving aids, such as a ripple mattress and sorbo rings, will help to prevent the development of pressure sores. When the patient is unable to attend to his own oral hygiene, the nurse should offer frequent mouth washes—particularly following meals—or attend to the cleaning of the patient's mouth personally.

Regulation of the bowels. A regular action of the bowels is desirable and in addition to the fibre in the diet, aperients may be required, e.g. liquid paraffin 15 ml with cascara elixir 75 ml; or syrupus sennae 15 to 60 ml.

Relief of pain. Analgesics may be ordered by the surgeon, e.g. aspirin 0.3 to 1 g, paracetamol 500 mg, if the pain is not severe.

Sedation. At night-time it may be necessary for a sedative to be ordered, e.g. Nitrazepam (Mogadon) 5 mg.

Antibiotics

When inflammation is due to invasion by bacteria it may be possible for the pathologist (or bacteriologist) to decide which is the organism responsible. There are available a great number of different chemotherapeutic agents, i.e. chemical substances which destroy or inhibit the growth of certain bacteria, and these may then be given in appropriate doses to the patient. If sulphonamides are taken by mouth, it is necessary to keep up a high level of fluid intake in order that the renal tract does not become blocked by their excretion. In addition, penicillin may be ordered, and, in the case of an adult, will usually be given by intramuscular injection or, in the case of children, may be ordered in rather higher doses by mouth. There are many other antibiotics, and information about these is given in the next chapter.

The administration of antibiotics by intramuscular injection is a frequent task for the nurse. Great care is necessary and an aseptic technique is essential. Disposable sterile syringes and needles are ideal for this purpose; they are produced commercially in clear plastic packs, having been sterilized by gamma irradiation, and everything is thrown away after a single use. When they are not available the syringe and needle are sterilized in an oven by infra-red rays at 180°C (356°F) for 20 minutes or in a high vacuum autoclave at 125°C (275°F) at a pressure of 32 lb per square inch over atmospheric pressure. Boiling syringe and needle in water at 100°C (212°F) for 5 minutes will not kill the spores of bacteria and organisms such as tetanus. Therefore special syringes should be kept for giving intramuscular injections only.

It is advisable for the nurse to wear rubber gloves, disposable where possible, when injecting antibiotics, in order to prevent the development of sensitivity to the drug, which may happen if it contaminates the hands. The cap of the bottle is wiped with spirit or Cetrimide 1 per cent and a volume of air, equal to that of the required dose of the drug, is injected through the rubber cap of the bottle containing the drug. When an ampoule is used the volume must still be checked as ampoules invariably contain an amount in excess of the prescribed dose. The drug is then drawn into the syringe, and in hospital the amount will require to be checked. Any remaining air is expelled from the syringe with the needle still through the rubber cap of the drug bottle. The needle, with syringe attached, is then withdrawn from the bottle, care being taken to support the piston so that no further air enters. Syringe and a new needle are placed on a tray, taking care to prevent the needle coming into contact with the sides of the tray as this may blunt it. The injection and prescription sheet are taken to the patient's bedside where the nurse makes sure that the name on the prescription sheet corresponds with that of the patient and explains about the injection before giving it.

The common sites for intramuscular injections are:

1   Lateral aspect of the thigh.
2   Gluteal region (the patient should lie in the prone position). The buttock is divided into four by two imaginary lines drawn at

right angles (Fig. 1.3). The upper and outer part of the upper and outer quadrant is chosen to avoid the nerve trunks and large blood vessels. Because of this danger, gluteal injection must be carefully sited.

3 Deltoid muscle (when the amount of fluid to be injected is small).

4 Pectoralis major. The patient's arm should be raised to shoulder level when using this site. The needle is thrust through the skin overlying the anterior fold of the axilla.

If frequent injections are given, the site should be changed each time.

The skin over the muscle area chosen is cleaned with an antiseptic, e.g. Cetrimide 1 per cent. The muscle tissue is held between the nurse's finger and thumb and the needle plunged into the tissue almost at right angles, about two-thirds of its length. In very thin people or children it is not necessary to push the needle so far into the tissue, but it is important not to introduce drugs for intramuscular injection into the subcutaneous tissue as they may cause a reaction. The needle should never be pushed in as far as the hilt in case it breaks off for it is then very difficult to extract.

The solution is delivered gently and slowly by applying pressure on the end of the piston. The butt of the needle should be held on to the syringe to prevent it becoming dislodged. The needle is then withdrawn quickly and the skin area massaged with a cotton wool

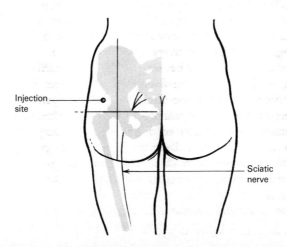

Fig. 1.3 Diagram to illustrate the injection site in the upper outer quadrant of the buttock.

swab for a few minutes to encourage the circulation of the blood to the part and to help deaden any pain.

The nurse should wash the gloved hands under running water, remove the rubber gloves and finally wash again under running water before drying the hands.

Nursing care

Rest may be provided by slings to support the hand and arm, e.g. large arm sling, clove hitch sling. Plaster of Paris bandages are sometimes applied to immobilize a limb and ensure absolute rest to the part. Splints of wood, metal or plastic material may be applied with a bandage so that a limb is kept at rest. When splints or plaster of Paris bandages are applied to an arm it is usual to support the limb by the use of a sling. If the leg is immobilized, the patient may be confined to bed.

It is the nurse's duty to observe that the blood supply to the part is not constricted by pressure. The extremities of the limb should be examined frequently for signs of venous congestion. The patient may complain of numbness of the part or the skin may be cold and appear white or blue in colour. The pressure should be relieved by the nurse if possible or reported to the doctor immediately. In bed the patient is supported comfortably with pillows, the part may also be elevated on pillows which are protected with plastic covers, or by the use of slings attached to a transfusion stand. The elevation of the part encourages venous return and lessens swelling. The lower limbs may be elevated on pillows or canvas slings attached to a Balkan Beam. The use of metal springs is recommended and gentle movements of the supported leg are encouraged both to stimulate the circulation of the blood and to prevent loss of muscle tone.

The free drainage of pus and serum from open wounds should be maintained and it may be desirable to nurse the patient with the inflamed area at a lower level, as in the case of inflammation of the middle ear (otitis media) when the patient should lie on the affected side with the back supported by pillows.

Care of the wound. A discharging wound may require the dressings to be renewed at intervals using aseptic technique. The surgeon may insert a drainage tube to allow the escape of pus and this is left in position until the discharge ceases. The nurse may be instructed to shorten the tube daily as the fluid from the deeper levels escapes; if the drainage tube is not stitched in position it should be turned every day to discourage granulation tissue forming around it. The wound and surrounding skin should be cleaned each time the dressing is renewed and Cetrimide 1 per cent in normal saline may be used. Other lotions which may be ordered include solutions of hypochlorite, e.g. Eusol or the more stable electrolytic hypochlorite, which are diluted half strength with sterile cold water. The hypochlorite solutions have an antiseptic action and also help to dissolve dead tissue. Peroxide of hydrogen should be diluted with cold sterile water and is used for dirty wounds as it helps to separate sloughs. After using hydrogen peroxide the wound should also be cleaned again with normal saline in order to remove any dead tissue and froth. Stronger antiseptics are not often used as they may also cause damage to healthy tissues.

Application of heat. Heat may be applied externally with a hot-water bottle which should be at a temperature of 82 °C or 180 °F and completely protected with a flannel cover. The nurse should watch carefully for any signs of the skin becoming mottled, when the hot-water bottle should be removed. An electric pad may also be used for applying heat, but should not be turned to 'high' and should never be left in position when the patient is sleeping or unconscious. Again, great care must be taken to remove the pad should there be any signs of the skin becoming mottled.

Hot wet packs may be ordered, especially for cellulitis. Generous gauze pads soaked in hot normal saline are applied as hot as they can be borne without blistering the skin and covered with cotton wool to retain the heat. They require frequent, often hourly, renewal. They are not often used because they make tissues soggy.

A further method of applying heat to an open wound is to immerse the inflamed part in hot saline baths 44 °C (110 °F) (some people are unable to stand this temperature and will require it cooler) for 5 to 10 minutes; the addition of fresh solution will be required in order to maintain the correct temperature. Aseptic technique is used and the wound cleaned and dried with cotton wool swabs before the dressing is applied at the completion of the treatment.

An infrared lamp may be employed to give dry heat to an inflamed area. It must never be placed closer than the prescribed distance, and is rarely ordered for more than 15 minutes at a time.

Short-wave diathermy may also be used, and this enables the deeper tissues to be heated; this technique, however, requires elaborate apparatus and the service of someone skilled in its use. The nurse must take great care when applying heat in any form so that the tissues are not burnt. Moist applications of heat are inclined to render the skin soggy and are not often used; the nurse should report to the doctor if the skin appears unduly moist.

Ulceration

A persistent breach in any epithelial surface is called an ulcer. The main causes can be grouped as follows; often more than one cause operates at the same time:

1 *Physical.* Pressure, e.g. bedsore or plaster sore, intense heat, cold, friction, chemicals, irradiation.
2 *Infection.* Acute infections, e.g. staphylococcal, may lead to local gangrene and ulcer formation. Chronic infection, e.g. syphilitic gumma, tuberculosis, fungal infection.
3 *Vascular Insufficiency.* Gangrene of skin follows arterial thrombosis secondary to atherosclerosis. Varicose veins and the sequelae of thrombosis of the deep veins of the legs are particularly prone to produce leg ulcers because of the waterlogging of tissues which accompanies venous stagnation leading to impaired nutrition of the skin.
4 *Sensory Loss.* Deficient sensation, e.g. as occurs in the peripheral neuropathy of diabetes, allows the individual to sustain injury without pain, and ulceration follows. Trophic ulcers on the sole of the foot arise because of anaesthesia of the overlying skin.

It is convenient to consider ulceration as passing through three stages. The first is *extension*, in which there is active destruction of the epithelium, e.g. bursting of an abscess. Discharge is copious, the floor of the ulcer is shaggy and there is a zone of acutely inflamed tissue surrounding it. In the second or *chronic* stage sloughs separate from the base of the ulcer, which becomes adherent to nearby structures, there is little discharge and the surrounding skin becomes fibrotic and often pigmented. The third stage is that of repair, the base of the ulcer becomes covered by velvety vascular granulations, the edge shelves and becomes less well-defined as the epithelium grows in.

Treatment

The treatment of any ulcer, acute or chronic, depends on finding the cause and dealing with it. Local treatment includes dressings, dealing with infection, discharge and sloughs, and measures to aid or speed healing such as rest in bed, splintage and supportive bandaging. On the whole, antibiotics are of little value in clearing up the infection on the surface of an ulcer, except in specific infections such as tuberculosis. If one type of organism is cleared from an ulcerated surface another type will usually replace it, frequently one resistant to the antibiotic used. In addition, skin hypersensitivity to locally applied sulphonamides and antibiotics is common. Mild chemical antiseptics are more useful, such as an aqueous solution of 1 per cent gentian violet or acriflavine 1 : 1000 solution. If there is a profuse discharge an antibiotic aerosol spray containing neomycin, bacitracin and polymyxin (polybactrin) is very useful in drying it up. The aim should be to make the surface of the ulcer clean and dry. Sloughs are usefully removed by gauze dressings soaked in half-strength hypochlorite solution (Milton). Adhesion of dressings is prevented by the application of special gauze impregnated with silicone (non-adherent dressings). Elevation of the limb and application of pressure dressings remove oedema. Some ulcers will heal if the cause is removed, rest provided and infection curbed. In some the defect is so great as to require plastic procedures, such as skin grafting, to speed healing.

Gangrene

Death of a portion of tissue large enough to be seen by the naked eye is called gangrene. Smaller groups of dead cells are referred to as *necrosis*. The piece of dead tissues is called a *slough* which, after separation, leaves an ulcer; so many of the causes of gangrene are the causes of ulceration. Gangrene is the term more often used to describe death of tissue from arterial occlusion. Gas gangrene is due to anaerobic infection (see next chapter); severe physical trauma, burns, frostbite and prolonged immersion in cold water may be followed by gangrene. *Diabetic gangrene* may be due to arterial disease, neuritis or infection or to a combination of these factors. Chemicals such as phenol, strong acids or alkalis may destroy skin, causing gangrene.

The terms 'wet' and 'dry' gangrene are more of historic than practical interest. The appearance of a limb affected by gangrene depends upon the amount of fluid present in it at the time of onset of the disease or injury, the speed of change and the incidence of infection. Where both veins and arteries become blocked by thrombosis it is possible for the limb to swell with oedema and also show gangrenous changes. Venous gangrene is a condition in which the veins of the leg alone become obstructed by thrombosis, producing gross swelling and death of tissue.

In dry gangrene typically a digit becomes shrunken and blackened and, so long as infection does not occur, the dead part may fall off to leave a slowly healing ulcer. The line of demarcation which delineates the gangrene is due to granulation tissue forming where the dead and living tissues join.

In wet gangrene more extensive necrosis occurs, allowing spreading cellulitis and infection with severe toxaemia.

When gangrene of the foot threatens, an emergency operation may be undertaken on the arteries supplying the lower limb in order to improve the blood supply (Chapter 19).

2
Infection, Immunity and Cross-infection

Infection

Infection is the entry of micro-organisms into the tissues of the body. These micro-organisms are most commonly bacteria, but may also be larger unicellular organisms such as the protozoa and moulds, or the smallest of all infectious agents, the viruses.

Micro-organisms or bacteria are to be found everywhere, in the air which we breathe, on our skin or on the objects around us which we touch. They are often classified according to their various characteristics; for example, if they are capable of growing on dead tissue they are called *saprophytes*, if on living tissue, *parasites*. Many are capable of both these faculties, for example *Escherichia coli* (*E. coli* or *B. coli*).

Historical background

It is usual to think of the modern study of micro-organisms as having started with the work of Louis Pasteur, who was commissioned to investigate the fermentation of wine and discovered that there existed on the skin of the grapes micro-organisms which we know as yeasts; these are capable of growing in the crushed grapes and converting the sugar to alcohol and carbon dioxide. He found that if sugar solutions were placed in vessels into which the spores could not gain access, no fermentation took place. It was an understanding of Pasteur's work in France which led Lister in Great Britain to appreciate that bacteria cause infection in wounds and in the body generally. It was he who propounded in 1867 the principles of wound infection, how the causative organisms could be identified and, finally, how they could be destroyed with antiseptics.

When micro-organisms enter the body and multiply rapidly, we speak of acute infection. When they invade the body but multiply only slowly, the infection is described as chronic; many acute infections later become chronic. Various attempts have been made to classify the bacteria which are harmful to man, and the most usual way is according to their shape. For example, spherical bacteria are called cocci, examples of which are *staphylococci, streptococci* and *pneumococci*. Rod-shaped organisms are called bacilli, such as *tubercle, typhoid* and *tetanus* bacilli. There are also other shapes such as spirilla, which are corkscrew-like in appearance, the *treponema* of *syphilis* is an example of this.

Portal of entry

Micro-organisms enter the body by various routes. Inhalation enables entry of bacilli causing whooping-cough and tuberculosis. Swallowing may allow the ingestion of the bacteria of typhoid fever. The skin when cut or abraded allows all manner of organisms to enter, but especially the staphylococcus and the streptococcus. Direct contact may be the portal of entry for some organisms, as in venereal disease. Viruses enter by all these routes, for example the virus which causes hepatitis can be taken in contaminated food.

Toxaemia

When bacteria have gained entrance to the body and started growing, they produce the changes described in the previous chapter on inflammation. At the same time the organisms are capable of manufacturing *toxins*, which are substances poisonous to the tissues. These toxins are usually subdivided into *exotoxins* and *endotoxins*. Exotoxins are noxious substances which are secreted by the bacteria and therefore enter the body tissues; endotoxins are poisonous substances which exist within the bacteria themselves and are only released by the disruption of those bacteria.

The presence of these toxins in the bloodstream causes the patient to feel generally unwell. It is usually easy for the nurse to recognise this because the patient appears listless and seems to have no energy. The skin loses its healthy glow, becoming sallow or even greyish. The patient may complain of a headache and aching pains in the back and limbs. Rigors (sudden chill with uncontrollable shivering) may occur. The reaction to this feeling of illness may be manifested by irritability and this is particularly so in children. There is anorexia and sometimes vomiting may occur. The kidneys are liable to be affected by the toxins so that the urinary output is lessened and albumin is present in the urine. Toxins may attack any organ in the body, while the infection itself remains localized. This is seen if a wound is infected with tetanus bacilli, when the liberated toxins may pass to the motor nerves of muscles causing stiffness and later spasm. Often the jaw muscles are the first to be affected; hence the descriptive name of lockjaw.

Nursing care in toxaemia

The treatment of a patient with toxic absorption will aim to help the body tissues to overcome the infection. Rest in bed is essential and sleep should be induced by making the patient comfortable. The sickroom must be well ventilated as fresh air is important. The patient should be encouraged to drink fluids in order to help the kidneys to excrete the toxins. A well-balanced diet, containing fresh fruit and vegetables, will be necessary. A gentle laxative such as liquid paraffin 15 ml with cascara elixir 7.5 ml or liquid paraffin emulsion 15−30 ml may be required.

Rigors. A rigor is a frightening occurrence, especially when experienced for the first time, and a nurse can do much to allay the patient's fear and anxiety by remaining with the patient and reassuring him that what he is undergoing is due to a normal bodily response to infection.

A rigor passes through three stages and the nurse, by recognising the signs of each, can take the appropriate action. During the first stage, the temperature rises, and the patient shivers uncontrollably and complains of feeling cold, is often nauseated and vomits, and complains of severe headache. The addition of warm blankets at this point will help to increase the comfort of the patient. When the second stage begins the patient complains of feeling hot and becomes restless and possibly delirious, although the temperature may still be rising. The blankets may be gradually removed. In the third stage, with the onset of heavy sweating, the temperature falls. During this stage the patient can be made more comfortable by sponging the skin, the nurse taking care not to allow the patient to become too chilled. As the rigor passes and sweating stops, the patient will require a change of bed linen and clothing and is allowed to sleep, since a rigor is commonly followed by a feeling of exhaustion.

Throughout the rigor, the pulse rate and temperature of the patient should be taken and recorded at regular intervals.

General hygiene. The care of the mouth is important and this should be kept fresh with mouth washes or cleaning at regular intervals as necessary. A daily blanket bath will be required and care of pressure areas must be given routinely while the condition persists.

Patients who are feeling ill, and toxic patients often feel very ill, need sympathy and understanding, therefore it is important for the nurse to have patience and exercise tact when looking after them.

Vaccination

It was Jenner who first noticed that dairy maids who had contracted a condition called *cowpox* were immune to *smallpox*, a disease which in the past used to kill or scar a great number of people in this country and all over the world. He discovered that cowpox was a very similar disease to smallpox but that cowpox, or vaccinia as its Latin name is, was a mild condition which evoked in the body the production of antibodies which were equally effective against smallpox. Thus if a patient is infected with vaccinia, or vaccinated, he has conferred on him by that very mild disease an immunity to smallpox. In like manner a patient can be given a vaccine prepared from dead bacteria, which, while not producing an attack of the disease, confers immunity by exciting the body's response to the toxins in those bacteria. Injections against typhoid are of this type.

Immunity

Immunity is the resistance of the body or its constituent tissues to invasion, especially by disease-producing micro-organisms. It is convenient to think of the body's defences against infection as being of two kinds. First, there are the white cells or leucocytes and it is the polymorphs which are mobilised first, so that the blood shows a rise in the total number of leucocytes from around 10 000 to 15 000 or much higher and the percentage of polymorphs goes up from around 60 per cent to 75 per cent or more. Second, there are the antibodies, which are gammaglobulins manufactured in the lymphocytes and lymphoid tissue (e.g. lymph nodes) in response to a specific antigen e.g. tetanus or chickenpox; there are therefore many different antibodies.

Immunity to infection may be general or specific, i.e. one patient may have greater resistance to infections as a whole than another. On the other hand, a patient may have a resistance to some particular form of infection. Some individuals possess a *natural immunity* to certain diseases, for example a baby is born with the mother's immunity and so it is very rare for the common infectious diseases like measles and chickenpox to be contracted during the first year of life. Most of us can recall acquaintances who have never developed an attack of mumps or chickenpox and yet they must have been exposed to this infection on many occasions. Natural immunity is inborn in such people.

Acquired immunity

This is immunity in an individual which may either develop as a result of an attack by a certain infection, or be conferred on him by some artificial means such as those described below. A good example of acquired immunity is the child who develops an attack of measles and is then resistant to that particular infection for the rest of his life. On the other hand, the person who has had chickenpox as a young child may in old age once more develop a mild attack of the disease, having lost the immunity which was acquired as the result of the first attack.

Increasing immunity

There are methods of artificially giving an individual some degree of immunity to certain organisms. The two main ways of doing this are as follows:

1   If the organisms which produce a disease such as typhoid fever are taken and destroyed and then a suspension of the dead bacteria is injected into a human being, its presence will call forth the defensive mechanisms of the body and produce immunity which may last for months or years. The patient runs no risk of developing the infection from the injection since the organisms have been destroyed, but the defence mechanism called forth gives them immunity to that disease and protects them should they swallow live typhoid bacilli.

2   The second method of inducing immunity in an individual requires the intermediate use of an animal. If into this animal is injected a small quantity of bacteria which produce a particular disease and if there are not sufficient numbers of that bacteria to cause more than a mild attack of the disease, then the defensive powers of the animal are called forth and the serum eventually contains an increasing quantity of immune bodies. The animal usually used is a horse, and the serum is obtained by taking a small quantity of blood from the horse and removing the red cells. The

serum can then be injected into a patient and such a technique is used
for protecting an individual against diphtheria. It has, however, to
be remembered that these techniques are not without danger. Some
individuals are particularly sensitive to the injection of serum and
may become severely shocked, a condition call *anaphylaxis*. This
condition is usually treated by the immediate injection of adrenalin.
Such a reaction to serum can be avoided if a minute dose is injected
first and a watch kept for any untoward symptoms before the rest of
the injection is made.

If immediate protection is required, for example in a patient with
a wound which may be infected with tetanus, the ideal treatment is
to give concentrated antibodies, which are injected in the form of
gammaglobulin. This preparation is, however, expensive and
though affording immediate protection it will only last for a short
time. Such immunity is *passive* as opposed to the *active* immunity
obtained by injecting dead bacteria and waiting for the individual to
manufacture his own antibodies.

To *summarize* then, immunity may be general or specific: this
specific form may be natural or acquired, and the acquired form
may be active or passive. This can be expressed diagrammatically as
follows:

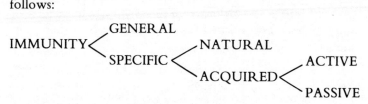

It is convenient at this stage to mention some of the commoner
acute chronic infections which may attack the body.

Acute infections

Staphylococcus aureus. This is one of the commonest causes of
acute infection in the body and is the organism seen in boils,
carbuncles and abscesses and frequently in acute osteomyelitis. The
pus formed is thick and yellow and causes such a reaction in the
tissues of the body that a membrane is formed around it (*pyogenic
membrane*) which limits the spread of infection.

Streptococcus. This organism is the cause of many sore throats,
tonsillitis and diseases of the middle ear. It also infects the lungs and
may invade open wounds. The pus produced is usually thin and

watery and the inflammatory process spreads widely in the tissues rarely forming a pyogenic membrane.

Clostridium welchii. This organism, one of a group of six, is the most frequent producer of gas gangrene, it is an anaerobe, which means that it is unable to multiply in the presence of oxygen. For this reason it usually starts multiplying in dead tissues, which, of course, are deprived of oxygen. The pus it produces has a particularly foul smell. The organisms are capable of producing spores which are singularly resistant to the usual forms of sterilization. The spores are typically found in woollen clothing and the soil.

Tetanus. The bacillus causing this disease, which is often called *lockjaw*, is an organism which develops in wounds contaminated by soil or occasionally clothing. The spores, which are the resting form of the organisms, are peculiarly resistant to antiseptics and heat. The typical symptoms of the disease are produced by the toxin of the organism entering the central nervous system and causing uncontrollable spasms. The incubation period of tetanus may be a long one, and the longer it is, the better is the prognosis.

Escherichia coli. This organism is normally found in the large bowel, but often escapes from there and causes infection in the urinary tract or in other sites in the body. It produces a distinctive fishy odour in the urine.

Pneumococcus. This typically infects the lungs, where it produces pneumonia. The organism is also found in other sites in the body and may infect any part of the respiratory tract.

Neisseria. The gonococcus causes infection (gonorrhoea), which is transmitted by sexual contact with infected persons. It causes *urethritis* and a urethral discharge in men and *salpingitis* in women.

Chronic infections

Chronic infections are often described as *granulomatous* because the progress of the infection is slow and accompanied by the production of much granulation tissue. Good examples are *tuberculosis, actinomycosis, syphilis* and *leprosy*.

Tuberculosis. The organism of tuberculosis is very resistant to antiseptics and may exist in a dried form for many months or years.

The development of the disease is dependent on the bacteria finding a suitable site in which to grow.

Actinomycosis. This disease is produced by the *ray-fungus* and the pus formed contains small yellow sulphur-like granules. The disease may occur in the neck, the lower small bowel or about the skin of the hands and is characteristically very chronic and accompanied by massive induration.

Syphilis. Syphilis is a venereal disease caused by *Treponema pallidum*, which is a spiral-shaped organism usually passed from one individual to another during sexual intercourse. For this reason the primary lesion of the disease is typically seen on the genitals, penis or vulva, where it takes the form of an ulcer with raised edges and considerable oedema, called a *chancre*. Occasionally a baby is born with the infection; this is called *congenital syphilis*, and if the child survives the following signs may be seen: lack of development of the hair and nails, a depressed nasal bridge with snuffles and a prominence of the frontal and parietal skull bones. In the adult the chancre is seen usually about 3 to 6 weeks after the primary infection has been contracted. The regional lymph nodes are frequently enlarged, and it is possible to demonstrate the organisms in the ulcer. After a few months the *secondary stage* of the disease appears. This takes the form of a mild fever with weakness and malaise, a sore throat and fleeting pains in the bones and joints. A rash appears all over the skin of the trunk; it is of a coppery brown colour. Finally, after a number of years the *tertiary stage* appears and can take many forms. There may be local areas of swelling and induration which tend to break down and ulcerate, these are called *gummas*. In addition, tertiary syphilis may attack blood vessels and the valves of the heart and typically produces lesions of the aortic valves and aneurysm of the aorta. When it affects the central nervous system a condition known as *general paralysis of the insane* occurs, which is often heralded by delusions of grandeur.

Antisepsis

A knowledge of the way in which micro-organisms are responsible for the infection of wounds and of the body generally, led Lord Lister to evolve a method of controlling this infection. He discovered that carbolic acid (phenol) was very potent in destroying bacteria, although in addition it destroyed, to some extent, the tissues with which it came in contact. He used this antiseptic, carbolic acid, to prepare or, as it used to be called, 'purify' the patient's skin and his hands before carrying out a surgical operation. In addition, when there was a carbolic spray in the operating theatre, he was able to open body and joint cavities and close them again, after which healing took place by first intention, that is, without suppuration. This was because the carbolic destroyed the organisms which are present in the air, especially in hospitals.

Antiseptic surgery. Previously it had been usual for most wounds to become infected, and so welcome was the sight of pus in such a wound, since it indicated that the body had mobilized its usual resources to deal with the infection, that it was frequently called *laudable pus*. Lister's introduction of the *antiseptic technique* heralded revolutionary changes and opened up the way for the enormous advances that surgery was to make in the next 50 years.

Aseptic surgery. It was apparent that it would be an even greater advance if, instead of killing the bacteria which had entered the wound, a technique was devised which prevented the bacteria from coming in contact with the tissues at all. Such a method is referred to as *aseptic surgery*, and today it is in common usage.

Ideally all patients due to undergo surgery are bathed immediately prior to receiving premedication, and the part of the body to be operated upon is shaved. In the operating theatre the site of the incision is prepared with an antiseptic solution such as Cetrimide in spirit or tincture of iodine, and sterile drapes are placed over the patient around the area to be operated on. All theatre personnel are attired in theatre clothing including special footwear and headwear. The surgeon and his assistants scrub their hands and wash their forearms with antiseptic soap solution and wear sterile gowns and gloves. All personnel in theatre wear a face-mask.

All instrumentation used is sterilized, as are the sutures, drains and wound dressings.

Such a technique allows the tissues to be freely exposed by the surgeon's knife and yet heal by first intention. In fact, if infection does take place after an operation under such conditions, it is necessary to investigate the procedure very thoroughly to find where the fault lies.

The surgery of infection

The use of antibiotics has removed most of the fears of infection. Septicaemia and pyaemia are rare today and when they do occur can usually be treated successfully. The surgeon, however, still has an important role to play in deciding when antibiotics should be used, which antibiotic is likely to be effective, when it should be abandoned and also when to drain for pus. It should be more widely known that not all infections require antibiotics and that although they can sterilize abscesses the pus has still to be evacuated, because it cannot be absorbed and unless drained will usually come to the surface and discharge spontaneously. One of the main disadvantages of using antibiotics is that they may be only partially successful and thus the infection is damped down but not rendered completely inactive. Thus a low-grade inflammation persists and this will encourage the formation of vascular granulation tissue and the whole disease process is made more chronic than it need be. In this way antibiotics can be abused as well as used.

The most important indication for using antibiotics is cellulitis, that is, inflammation spreading in the tissues, which may resolve or go on to pus formation. Cellulitis can be associated with lymphangitis and lymphadenitis and it is in these conditions that chemotherapy can be so successful.

Acute abscesses. An acute abscess is a collection of pus surrounded by a zone of inflammation. Most abscesses tend to enlarge along the tissue planes because these offer the least line of resistance. In some tissues and especially the breast, the abscess cavity becomes loculated and if only one part of it is drained the rest will continue to give trouble. The reason for delay in healing in some abscesses is that the walls have become too rigid to contract, as in bone, there may be a foreign body present such as a non-absorbable suture, or there may be some other underlying disease such as neoplasm.

An abscess causes throbbing pain and overlying it will be a brawny swelling, tenderness and oedema. When pus forms, fluctuation can be elicited if it is near the surface. There is fever and leucocytosis, 15 000 to 40 000 white cells per mm^3. As soon as the surgeon diagnoses that pus is present he arranges to drain it. An incision is made over the site of maximum tension, all the loculi within are broken down to leave a single cavity and then when the pus has been mopped out and some of it sent to the laboratory for bacteriological examination, a drainage tube or tubes are inserted.

Chronic abscesses. This type of abscess also contains pus but often there is little evidence of inflammation around it. Tuberculosis is one of the organisms which causes a very low-grade type of inflammation and the abscess so formed is referred to as a *cold abscess*. In this type of infection there is no urgent need for drainage and it is more important to diagnose what the organism is and then give the specific chemotherapy for it. A *sinus* is a narrow track, blind at one end, lined by granulation tissue. It usually leads from an abscess cavity to the skin or some other body surface. A *fistula* is a narrow track which joins two epithelial surfaces, e.g. fistula-in-ano, which joins the anal canal to the skin in the perineum. The causes of sinus and fistula are similar: the continuous passage of secretions and pus and the eventual epithelialization of the lining all prevent spontaneous closure.

Chemotherapy

Sulphonamides. This group of drugs exerts its action mainly by inhibiting the growth of susceptible organisms and it is therefore correct to describe the sulphonamides as bacteriostatic. There are a great many sulphonamides in general use, each having been evolved for its action against certain types of bacteria. The main disadvantage of these drugs is their toxicity which manifests itself in three ways: *anuria* due to blockage of the renal tubules by crystals of the drug; a rash accompanied by *fever*, the whole condition resembling measles; depression of the polymorphonuclear leucocytes to produce *agranulocytosis*. Therefore patients taking these drugs are encouraged to drink plenty of fluids to prevent blockage in the tubules of the kidneys and are warned to stop taking the tablets and report to their doctor if they develop a sore throat and feel feverish, since these are usually the first signs of agranulocytosis.

Penicillin. In 1925 Alexander Fleming noticed that one of the culture plates in his laboratory, upon which staphylococci were growing, showed inhibition of growth where there had been contamination by the mould *Penicillium*. In 1940 Howard Florey and his colleagues at Oxford, with the support of Lord Nuffield, directed their energies to make penicillin, which then became available for injection into human beings. Penicillin was thus the first antibiotic to be used on a wide scale and it is remarkable how few complications it produces. Penicillin still remains the safest of all this group of substances and this is also true for the newer penicillinase-tolerant pencillins. Some patients become hypersensitive and develop troublesome skin rashes. Sensitivity is common in nurses giving injections of penicillin and therefore they should always use rubber gloves when making up or giving such injections.

Table 2.1 shows many of the commoner antibiotics at present in

Table 2.1

Infecting agent	First choice of antibiotic	Alternatives
Staphylococcus		
non-penicillinase-producing	Penicillin	Cephalosporin
		Vancomycin
penicillinase-producing	Ampicillin	Cloxacillin
Streptococcus		
haemolytic	Penicillin	Erythromycin
'faecalis'	Ampicillin	Cloxacillin
Esch. coli	Sulphonamide	
urinary	and Trimethoprin	Ampicillin
non-urinary	Gentamycin	Kanamycin
		Cephalosporin
Pseudomonas	Gentamycin with Carbenicillin	Polymyxin
Proteus	Ampicillin	Chloramphenicol
	Kanamycin	Tobramycin

use against infecting micro-organisms. This list of antibiotics is always being added to. In addition to the untoward effects of sulphonamides and penicillin mentioned above it should be added that almost all antibiotics may produce depression of the bone marrow with occasionally fatal results. Chloramphenicol if given in repeated courses to children is especially liable to produce destruction of the marrow with a fatal outcome. In addition, all the broad-spectrum antibiotics taken by mouth reduce the number of organisms in the bowel and this can lead to nausea, vomiting and diarrhoea. Occasionally the diarrhoea changes to a fulminating enterocolitis which is due to an antibiotic-resistant staphylococcus and may kill the patient.

Cross-infection

Sepsis due to cross-infection has become a major problem in surgical wards and an infection arising in clean surgical wounds may lead to a prolonged stay in hospital, danger to other patients and even, rarely, death. 'Clean operations' are those in which infection should not happen, for example hernia operations. Where control of sepsis in hospital is good the incidence of infection in such clean wounds should be no more than 2 to 5 per cent. It is of course not always easy to define wound sepsis; often there may be a little redness around a wound and the patient leaves the hospital only to return to the outpatient department a week or two later discharging pus.

The increase in hospital sepsis has arisen because of increasing reliance on antibiotics and slackening of standards of sterility in the ward and operating theatre. In addition, in the last twenty years there has been an ever increasing load of surgical operations performed in hospitals which were built for much less busy conditions. When antibiotics were first introduced they worked with an almost magical effect, but as the sensitive organisms were killed off, resistant strains developed, especially in hospitals, and thus new and far more difficult infections are now the rule.

A striking example of the way in which nasal carriage of staphylococci spreads in hospital is its incidence in nurses in training. Only 20 per cent of nurses entering a preliminary training school from civilian life carry staphylococci in their noses, but after three months in hospital the incidence rises to 80 per cent and a high percentage of the organisms are resistant to both penicillin and tetracycline. Clearly it is impossible to eliminate these, but it is important to have careful sterilizing procedures and wound care both in ward and operating theatre so that wound infection does not occur. The spread of infection in a hospital is a vast problem, it will be considered here under the following six headings.

1 The patient
2 The patient's attendants
3 Central sterile supply department (CSSD)
4 Operating theatre
5 The wards
6 Control of infection.

The patient. Patients may bring infection into hospital, this is more likely if they have been in hospital before. A cough producing virulent organisms in the sputum is particularly suspect and the patient should be isolated. Extensive skin preparation is not usually carried out before operation and most surgeons accept a moderately wide shaving of the area and a shower or bath with soap containing hexachlorophene. If boils are present, operation should be delayed.

The patient's attendants. No nurse or doctor who has an active cutaneous infection like a boil or pimple should attend a patient. Before any kind of handling of dressings or wounds the hands should be thoroughly washed with a soap containing hexachlorophene to reduce the number of organisms on the skin. It must be remembered that it is not effective in much depth and that the reduction is quite short lived. If greater protection is required then rubber gloves must be worn. The commonest mode of cross infection is by contact, so the handling of wounds should be minimized and a non-touch technique should be used for all dressings.

CSSD. Control of infection in hospital has been made easier by the establishment of the Central Sterile Supply Department. In this the dressings, instruments and syringes are sterilized and packed before delivery to the wards. Special packs are prepared for such things as intravenous cutting down, tracheostomy and catheterization. The use of disposable plastic and paper has simplified many procedures. Much of the sterilization is done in hot-air ovens and high-pressure autoclaves. Many of the plastic materials like catheters come straight from the manufacturer enclosed in polyethylene packs sterilized by gamma-radiation.

In recent years it has been discovered that some of the autoclaves used in operating theatres are inefficient and these have been replaced by modern automatic ones.

The operating theatre. It is common practice for all people entering the theatre suite to wear the theatre clothing provided, which includes boots or shoes and a hat and face mask. The majority of patients are taken to theatre on a special trolley and clean blankets are provided for each patient. If a patient is taken to theatre in their own bed, the use of fresh linen is recommended. Clean anaesthetic equipment is used for each patient and sterilized following use.

The ventilation in operating theatres should be filtered humidified air which is introduced at a greater pressure than that of the adjoining rooms so that the flow of air is always outwards from the theatre. Thus infected air from the wards, corridors and lift shafts is not sucked in to the operation area.

The operating theatres should be thoroughly cleaned daily and a regular programme for equipment maintenance and wall washing is recommended.

The wards. One of the major risks in the ward arises when dressings are changed, so this should be kept to a minimum and preferably carried out in a special room properly ventilated and set aside for this purpose. Where this is not possible, wound dressings should be carried out at a suitable time of day; not during bed-making or at meal-times for example. The dressings come pre-packed and sterilized from the CSSD and as far as possible all materials are disposable. Instruments when contaminated are put into paper bags and returned to the CSSD for further cleansing and sterilization.

Dust must be kept to a minimum by using oiling on the floors and vacuum cleaners rather than brooms and dusters. Wollen blankets should be replaced as far as possible with cotton ones which are dust free and can be boiled. All drainage systems should be closed, that is if urine is being collected by catheter it should pass into a bottle which is properly closed from the outside air.

Control of infection. Most hospitals today have a cross-infection committee upon which a bacteriologist and representatives of the medical and nursing staff meet at regular intervals to review the amount of cross-infection occurring and what steps should be taken to control it.

Each ward has its *sepsis book* in which it records any infections that occur in patients while in hospital. The use of the side rooms for isolating patients is controlled by this committee and arrangements made for the proper fumigation and cleaning of rooms and bedding after infected patients are discharged.

3
Shock and Haemorrhage

Shock

Shock is a difficult term to define because it has been applied to so many clinical states including the effects of blood and plasma loss, severe infection, anaphylaxis, adrenal failure and toxaemia. All of these may produce a similar clinical picture with the following features: low blood pressure or hypotension, rapid pulse or tachycardia, pallor, cold sweating extremities, subnormal temperature, rapid respiration, thirst, scanty concentrated urine, restlessness and alertness.

Surgical shock, no matter how it is produced is the result of insufficient blood, and therefore of oxygen, perfusing the cells in the tissues.

Undoubtedly the commonest cause of shock is loss of blood which has taken place rapidly; severe tissue injury such as a fractured femur occurring in a road accident can lead to a very great loss of fluid into the tissues; and the third important cause of shock is burns and scalds. One often reads of somebody receiving a severe shock, associated for example with bad news. This is a different use of the word shock, but in fact nervous factors do enter into the production of shock, and it is known that the individual who is physically tired or exhausted or working under great mental strain is more readily precipitated into a state of shock than a normal healthy person. Painful nervous impulses are an important contributory cause of shock.

Types of shock

The normal adult's blood volume is between 5 and 6 litres although only one litre will be found in the arterial system at any one time. Each heart beat puts out about 80 ml of blood and the systolic pressure in the main arteries is about 120 mm Hg. On the venous side pressure falls to a few mmHg and the body is geared to maintain good tissue perfusion. If arterial pressure falls, the blood vessels in the muscles, splanchnic area and skin contract due to the action of the sympathetic nervous system and the secretion of adrenal hormones, the heart beats faster and its output per beat may rise.

There are thus a number of different ways in which shock can be produced and in order of frequency of occurrence they are as follows, always remembering the likelihood that in any shocked patient probably more than one factor will be responsible.

1 Hypovolaemic (oligaemic) shock is due primarily to loss of blood volume, e.g. severe trauma and burns.
2 Cardiogenic shock occurs with damage to the heart, e.g. myocardial infarction.
3 Neurogenic shock is due to temporary or permanent injury to the nervous system and loss of blood-vessel tone, e.g. spinal anaesthesia.
4 Septic shock results from toxins damaging the capillaries so that fluid enters the tissues, the small vessels are paralysed and the myocardium may suffer, e.g. gram-negative septicaemia.

Symptoms and signs

Despite the fact that shock is a difficult term to define, the picture which it presents can be readily recognized and clearly described.

The patient is anxious and distressed, the face is pale or even greyish and the skin feels cold and moist. The tip of the nose and the lobes of the ears are peculiarly clammy. The pulse is fast and of poor volume and if the blood pressure is measured it is found to be lowered. The respirations may at first be more rapid and are often shallow, but as the patient becomes increasingly shocked, due to lack of circulating blood, so the breathing becomes deeper and eventually may show the phenomenon known as *Cheyne–Stokes* respiration. In this condition the patient takes a number of very deep breaths and this so washes out the carbon dioxide from the circulating blood that the respiratory centre in the medulla loses its stimulus and breathing stops. As carbon dioxide accumulates and its level rises again, breathing is initiated once more and this intermittent pattern of a number of deep breaths followed by a period of arrested breathing, or apnoea, is a bad prognostic sign.

Because there is a great loss of fluid from the effective part of the circulation and possibly from the body as a whole, there is usually marked thirst. Strangely enough this is accompanied, in severe cases, by vomiting and a typical example is the small child who, having suffered widespread scalds or burns, is quite unable to retain any fluid taken by mouth because it is immediately vomited back again. Finally, in its severest form, there is great loss of strength and the muscles may be hypotonic or even relaxed. Eventually, if the blood pressure falls low enough the individual faints, in other words loses consciousness.

Treatment

The first and most important duty of anybody caring for a shocked patient is to *reassure* the individual. There is no doubt that the nervous element in shock is an important one and if the patient's confidence can be gained it will help to break what may become a vicious circle of falling blood pressure and increasing shock. At the same time the patient should be made to *feel warm* with dry warmed blankets and care should be taken not to overheat the bed clothes because then the patient may sweat and lose even more fluid.

The next and by far the most important way of raising the blood pressure and therefore combating shock is to *replace the fluid* lost whether it is blood or plasma, as described above, checking the result by the central venous pressure catheter if it has been inserted. Details of finding the right blood group are described later in this chapter. Suffice it to say now that an intravenous infusion is set up as quickly as possible, usually with Ringer's saline and lactate in the first place, and this is replaced as soon as possible by compatible blood. If the main loss of fluid is plasma, as occurs in burns, then plasma is the right fluid to give. Alternatively dextran, which is a large molecule sugar-like substance, can be given intravenously. New preparations are appearing, recently, hydrolysed starch and a fluid gelatine have been on clinical trial. None should be given until blood has been taken for grouping since the presence of these plasma expanders, as they are called, interferes with this.

When a patient is severely shocked, two major problems arise: how much intravenous fluid to give and how quickly to give it. These questions are usually answered by setting up a central venous pressure catheter. Through a needle in a forearm vein a long nylon catheter is threaded until the tip is in the termination of the inferior vena cava (IVC) or right atrium. A water manometer is connected and the level above the junction of manubrium and sternum should be 2−8 cm of water. The intravenous fluid is then run in through the catheter until the pressure is achieved. A catheter in the IVC allows the fluid to be run in much more quickly than through a peripheral vein. By this time the patient will probably have been transferred to the Intensive Care Unit (ICU) and frequent ($\frac{1}{4}$ and $\frac{1}{2}$ hourly) recording of pulse, blood pressure and respiration rate will be possible. A glance at the chart then gives an excellent idea of progress.

Since the causes of shock are almost always painful ones, e.g. fractures and extensive soft tissue lacerations, the use of a drug which will *relieve pain* may well serve a double purpose, allaying the patient's anxiety and diminishing noxious impulses from the damaged tissues. For these reasons the injection of morphia is perhaps one of the most useful therapeutic measures available. The drug is given according to the age and weight of the patient and the usual dose for a healthy young adult is 15 to 20 mg. It is important that the dose should *not* be repeated if there is no immediate improvement, because it may mean that the peripheral circulation is so sluggish that the drug has not been carried properly into the blood stream and for that reason when the shock begins to wear off, the drug will be absorbed. Morphia is especially beneficial as it is the best of pain relievers and also induces a euphoria, or peace of mind, which is extremely helpful under these conditions.

The use of *oxygen* to relieve cyanosis is greatly helped when the gas is piped to the bed-side, it is only necessary to connect it with some kind of wash-bottle or flow-meter so that the speed of delivery is regulated and the oxygen humidified and then a mask is placed over the nose and mouth. A satisfactory concentration is usually provided by a flow of around 5 litres per minute. It must be remembered that oxygen is a drug and should be administered correctly and with care. Some patients cannot tolerate a mask and then probably the advantage of the oxygen is outweighed by the discomfort it causes, or an oxygen tent must be used. If breathing is still inadequate a tracheostomy is performed and the lungs rhythmically inflated with a respirator such as the Blease.

If septic shock occurs the clinical presentation may be puzzling since the arms and legs often feel warm because toxins paralyse the capillaries, which then dilate. In addition to all the measures described above antibiotics must be given. This will be done by intravenous infusion and a broad spectrum type will be used until the laboratory, as a result of incubating pus or blood culture, can say what is the best drug to use.

Haemorrhage

Haemorrhage is a word derived from the Greek and means loss of blood. It is convenient to distinguish between the kinds of bleeding which occur from different varieties of blood vessels. *Arterial bleeding* is usually bright red in colour, the blood comes in spurts and under pressure and it may be of considerable quantity if the vessel divided is a large one. *Venous bleeding* is usually dark and the blood tends to well up out of the vessel, although the loss can be severe when one of the larger veins is damaged. *Capillary bleeding* is merely an ooze—the sort of bleeding one sees when the skin is abraded by a fall on a rough surface. The blood soon clots under normal conditions and the loss is therefore minimal.

Symptoms and signs

If a patient loses a small quantity of blood he is probably only inconvenienced by it, but if the loss of blood is great in volume and especially if it occurs rapidly, then a state described as shock appears. The patient goes pale and comes out in a cold sweat; this is most noticeable in the lobes of the ears and also the tip of the nose, which become cold and clammy. The blood pressure falls and the pulse rate rises, so that if felt at the wrist it is of low tension and fast. The patient usually complains of thirst and is often restless. If the blood loss is very severe, air hunger may occur. In this condition the patient does not have enough circulating blood to convey oxygen to the brain, so that the respirations are gasping in type. Finally, the loss of blood may be so great that the individual is rendered unconscious or faints.

Under normal circumstances the bleeding comes to an end when the fluid clots, and it is therefore necessary to digress for the moment on the subject of blood clotting.

Clotting and its mechanism

When the tissues are injured, a substance called *thromboplastin* is released from the damaged cells, and activates a substance, called *prothrombin*, circulating in the blood to form a *thrombin*. If enough calcium is present in the blood, a clot or thrombus is formed. A knowledge of these factors helps one to understand how blood is stored for transfusion. If sodium citrate is added to the blood, the calcium is rendered inactive and the blood cannot clot. When blood is taken for transfusion it is usually run into a bottle containing a solution of citrate and the blood remains fluid until it is required for giving to another patient. In addition to prothrombin another substance called *heparin* is also present in the blood and helps to keep it fluid; both of these substances are manufactured in the liver. Thus thrombin assists in the clotting of blood while heparin keeps it in the fluid state. Prothrombin is formed from the vitamin K which is absorbed from the gut in the terminal ileum and thus it may be deficient in patients suffering from malabsorption. When a patient is lacking vitamin K, such as in obstructive jaundice, it may be given by injection so that the blood clots normally. Platelets or thrombocytes also play a part in the arrest of bleeding. Platelets aggregate at a site of injury and release *serotonin*, which causes vasoconstriction. The platelet aggregation forms a plug which is of particular importance in the arrest of capillary bleeding. Fibrinogen is a natural constituent of the plasma, but only changes into fibrin once thrombin is formed.

To simplify:

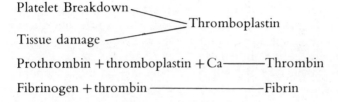

Platelet Breakdown
Tissue damage
Thromboplastin

Prothrombin + thromboplastin + Ca———Thrombin

Fibrinogen + thrombin —————————Fibrin

The above simplified account of blood clotting necessarily omits much detailed and important additions to knowledge in recent years; no less than 13 factors, necessary for normal clotting have now been isolated. Their importance is illustrated by Factor VIII, the antihaemophilia one, which is injected into patients with haemophilia so that they can undergo surgery. An entirely different cause of failure to clot normally is afibrinogenemia—lack of fibrinogen—sometimes due to severe infection and also, rarely, inherited. It is treated by giving freeze-dried fibrinogen.

Anticoagulants. If for some reason it is necessary to hinder clotting or thrombosis in a patient, this can be achieved by giving substances such as *dicoumarol* or *ethyl biscoumacetate* which prevent the liver from manufacturing prothrombin and thus stop the blood from clotting. Dicoumarol was originally discovered because it was noticed that cattle eating spoiled sweet clover sometimes died from a bleeding disease. Research carried out to discover the cause of the bleeding, led to the discovery of a substance like dicoumarol in the spoiled clover.

It is also necessary under certain conditions to prevent the clotting of blood by means which take effect more quickly than is the case with dicoumarol. Under these conditions 5000 to 15 000 international units of *heparin*, which is rapidly destroyed in the body, can be injected into a vein every 4 to 6 hours and the blood prevented from clotting. A substance, *protamine*, when given intravenously, immediately neutralizes heparin.

The term *clotting time* is a useful one as it gives an indication of how long the patient's blood requires to clot. Sometimes the laboratory reports this in the form of *prothrombin time* or a *prothrombin index* relating the patient's blood to what is considered normal. Clotting time must not be confused with *bleeding time*. Prolonged bleeding time is mainly due to an inability of the blood vessels to retract when damaged.

Treatment of blood loss

The treatment of a patient with haemorrhage falls normally into two parts: first aid, which is usually carried out before the patient is moved, and second aid or definitive therapy, which must be done in a doctor's surgery or hospital.

When patients are bleeding or have lost a quantity of blood, the first thing they need, in addition to the bleeding being stopped, is reassurance. They are mentally upset and this anxiety worsens the changes already produced by having lost blood. In addition they are almost certain to be in pain; the drug which is usually prescribed to control the pain and anxiety is morphine. This can only be given when ordered by a medical practitioner, but is one of the most important single factors in treating haemorrhage.

Control of bleeding

Elevation. Venous bleeding can be readily controlled either by elevating the part of the body from which the blood is flowing or by firm pressure applied locally over the bleeding point. So long as the damaged vein is raised to a point higher than the heart, blood will not flow from the wound. A patient with varicose veins who ruptures one of them is immediately laid down and the leg raised to stop the bleeding.

Pressure. A firm pad and bandage will also control venous bleeding. Loss of venous blood can be serious when one of the major veins such as the inferior vena cava is torn at operation.

Tourniquet and pressure points. Control of arterial bleeding is more difficult, and the loss of blood may be serious. Local pressure over the bleeding point may in itself be inadequate and this is usually the case. However, when it is not possible to keep up the pressure manually, a *tourniquet* is employed. This consists of a pad and an adjustable strap which allows pressure to be brought to bear on a limited area. For proper use it has to be applied to one of the limbs because it is not possible to tie a tourniquet on the head or trunk. With a knowledge of anatomy it is possible, in most cases, to apply pressure to the main artery between the injury and the heart. For example, if the bleeding is in the front of the thigh, it is possible to apply firm pressure, which must be maintained, to the femoral artery at the groin and so control the bleeding. Such *pressure points* (Fig. 3.1) are found where large vessels run fairly near to bones because it is by counter pressure on something firm that it is possible to compress an artery. Fig. 3.1 shows the main pressure points in the body and these should be memorized since if they are to be used at all, it will be in an emergency. If a tourniquet is applied, the patient should not be left until medical help arrives. Every 15 minutes the tourniquet should be slacked off and only reapplied if bleeding is severe. If this is not done the tissues will become gangrenous from loss of blood. Usually clotting will seal off a vessel in a comparatively short time and this applies even to large arteries so long as they

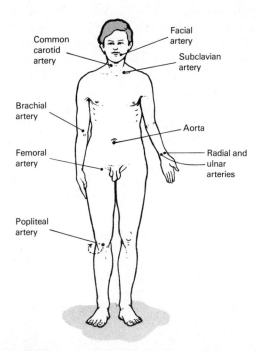

Fig. 3.1 Pressure points.

are not cleanly cut. Any vessel which has been cleanly severed needs to be clamped and tied.

Transfusion

The first-aid measures for controlling haemorrhage have been discussed above, it is now necessary to describe the definitive treatment of haemorrhage. This consists of replacing the blood lost and properly securing the bleeding vessels. The replacement of blood is called *transfusion*; this refers to the original method of giving blood to a patient, which was by transferring it directly from one individual to another. Today this is very rarely done because it is found much more convenient to take the blood from a donor and store it, so that it is ready for immediate use when required by a patient who has lost blood. This is then properly called the *infusion* of blood, but by long usage the term transfusion is still employed.

Blood groups. It is necessary to know whether the blood is suitable for the patient before giving a blood transfusion. The red cells can be divided into four main groups as regards their behaviour when mixed with the serum of another individual. Similarly the serum of the population is divided into four main groups, and a knowledge of these is necessary so as to avoid an incompatible transfusion. When blood is taken from a donor and given to a patient the important factor to consider is the compatibility of the red cells of the donor with the serum of the recipient. In Table 3.1 it will be seen that the international classification of *blood groups* describes four varieties of cell factor; AB, A, B, and O. The serum factor is also shown in the table which thus demonstrates how to determine to what group the cells of a patient belong. It is only necessary to have serum from

Table 3.1

Blood Group	Cells containing antigen:	O	A	B	AB
O	Serum contains antibodies Anti-A, Anti-B	−	+	+	+
A	Anti-B	−	−	+	+
B	Anti-A	−	+	−	+
AB	None	−	−	−	−

Where + = agglutination and − = compatible

the two groups A and B in order to decide the group to which the individual's red cells belong. Should the wrong red cells be given to a recipient, then the cells will *agglutinate*, or aggregate together and form clumps. In the circulation such clumps of red cells cause blockage in the kidneys and other parts of the body, with intense pain in the back, haematuria and eventually coma and, if the transfusion is not stopped in time, death. It is therefore desirable to transfuse a patient with blood of the same group as his own. However, if the correct group is not available, Group O may be given to any of the other three groups—hence its name as the 'universal donor'. A and B may be given to AB but not to O. AB blood can only be given to an AB recipient.

An AB patient can receive blood from any group and is known as the 'universal recipient'.

Rh factor. In recent years many other factors which affect transfusion have been discovered in the blood, one of the most important being called the *Rh Factor*, or rhesus factor. This gets its name from the fact that it was first discovered in certain monkeys of the Rhesus species. In this country about 85 per cent of the population have the Rh factor and their blood is said to the Rh positive, the remaining 15 per cent are said to be Rh negative, but if they are given blood from individuals of the former group, then they can become sensitive to the Rh positive red cells and this may lead to severe reactions. For example, if a mother who is Rh negative has a husband who is Rh positive, she may have a Rh positive baby; because of this induced sensitivity such a baby may be born with anaemia and jaundice, and in order to prevent the baby's death it may be necessary to give an *exchange transfusion*, which means draining off most of the baby's blood at birth and replacing it with Rh negative blood. The Rh negative blood will not be destroyed by the antibodies which have been passed to the baby from the mother. Meanwhile the mother is given an injection of gamma globulin which contains a concentration of antibodies active against the antigen in the baby. By this means she can have a normal pregnancy next time.

Rh positive individuals cannot form rhesus agglutinins, therefore they may receive Rh negative blood, but Rh negative individuals should not be transfused with Rh positive blood.

Stored blood. In this country, blood is usually given voluntarily by donors. The blood is prevented from clotting by adding it to a citrate solution in plastic containers holding approximately

450 ml, called one *unit* of blood; it will keep for at least 28 days if stored in a refrigerator at 4 °C and it can then be used as required. It is most important to check the blood group marked on the container with that of the patient and it is necessary to see that the filter and drip chamber are in proper working order. Blood is given through plastic disposable giving sets, which are less likely to produce febrile reactions or thrombophlebitis than those that were used formerly. Unless the blood is required in extreme urgency it is essential that it should be *cross-matched* with the patient's own serum before transfusion. Aseptic precautions should be observed in order to avoid introducing infection into the patient. In addition, the blood should be allowed to reach room temperature before it is given, but on no account should it be heated by standing it in hot water as this may destroy some of the red cells. Where blood is required to be given in large quantities over a short period of time, special equipment is available in most modern operating theatres and intensive care units for this purpose. If large amounts of cold blood are given too rapidly, they may cause a severe temperature drop and lead to ventricular fibrillation.

Blood preparations. Apart from whole blood, used to treat massive haemorrhage or shock, there are several other preparations of blood components available which allow specific blood replacement therapy. The most commonly used are:

(Packed) *Red Blood Cells.* This is the transfusion of choice to improve haematocrit or haemoglobin level. It is indicated for chronic anaemia or chronic blood loss where anaemia is not accompanied by a significant decrease in blood volume, and where an increase in blood volume is undesirable.

Platelets. Transfusion of platelets is indicated where the platelet count is below 10 000 and for those patients with a bleeding problem whose count is below 20 000, to prevent haemorrhage or provide maintenance.

Plasma protein fraction (PPF), *Haemaccel* and *Dextran 70 in N Saline.* These are plasma volume expanders which are chosen for use whenever plasma is indicated to restore or maintain blood volume in a patient with hypovolaemia without acute blood loss.

Technique. An intravenous needle is inserted through the skin, a plastic cannula passed through it and the needle withdrawn. Veins of the arm are preferred, especially those near the wrist; veins in the leg should be avoided for transfusion, because deep vein thrombosis is a risk and the patient's movements are restricted. If a transfusion must be given rapidly a Martin's pump is clamped to the drip stand. The flow of blood is speeded by the pressure of an eccentric cam rotating and pressing on the tubing of the giving set.

The transfusion may slow down because the infused blood is cold and viscous and the vein goes into spasm. A warm pad over the vein may relieve this. The height of the bag may be raised to increase the head pressure. A transfusion may stop because a haematoma forms or the needle slips out of the vein. Immediately this happens the clip on the tubing should be closed and the doctor sent for.

Care of patient receiving a blood transfusion

The nurse should monitor and record temperature, pulse, blood pressure and respirations at regular intervals throughout the transfusion. The transfusion should be given at the rate ordered by the doctor and all blood should be carefully checked by a trained nurse or doctor, for the correct grouping, name and date of expiry. Cold blood should preferably be warmed before transfusion or transfused through a warming apparatus. The site of infusion should be inspected for any developing soreness, and the infusion resited if the vein becomes sore or blocked. It should be resited in any case every two or three days.

An observant nurse will immediately recognise any signs of transfusion reaction and initiate the appropriate course of action, while remaining calm and not alarming the patient. Some patients receive transfusions over a long period of time and the nurse must be alert to their temporary inability to help themselves with some personal needs, such as washing, brushing their teeth, combing their hair or cutting up their food at meal times.

Reactions to transfusion. These are due to transfusions with blood of the wrong group, transfusion with infected or haemolysed blood, or faulty infusion apparatus. Some patients who have certain blood disorders, e.g. leukaemia, seem to have reactions unexplained by the above reasons.

Signs and symptoms. Transfusion reactions often develop within minutes of the transfusion having started. Fever, with a slight rise in temperature 37.2−37.7°C to severe rigor 40.5−41.1°C, headache, cyanosis, dyspnoea, substernal or low back pain, urticaria may also appear. Complete or partial reduction in urine volume tends to develop later but together with pain in the loins is an important

observation as it may indicate renal damage. Jaundice, which will
not be immediately evident, may follow in a few days if there has
been haemolysis, or in a few months if the serum of the donated
blood contained a virus of hepatitis.

Operative treatment

The proper control of haemorrhage cannot be said to have been
achieved until the bleeding points have been suitably tied off. This
can usually be done only by giving the patient a general anaesthetic
or an injection of local analgesic, cleaning the wound by excising
dead and soiled tissue and finally clamping and tying off the
bleeding vessels with ligatures. Such an operation may be a matter
of great urgency, as when the spleen has been ruptured in a road
accident and the patient is bleeding to death internally, the blood
entering the peritoneal cavity. An ectopic pregnancy may rupture
and cause exsanguination in a similar manner. In such circumstances
it is necessary to give an immediate transfusion of blood and the
patient is then anaesthetized as soon as possible so that the bleeding
may be arrested at operation. It may be possible to collect the blood
from the peritoneal cavity and give it back to the patient.

Special applications

Under certain circumstances special techniques may be necessary to
control bleeding. For example, when a tooth socket continues to
bleed, due to some blood disorder, the local application of adrenalin
1 part in 1000 on a gauze pack may be efficacious. The latter acts by
causing constriction of the small blood vessels and is especially useful
for controlling oozing from a raw surface. Similarly, during surgical
operations, oozing from a wide area may be stopped by the
application of gelatine foam or oxycellulose gauze, both of which
are haemostatic and later absorbed by the tissues. If the patient has
haemophilia an injection of antihaemophiliac globulin (Factor VIII)
is given.

Conditions predisposing to bleeding

Haemophilia. There are various disorders which cause the patient
to lose an excessive amount of blood from what is otherwise a trivial
injury. Haemophilia, which has been mentioned already, is one of
these. It is a rare disease, found almost exclusively in males but it is
handed on by the mother. Even trivial injury may cause a fatal

haemorrhage in a haemophiliac, and often there is bleeding into a joint (*haemarthrosis*), into the bowel, or into the subcutaneous tissues. It is treated with AHG (antihaemophiliac globulin).

Purpura. In purpura there is a lack of platelets in the blood. These tiny cells are necessary for clotting and when their number is diminished from the normal, which is 200–300 thousand per mm^3 of blood, bleeding occurs. There are a number of causes of purpura, some are congenital, others are due to taking toxic drugs and to allergy.

Jaundice. Jaundiced patients show an increased clotting time, and the bleeding from such patients, if they are subjected to operation, may be excessive. In their case, however, it can be suitably controlled by giving vitamin K by mouth or by injection. It is usually necessary to give it by injection because the normal vitamin K produced in the bowel cannot be absorbed in the absence of bile salts.

Types of blood loss

Haemorrhage may be classified according to the site from which blood is lost. The following is a list of some of the terms in common usage:

1 *Epistaxis*, bleeding from the nose.
2 *Haemoptysis*, spitting up of blood from the lungs.
3 *Haematemesis*, blood vomited from the stomach or oesophagus; it often resembles coffee-grounds due to the action of the acid in the stomach.
4 *Haematuria*, blood from the urinary tract which is voided in the urine.

It is the nurse's responsibility to report haemorrhage immediately, so she must be constantly observant of any signs or symptoms of bleeding occurring. *External bleeding* may be obvious, as from an open wound or abrasion, from an orifice such as the nose (epistaxis), the ear or the vagina.

Blood coughed up from the lungs (haemoptysis) appears as bright red froth or is mixed with the sputum. This should be saved for inspection by the surgeon.

Blood which is vomited (haematemesis) may be brown and similar to coffee grounds due to the action of the gastric juices on the blood. If copious, however, the blood may be vomited in an unaltered condition and should always be kept until it has been seen by the surgeon.

Bleeding from the stomach or intestines (melaena) may be present as a dark tarry stool in which the blood has been altered in its passage through the alimentary tract. Medicines containing bismuth, iron or manganese may cause the faeces to appear dark in colour and should not be mistaken for melaena. This is why dark stools must be kept so that they can be tested for blood if necessary. Bleeding from the lower part of the alimentary tract may appear as bright blood in the faeces.

Occult blood is a term used to describe blood from the alimentary tract which is passed in the faeces and is not discernible to the naked eye. Chemical tests may be carried out in the pathological department to prove the presence of occult blood in the stool. A meat-free diet and the exclusion of green vegetables for three days prior to the collection of the specimen of faeces is necessary to enable these tests to be accurate.

Haematuria. Smoky urine may occur with slight bleeding from the urinary tract, while severe bleeding is indicated by a bright red or even dark red colour. It may be possible to note whether the blood appears at the beginning of micturition, the end of micturition or is intimately mixed with the urine. This information helps one to determine from which part of the urinary tract the blood is coming. A specimen of urine may be required for microscopical examination in order to determine the presence of blood cells, this being the most reliable test for haematuria. The nurse may be required to carry out chemical tests for this. After operation on the urinary tract when there is intermittent or continuous drainage from the bladder, it is advisable to save specimens of blood-stained urine at regular intervals, e.g. quarter- or half-hourly, so that the progress of the bleeding may be estimated.

Reactionary haemorrhage may occur after any operation as the blood pressure rises within the first twenty-four hours and the nurse should observe the bandages frequently in case this happens. A bright red stain will be seen if fresh bleeding occurs, while stale blood on the bandages appears brownish. Sometimes there is an ooze of serum through the dressings and this shows as a yellow or slightly blood-stained area.

Secondary haemorrhage, being due to sepsis, occurs about the seventh to tenth day following operation and is usually preceded by a small warning or premonitory bleed. A stain on the bandages at this time may indicate pus, which can give a yellowish stain in staphylococcal infection, or may be mixed with blood to give a brownish colour. Streptococcal infection develops thin watery pus while bacillus pyocyaneus pus has a typical greenish-blue colour. If pus is present there is usually a foul odour. A nurse with a keen sense of smell may find this a great asset as she learns to recognize distinctive odours, e.g. *Bacillus welchii*, haemolytic streptococci, *Bacillus pyocyaneus*.

Internal haemorrhage is something which the nurse should be able to recognize. The patient is *restless* and worried, the skin *pale* and cold and there may be sweating. There is a *rise of pulse rate* which if taken at frequent intervals is found to go on increasing, eventually becoming irregular. The breathing is rapid and gasping in type, the blood pressure low. The patient may complain of thirst and dizziness and typically feels light-headed and cold. If left untreated, collapse follows and the patient becomes unconscious.

Nursing care

The patient must be kept at rest with the head low, and if there is severe external bleeding, first aid should be given urgently to stop the flow of blood. If the bandage is stained, the nurse should cover the area with sterile dressings using an aseptic technique and apply fresh bandages very firmly. A message should be sent to the surgeon indicating the amount of the bleeding and the condition of the patient.

The patient will be frightened, and the nurse must remember that this tends to increase the degree of shock. The nurse's actions should be purposeful and, although quick action is essential, gentle, her attitude should aim to give the patient reassurance. Apparatus for administering oxygen should be brought to the bedside and used if the patient has sighing respirations. When morphia is ordered by the surgeon it is given and in hospital must be checked with the prescription sheet as it is drawn up into the syringe. It is then taken to the bedside and further checked to make sure that the drug is given to the correct patient. If morphia has not already been ordered, the nurse should have the prescription sheet of the patient ready and be prepared to give an injection of morphia as soon as the doctor arrives and writes such instructions.

Preparations should also be made for giving blood, as a transfusion or an infusion of intravenous fluid will almost certainly be called for if the haemorrhage is at all severe.

The nurse's further duties will depend on the course decided by the surgeon. It may involve preparing the patient for the operating theatre, where treatment will be carried out to stop the bleeding. If an anaesthetic is *not* to be given, fluids by mouth should be encouraged, so it is important to find out first if surgery is contemplated. The nursing care not only includes assisting the surgeon, but also giving a careful report and anticipating the patient's requirements if urgent treatment is called for.

4
Fluid and Electrolyte Balance and SI Units

Probably the most important single factor which has made modern surgery safe is a greater knowledge of the fluid and electrolyte requirements of the body together with a proper understanding of the nutritional needs. This knowledge is necessary in order to prepare patients for surgery and also to recognise and correct postoperative deficiencies.

Normal body fluids

The nutritional requirements of the patient who is about to undergo a surgical operation are primarily:

1 Water
2 Salts
3 Carbohydrate
4 Protein
5 Vitamins and iron

Far and away the most important of these are the water and salts because deficiency or excess of either can have disastrous effects. Carbohydrate, protein, vitamins and iron are more important from the long-term point of view and do not require urgent and rapid correction.

The normal healthy adult, who is generally considered to weigh 70 kilograms, contains approximately 60–70 per cent of his body weight in water, the total varying with sex and age. This water is distributed through two main compartments: the *extracellular* fluid, which is made up of the plasma and the fluid between cells, and the *intracellular water*. The partition of water in the human body can be roughly expressed as in Fig. 4.1. Each of the fluid compartments and all the secretions of the body except urine and sweat have the same osmotic pressure even though their composition varies. They are described as being normally isotonic (expressed as N for normal)

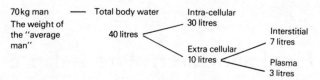

Fig. 4.1 The partition of water in the human body.

and this is osmotically equivalent to a 0.9 per cent solution of saline.

The principal ion which exerts this osmotic pressure in the extracellular fluid is sodium, but chloride and bicarbonate exert a lesser effect. The principal ions in the intracellular fluid are potassium and phosphate. The measurements of the concentration of these salts are expressed in millimoles per litre. The molecular weight of an element is the smallest part into which the element can be divided and moles are used, rather than grams, because ions interact with each other proportionally to their molecular weights and not according to their masses or weight in grams. The amount of salts in the various body fluids are expressed in millimoles rather than moles because amounts measured are so small, a millimole being a thousandth part of a mole.

Acid and base in the body are very carefully balanced by a system of buffers to produce a constant normal reaction, which is expressed as a hydrogen ion concentration or pH of 7.4. These buffers are combinations of a weak acid and base and the most important one in the blood plasma is the bicarbonate. Thus in a diabetic patient, who is unable to metabolize sugar properly, the ketosis which develops is at first buffered in this way. A measure of this mechanism is the estimation of bicarbonate and the standard bicarbonate is the concentration in fully oxygenated blood when the level of carbon dioxide is normal.

Table 4.1

	SI units
Sodium	138 to 145 mmol/l
Potassium	3.5 to 5.0 mmol/l
Chloride	96 to 104 mmol/l
Urea	3.3 to 6.6 mmol/l
Standard bicarbonate	21 to 25 mmol/l
pCO_2	34 to 46 mmHg
Protein	60 to 74 g/l
Urine specific gravity	1.006 to 1.036

The body is so skilful at buffering and adjusting generally to increases or deficiencies in the various ions that it is only when they are grossly altered that changes appear in the blood and are revealed by laboratory tests. Indeed electrolyte measurements are most valuable when repeated at intervals in order to show the general trend or change that is going on. The normal range of concentrations is given in Table 4.1.

Normal fluid balance

The normal intake of fluid in a 70 kilogram man in a temperate climate is approximately as follows:

Daily Intake		Daily Output	
Fluid in drinks	1500 ml	Urine	1400 ml
Fluid in food	1000 ml	Insensible fluid loss	1000 ml
		Faeces	100 ml
	2500 ml		2500 ml

The insensible loss is continuous under all circumstances and is the moisture which escapes in the breath and from the surface of the skin. Clearly in a tropical country this will be greatly increased and then the loss in the urine will be proportionally less.

Dehydration

The commonest disorder of fluid balance which has to be treated is dehydration. This can be due to a diminished fluid intake or more commonly to increased loss especially from the gastro-intestinal tract such as occurs with vomiting, diarrhoea or gastric aspiration and the loss which occurs from the circulating blood volume due to haemorrhage and shock. The type of fluid lost in these different conditions is necessarily in different proportions. In severe vomiting there will be loss of water, chloride and potassium. The pH of the blood will fall, the bicarbonate rise and thus more bicarbonate will be excreted in the urine. With continued vomiting the serum potassium will fall and as a result of the dehydration due to loss of water, the level of urea will rise. Potassium deficiency is called hypokalaemia and must be corrected by its replacement in the infusion fluid.

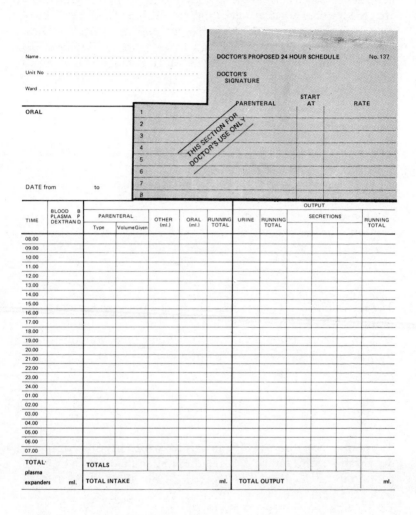

Fig. 4.2

Losses of water and salt or loss of blood volume due to haemorrhage lead to a reduction in the volume of circulating fluid with a resulting low blood pressure and decrease in the output of urine. Continued loss of water and salt produces a picture of dehydration in which there may not be great thirst but the tongue is dry, the skin is inelastic, the blood pressure low and the urinary output minute or non-existent. Although the electrolytes may have been greatly depleted the blood levels may be high, because the loss of water leads to concentration of the circulating fluid, a condition referred to as haemo-concentration.

Postoperative management

It is most important that a very careful record be kept of all the fluid which the patient loses and which is replaced by intravenous, oral or other route, so that an estimate can be made of what is necessary to keep the patient in good fluid balance. This is done by recording all the intake and output on a fluid-balance chart, a typical example of which is given in Fig. 4.2.

Central venous pressure is measured by the anaesthetist during operations which involve a great deal of blood loss and in cases of severe injury. This is the measurement of pressure in the right atrium and indicates any change in blood volume. It is of value in the postoperative period to give warning of the overload of the circulatory system by over transfusion as this can cause heart-failure. It is also an excellent route for introducing blood or other fluids into the circulation.

All patients after a surgical operation will be a little dehydrated because intake by mouth even in the normal individual may have been restricted and there may be very little secretion of the urine in the early postoperative hours. Other losses may occur, which are not at once apparent, such as pooling of fluid in the gut or in the tissues, especially in the extracellular space. Thus a careful record must be taken and a clinical examination may reveal dry tongue and inelastic skin and poor circulatory tone, which denote dehydration. Serum electrolyte and urea estimations will be of value in helping to estimate what is going on. If there has been great fluid loss before the operation or if much fluid has to be aspirated by nasogastric tube after operation, intravenous therapy is essential. Any patient on intravenous therapy for more than three days should have the serum electrolytes measured and in addition haematocrit and plasma protein estimations, to give an index of haemo-concentration. The specific gravity of the urine is also of value but it must be remembered that there may be kidney damage so that repeated estimations are necessary to record progress. The common deficiencies are of water, chloride, sodium and potassium. From a study of the fluid-balance chart and the laboratory reports on the levels of the electrolytes in the blood it is possible to estimate what is required to make up the balance and the corresponding number of bottles of intravenous saline of varying strength and possibly potassium supplements will then be given.

SI units

In 1976 a new system of measurement was introduced in the UK and EEC countries but not in the USA. For those who were familiar with the old units the main changes are outlined here. These new units will have the initials SI (Système International).

The basic SI units are as follows:

Physical quantity	Name of SI unit	Symbol
length	metre	m
mass	kilogram	kg
time	second	s
electric current	ampere	A
thermodynamic temperature	kelvin	K
luminous intensity	candela	cd
amount of substance	mole	mol

The common units mostly likely to be encountered are given in Table 4.2.

Nutrition

In addition to the requirements of water and salt, other deficiencies must be corrected as they arise and also before operation, if this is possible. The commonest nutritional problem in surgery results from starvation such as occurs with obstruction to the oesophagus or pylorus, or from the losses resulting from severe diarrhoea as in ulcerative colitis. If time allows, replacement of carbohydrate, protein, iron and vitamins over a period of a week or ten days will enormously improve the state of the patient and make the chance of a successful operation much more likely. If, however, time does not allow this, then the replacement of salt and water is dealt with by means of an intravenous infusion in the hours before the patient goes to the operating theatre.

Table 4.2

		Old units	SI units	Normal range in SI units
P	Albumin	g/100 ml	g/l	36−53 g/l
P	Bilirubin	mg/100 ml	μmol/l	5.0−17 μmol/l
P	Calcium	mg/100 ml	mmol/l	2.15−2.65 mmol/l
P	Chloride	mEq/l	mmol/l	96−104 mmol/l
S	Cholesterol	mg/100 ml	mmol/l	3.9−7.8 mmol/l
P	Creatinine	mg/100 ml	μmol/l	44−160 μmol/l
B	Glucose	mg/100 ml	mmol/l	3.0−5.3 mmol/l (fasting)
S	Iron	μg/100 ml	μmol	10−34 μmol/l
S	IBC	μg/100 ml	μmol/l	36−77 μmol/l
P	Magnesium	mg/100 ml	mmol/l	0.7−1.1 mmol/l
P	Total Protein	g/100 ml	g/l	65−80 g/l
P	Phosphate (as P)	mg/100 ml	mmol/l	0.8−1.55 mmol/l
P	Potassium	mEq/l	mmol/l	3.5−5 mmol/l
P	Sodium	mEq/l	mmol/l	138−145 mmol/l
S	Triglyceride (as tripalmitin)	mg/100 ml	mmol/l	0.5−1.9 mmol/l
P	Urate	mg/100 ml	mmol/l	0.1−0.4 mmol/l
P	Urea	mg/100 ml	mmol/l	3.3−6.6 mmol/l

P—Plasma
S—Serum
B—Blood

Haematological values

	Old units	SI units	Normal range in SI units
Haemoglobin	g/100 ml	g/dl	14.8 g/dl
Haematocrit	%	none	45 m/%
MCH	pg	pg	27−32 pg
MCHC	%	g/dl	33 g/dl
MCV	μ^3	fl	78−94 fl
RBC	$\times 10^6/mm^3$	$\times 10^{12}/l$	4−6 $\times 10^{12}/l$
WBC	$\times 10^3/mm^3$	$\times 10^9/l$	3−8 $\times 10^9/l$

The most satisfactory way of assisting a malnourished patient, who can usually take only a fluid diet, is to give a high calorie preparation such as Complan* which contains all the essential ingredients including vitamins and iron. Alternatively, the patient's complete diet can be processed in a food mixer or blender and the resulting fluid given via a Ryle's tube into the stomach. When the oral route cannot be used, help is obtained by using intravenous alimentation. Intravenous preparations are now available containing all the essential fat, carbohydrate and protein which the patient needs so that he can be kept in good nutritional balance entirely by

*Manufactured by Glaxo.

the intravenous route and thus where there are fistulas into the bowel and the wasting process prevents healing, the vicious circle can be broken.

As soon as the patient can take fluid and food by mouth this is far and away the best and also the safest method of administering what is required. Enthusiasm for intravenous therapy must never be allowed to jeopardize the use of the normal route by which we daily take our food and fluids.

5
Burns and Scalds; The Hand

Burns and scalds

Burns and scalds kill more than 700 people each year in England and Wales. Children under three years and older people over 65 make up a large proportion of those who die. In the majority of these deaths the accidents which led to them could have been prevented. Such measures as the enforcement of safety guards for all fires, the use of flame-proof material for children's clothes, especially pyjamas, discouragement of the wearing of nightdresses by little girls and close supervision of children in rooms containing fires could all help to reduce the appalling amount of disfigurement and death which burns cause. Widespread propaganda is necessary and everybody should be made aware of the problem and how they can help. For example, old people have to be watched when they sit near a fire for they may fall asleep and tumble forwards and their clothes be set alight. Children cannot resist pulling at attractive tea cosies or the handles of saucepans on stoves and they should therefore be watched most carefully when exposed to such hazards. A surprising number of burns could be avoided by banning the sale of fireworks. It is not only that people die as a result of preventable burns but also it has to be remembered that there is the misery of prolonged and painful invalidism, repeated plastic operations and dressings that have to be performed to correct scarring.

When a fire breaks out in a closed space, smoke and fumes are produced, especially from the combustion of synthetic materials. Asphyxiation due to these noxious gases may prove more lethal than burning because of the development of pulmonary oedema.

Types of burns

A burn can be defined as the destruction of tissue by dry heat and a scald as destruction by moist heat. Burns are best classified in terms of their depth for this is what will decide the course they take and the kind of treatment necessary.

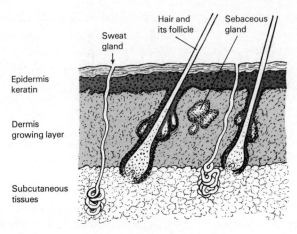

Epidermis
keratin

Dermis
growing layer

Subcutaneous
tissues

Sweat
gland

Hair and
its follicle

Sebaceous
gland

Fig. 5.1 Diagrammatic cross-section through skin.

Burns are *superficial* (1st degree) or *deep* (2nd degree). Complete charring is sometimes referred to as 3rd degree. Superficial burns are those in which there is reddening and blistering of the skin which should heal in a few days to two weeks without any scarring. Deep burns may be *partial thickness* or *full thickness*. In partial thickness burns the destruction of the germinal or growing layer (Fig. 5.1) is incomplete and thus regrowth of skin can occur from the islands of germinal epithelium which remain. In addition, the sweat and sebaceous glands dip down below the basal layers of the skin and from their epithelial covering regrowth may occur. However it will be very much delayed by infection. Full thickness burns involve destruction of tissue at least beyond the germinal layer of the epidermis. Thus no regrowth of skin is possible in the burnt area and healing, which can only take place from the nearby less damaged skin, is slow and complicated by scarring and contracture.

Complications

The complications of burns are best considered as *general*, i.e. those which affect the patient as a whole, and *local*, due to changes in the tissues which are actually damaged by heat.

General effects. The most important general effect of a burn is the exudate of plasma, that is the water, electrolytes and protein that leaks out from the dilated and damaged capillaries at the site of injury. The amount of exudate is proportional to the extent of the burn and if this is large, then because of the loss of fluid there will be a fall in blood pressure and a reduction in the circulating volume of blood with concentration of the cellular part of the blood, referred to as haemo-concentration. The loss of exudate is greatest in the first 8 hours after burning and slows up at about 48 hours.

If the burns are very extensive and deep, destruction of the red cells may also occur, so that when the blood volume has been restored by infusions of plasma or saline the patient will be anaemic. Other causes of anaemia in burning are due to infection of the burns, when the resultant toxaemia destroys the red cells, and malnutrition because it is often difficult to get a burnt patient to take a satisfactory diet.

Nausea and vomiting are particularly common after burns, especially in children and often make it necessary to provide the patient's requirements by the intravenous route. Such patients are severely dehydrated and in addition are depleted of nitrogen because of the protein loss in plasma exudate. Subsequently there is a failure to take food by mouth and the additional nitrogen loss by the body in the period after injury. The loss may be aggravated by fever and infection. Patients suffering from malnutrition in this way will show very slow healing of the tissues and skin grafts are not likely to 'take'.

Local effects. The local effects will depend on the severity of the heat and the extent of the area to which it is applied. The least that can happen is erythema and blistering and the worst, complete charring. Between these two there is every degree of depth of burn and it can be very difficult to assess what the depth is. In partial thickness burns it is usual to see most of the changes of inflammation, but in full thickness the dead tissue cannot respond in any way. As the dead tissue separates, the raw surface remaining forms an excellent culture medium for bacteria and this is one reason why it is very difficult to exclude infection from burns, especially by cross-infection from other patients and staff. One of the worst offenders is *Pyocyaneus aeruginosa*, which forms greenish pus with a musty odour and is resistant to most antibiotic treatment.

From about the second to the fourth week the dead areas separate leaving pink granulation tissue exuding serum or sometimes pus. In places, islands of regenerating skin appear, in other parts healing can only occur from the edge inwards. Unless skin grafting is carried out the end result is scarring.

Electrical burns are always full thickness but occur over a very limited area. Because of this it is often best for them to be excised immediately after they have occurred.

Scalds and burns affecting the head and neck carry a special risk because if the mucous membrane lining the nose and throat becomes oedematous the patient cannot breathe and only a tracheostomy will provide relief.

A common and lethal complication of fire inside a building is the inhalation of smoke and especially fumes at a high temperature. The resultant tracheitis, bronchitis and subsequent pulmonary oedema may be rapidly fatal unless relieved by oxygen therapy. In severe inhalation problems and asphyxia it may be necessary to perform an urgent tracheostomy and use a respirator.

Finally, on the subject of complications it must be added that burns may cause quite severe mental changes. In children especially, it is not uncommon for them to wake up with nightmares for at least a year after the accident often reliving the terrifying experience through which they have passed. Great patience is required in handling such children, but fortunately their terrors are almost always forgotten in time.

Treatment

First aid. When seeing a burn for the first time it is most important to assess its severity and decide whether or not hospital treatment is necessary. Minor burns which are superficial require only the application of a sterile dressing followed by inspection every few days until healing has occurred. The local pain can be severe and non-greasy applications, often containing anti-histamine substances, are available which are excellent for this. Severe burns should be covered by sterile towels and the patient sent to hospital. No attempt should be made to dress such injuries with antiseptics, antibiotics or any other more homely application, because it may delay the proper treatment in hospital.

Fluid replacement. The need for fluid replacement following burns depends on the extent and the depth of the burn and also the degree of shock as measured by the fall in blood pressure and evidence of poor circulation. If the burn involves more than 15 per cent of the body surface intravenous therapy will be required. Wallace's 'rule of nine' (Fig. 5.2) gives an easily remembered guide to the areas making up the total body surface. Eighteen per cent is allowed for the front and the back of the trunk, 9 per cent for each upper limb, 18 per cent for each lower limb and 9 per cent for the face. Fig. 5.2 shows this simply and the amount of fluid the patient will require intravenously can be calculated directly from the

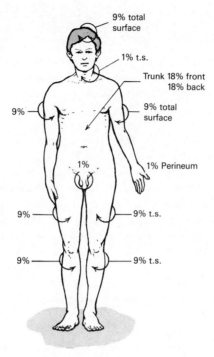

9% total
surface

1% t.s.

Trunk 18% front
18% back

9% total
surface

9%

1%

1% Perineum

9% — 9% t.s.

9% — 9% t.s.

Fig. 5.2 Wallace's Rule of Nine—each area is given in per cent of total body surface.

percentage of the body surface involved. Very approximately it can be said that 2 ml of fluid is needed for each 1 per cent of body surface area burnt, per kilogram of body weight. Half of this volume is usually given immediately as dextran or saline and the remainder as plasma and blood. The infusion is given rather quickly over the first 8 hours and much more slowly thereafter. If the patient is vomiting then additional fluid is required to make good this loss.

When more than 20 per cent of the body surface is burnt and especially if some of the burns are deep, half of the fluid given is in the form of plasma and the other half shared between blood and saline. The progress of resuscitation is measured by the improvement in the general well-being of the patient and the slowing of the pulse rate and rise in blood pressure. An adequate output of urine is an excellent sign of satisfactory treatment and the return of the haemoglobin level and the electrolyte values to normal are likewise good signs.

Pain is best treated by giving morphia, the dose of which depends

on the body weight and if the patient is in great distress the doctor
may decide to give the first injection intravenously.

Local applications. The overriding considerations in treating
burns are to prevent infection and to encourage healing. Two main
techniques have evolved, *open* and *closed*. In the open or *exposure*
method the patient is nursed in an isolation cubicle lying on sterile
sheets and in a warm, dried, filtered air which encourages a
coagulum to form over the raw areas. Infection is discouraged by
strict nursing technique and by spraying the burned areas with
antibiotic powder which forms a crust. This method is well suited to
widespread burns and scalds of the trunk and limbs, but is not used
for the hands and face because the immobility produces fibrous
contractures with a mask-like face and immobile fingers.

The closed or *pressure dressing* method consists of a layer of open
mesh paraffin gauze covered by gauze, wool and crepe bandages.
The fingers and face, however, are best left covered only by the non-
adhesive gauze or tulle gras and antibiotic-containing cream. A
water-miscible cream containing 1 per cent of silver sulphadiazine
or mafenide is often used as it is antibacterial, reduces exudate and
does not delay healing.

A third technique for the treatment of burns which are limited in
area but deep is by primary excision and grafting. It is best suited to
deep local burns of the hands, usually electrical burns.

Antibiotics. Antibiotics are always required in the treatment of
burns and can be given locally or systemically or both.
Unfortunately bacterial resistance is quickly acquired and therefore
a change of antibiotic is often necessary. Locally administered
antibiotics may have to be discontinued because hypersensitivity
develops.

Skin grafting. Whenever the full thickness of the skin is destroyed
the sooner it is grafted the better will be the result, not only from the
point of view of recovery of the patient, but also for functional
reasons and for a good cosmetic effect. As soon as it is clear that there
is no ingrowing of skin from the edges or that there are no small
islands of regenerating epithelium in the burned area, an attempt
should be made to obtain as healthy granulation tissue as possible in
preparation for grafting. This is unlikely to be successful unless the
patient's nutrition is adequately maintained; a good balanced diet is
most important and oral feeding with protein supplements such as
Complan with vitamins and iron is useful. Anaemia has to be

corrected by blood transfusion. The area to be grafted must be free from infection and the granulations should be firm, dry, flat and of a dark pink colour. If there is much dead tissue and slough present, this can be removed with applications of sodium hypochlorite (Milton) or repeated immersion in baths.

Skin grafts are either full thickness or partial thickness. Full thickness grafts are only used for cosmetic reasons, as on the face, or where they will have to withstand hard wear as in the hands. They need to 'take' their blood supply with them and this can be achieved by microsurgical technique, anastomosing the artery and vein to a nearby blood supply or swinging a flap on a vascular pedicle and later detaching it. Split skin or partial thickness grafts are much more useful since they can be used to cover large raw areas; very thin grafts leave practically no scarring in the donor area but are not thick enough to withstand trauma or hard wear. The thicker the graft is cut the more noticeable is the subsequent discoloration and irregularity of the donor site.

The split skin graft is cut with a special (Humby) knife which resembles a long razor with an adjustable roller in front of the edge to regulate the thickness of the graft. A board (Gabarro) is held firmly on the skin in front of the knife and the skin is stretched by an assistant to aid the process. An electrical (Padget) dermatome may be used where big areas of skin are to be cut. The commonest site for taking grafts is the inner side of the thigh and very thin grafts may be repeatedly cut from the same area at intervals of a few weeks. In young girls the buttocks are chosen since any discoloration or scarring is less likely to show in later years.

If large areas of burned skin need to be replaced the technique of mesh grafting makes a little skin go a long way. Multiple parallel rows of small slanting cuts are made in the graft with a mesher and the skin can then be stretched, to four or five times its size and stitched in place, it then resembles a string vest and the holes are rapidly epithelialised by spread from the edges of the graft. Most skin grafts require anchoring with stitches and are then covered with paraffin net, tulle gras or other non-adhesive dressing; wool and firm bandaging holds it in position. When large areas need to be covered and the patient has no suitable donor sites, skin from other patients or animals (usually the pig), so called xenografts, may be used for temporary cover. They are all rejected in weeks or months. If more skin is cut than is immediately needed, the excess can be banked for up to 3 weeks at 4 °C wrapped in saline gauze. At much lower temperatures it may be stored in glycerine for some months.

If the burned area is covered with unhealthy sloughs and is slow to granulate the patient is anaesthetized in the theatre and desloughing is followed by immediate skin grafting.

Nursing and rehabilitation

The care of patients with extensive burns is one of the biggest challenges that the hospital has to meet and it is on the nursing staff that most of the load falls. The patient, who immediately before was well and active, suddenly has to adjust to complete dependence on the nursing staff. Often anxiety and depression are increased by the knowledge that the accident could have been avoided and there is the added distress of knowing that some degree of disfigurement and disability are inevitable and that recovery may well take many months. In such circumstances the nursing care must be not only skilful but tempered with sympathy, compassion and patience.

When burns are very extensive and deep it is ideal, if the patient is well enough to be moved, to transfer him to one of the specialised regional burns units which have now been set up in many countries. The highly specialized skills and expertise available more than compensate for the lack of convenience for visits by relatives and friends.

Patients who have extensive burns are best nursed in cubicles with glass partitions so that they can be observed by the staff without being disturbed and the risk of infection is lessened. The temperature inside the cubicle should be maintained at 15 to 18 °C and can conveniently be raised to 20 to 24 °C when the exposure method is being used. Anyone entering the cubicle should wear a mask and preferably a sterile gown. Bed linen should be sterile and changed frequently and any mattress or pillow should be protected by a plastic cover.

The nourishment of such patients is particularly important and they must be encouraged to drink plenty of fluid. It is advisable to give these drinks at definite intervals at first to ensure a steady intake. It is similarly important to keep a careful record of the amount of fluid taken and the urinary output. A high calorie, high protein diet containing adequate vitamins is essential and the basis for this will be milk, eggs, meat and fish with adequate amounts of fresh fruit or fresh fruit juice.

The general hygiene of the patient is particularly important and mouth washes are necessary; if the eyes are sore, drops of castor oil are soothing. Sedatives will be necessary, especially at night time, and Nitrazepam (Mogadon) 5 mg may be ordered and Paracetamol (Panadol) tablets, one or two crushed in water.

As the patient begins to feel better it is very important that an interesting pastime be encouraged and the assistance of an occupational therapist is ideal. As healing progresses the physiotherapist will be asked to help with exercises designed to prevent deformity or muscle contracture and the nurse must be prepared to encourage the patient to carry out these movements when the physiotherapist is not present. Patients often worry a great deal about disfigurement and they can be reassured that the excellent results obtained by plastic surgery will correct this.

The hand

The largest part of hand surgery deals with infections and this is confirmed by the number of attendances at the emergency department of a district hospital, where between a quarter and a third will be found to be for septic hands.

Sepsis of the hand

Infection of the hand almost always follows injury and the commonest organisms are the staphylococcus and, more rarely, the streptococcus. Both before and after operation support of the hand in the proper way is important in relieving pain, helping localization of infection and preventing permanent damage. The hand and forearm should be supported on a light plaster of Paris slab in the position of function with a little dorsi-flexion at the wrist and a little flexion at the interphalangeal joints. The whole arm should be placed in a sling.

Chemotherapy is always ordered when there is cellulitis and lymphangitis. Penicillin as procaine penicillin up to 1 g a day intramuscularly is given for 5 days. If the organisms appear resistant, after 48 hours and guided by the laboratory report on sensitivity, a suitable antibiotic is prescribed. If pus is present, or as soon as it forms, the correct treatment is incision and drainage; antibiotics will only be of use to control spreading infection. Septic fingers are extremely painful and the patient must be given analgesics to take home and use, especially at night time. Calcium aspirin 300 to 600 mg, codeine 30 to 60 mg and paracetamol 500 mg, or Distalgesic tablets are useful.

Operations

All operations on fingers and hands require anaesthesia and a very satisfactory method is a local block at the root of the finger. Adrenalin is never added to the solution for fear of producing spasm of the digital arteries with resultant gangrene of the finger. The incision is usually made over the maximum bulging, but the finger tip is avoided as far as possible because the subsequent scar would interfere with function. Drains are rarely necessary. If the abscess is large or complicated the surgeon may require a general anaesthetic and a tourniquet on the arm so that a bloodless operation field is obtained. Dressings are changed as frequently as possible, the hand being supported on a light plaster slab. Active movements are encouraged and supervised by a physiotherapist from the very start.

Paronychia

This is infection beside the nail and usually starts where unhealthy skin overhangs the nail or nail bed. The area is unroofed and it is rarely necessary to remove all the nail.

Pulp space infection

This is probably the commonest, certainly the most painful and possibly the most serious, finger infection. The pulp, which constitutes the finger tip, consists of fatty tissue with tough fibrous septa and thus pressure leads to necrosis and drainage incisions have to be generous. Incisions are usually sited to one side of the finger so that there is subsequently no scar to get in the way of fine movements.

Osteitis

If the infection involves the bone then it will not clear up until the dead bone or sequestrum is removed. It is one of the commonest causes of chronic infection in the hand.

Other infections

Tenosynovitis is infection of a tendon sheath and fortunately is rarely seen. The patient has great pain and is toxic because the pus is confined within the fibrous sheath. It spreads readily in this space and therefore needs to be thoroughly drained; penicillin may then be injected into the space inside the sheath. *Palmar space infection* is not common and occurs in the loose tissue planes often causing oedema and swelling on the dorsum of the hand as well. *Web infections* are usually due to small foreign bodies being driven into the web between two fingers and are drained by incisions made directly over the swelling.

Injuries of the hand

Injuries to tendons are common in the hand because they are near the surface and they are especially liable to damage at the wrist. The extensor tendons may be divided anywhere along their length; they are readily repaired by suture and usually heal well. If an extensor tendon to a finger is not repaired a *mallet finger* results but this is not a severe disability.

Flexor tendons may also be divided at any place in the finger or wrist but on the whole they tend not to heal so well. It is important that they are rested immediately after repair, and subsequently skilful supervision of active and even passive movements is necessary to obtain a good functional result. Where the little finger is severely damaged by tendon injury it is often better to amputate the finger because its presence may impede movements in the rest of the hand.

Much surgery of the hand today is reconstructive, as in the replacement of crippled finger joints with plastic prostheses in rheumatoid arthritis. This is primarily the responsibility of the orthopaedic surgeon as is the care of nerve injuries described below.

Nerve injuries

Median nerve. Division of this nerve at the level of the wrist leads to paralysis of the small muscles of the thumb, the lateral two lumbricals and loss of sensation of the $3\frac{1}{2}$ fingers on the radial side of the hand. Abduction of the thumb is not possible, i.e. it cannot be carried up in a plane at right angles to the flat of the hand. The nerve can be repaired by suture and the hand supported until function has returned. The *carpal tunnel* syndrome represents a specialized form of median nerve injury. Division of the transverse carpal ligament frees the nerve and allows it to function properly.

Ulnar nerve. Division of the ulnar nerve at the wrist paralyses the muscles of the hypothenar eminence, the interossei and the medial two lumbricals. There is anaesthesia of the little finger and half of the ring finger. The hand takes up a typical clawed position with the little finger most flexed and the others affected in lessening amount; if the injury is not successfully repaired the clawing eventually becomes permanent.

In *Dupuytren's contracture* of the hand the palmar fascia becomes thickened and contracts. The little finger is slowly pulled down into the palm in severe flexion to be followed by the other fingers in turn. Toes may be affected in the same way and the cause of the condition is not known. Surgical correction by excision or multiple incisions of the fibrous tissue allows the fingers to be straightened.

6
Neoplasms and Tumours

The word tumour, derived from the Latin 'tumor' meaning a swelling is used to describe any abnormal mass of tissue and it may take the form of a simple new growth, a malignant growth or even a swelling due to inflammation. In this chapter, however, we are concerned with tumours produced by new growth or neoplasm and not as the result of inflammation. It is possible to classify tumours into two large groups: simple and malignant.

A *simple tumour* is a local overgrowth of the tissues, usually of one particular kind of cell and does not kill the host in which it arises. It is usually *encapsulated* because by increasing in size, it presses on the surrounding tissues which become condensed, especially the connective tissue, and a distinct covering, or capsule, is thus formed. For this reason a simple tumour can usually be enucleated or shelled out from its capsule and if completely removed it does not recur. Simple tumours neither infiltrate the surrounding tissues nor spread via the lymphatics or blood stream, but remain strictly localized.

A *malignant tumour* is also a local overgrowth of tissue, but it may spread in various ways: it may infiltrate the surrounding tissues; clumps of malignant cells may be carried via the lymphatics and produce growths in the lymph nodes; malignant cells may pass into the blood stream and lodge in distant parts of the body giving rise to additional tumours, called *secondaries or metastases*. In addition, a malignant tumour, unless treated, will usually continue to grow until it destroys the host. It is difficult to give an accurate definition of a malignant tumour, but probably the best is that given by the pathologist R. G. Willis: 'A tumour is an abnormal mass of tissue, the growth of which exceeds and is incoordinated with that of the normal tissues and persists in the same manner after cessation of the stimuli which evoked the change.'

Simple tumours

Simple tumours are very common, especially on the skin, and there must be few amongst us who cannot boast at least one *papilloma*, that is a warty excrescence, or a pigmented naevus, i.e. a mole. Probably the commonest tumour seen in children is the *haemangioma*, which is a local overgrowth of blood vessels. It may be made up of capillaries, the so-called strawberry birth-mark, or of larger vessels when it constitutes a cavernous haemangioma. Tumours of lymph vessels are called *lymphangiomas* and may occur in the neck region in infants, when they are referred to as *cystic hygromas*. In each case the local overgrowth of tissue is benign and does not usually spread beyond a strictly demarcated limit. Sometimes simple tumours are made up of more than one kind of tissue, as for example in the neurofibroma, which may be multiple and which is made up of nervous and fibrous tissue. Most of these tumours are given Latin names describing the kind of cells of which they are composed: appended is a list of some of the common ones although there are a great many others, tumours having been described as arising in every tissue of the body:

Adenoma, gland tissue   *Myoma*, muscle
Angioma, blood vessel   *Neuroma*, nerve tissue
Chondroma, cartilage   *Papilloma*, epithelium
Fibroma, fibrous tissue   *Osteoma*, bone
Lipoma, fatty or adipose tissue

Treatment

Simple tumours usually require surgical excision and since such tumours do not infiltrate, it is possible to *excise* (cut out) or *enucleate* (shell out) them completely and they do not recur.

There are three good reasons for removing such tumours: they may be unsightly, they may cause disability of one kind or another by pressure on the surrounding tissues, and they may eventually undergo a malignant change if left.

Malignant tumours

Causes of malignancy

The cause of malignant disease is not known, but some of the factors which encourage its development are listed below. It must not be forgotten that cancer is not one disease, but a great multiplicity of diseases and there are many contributory causes.

Age. Carcinoma is rare in the young, it occurs more commonly after the age of 40 and two-thirds of those dying from cancer in the British Isles are over the age of 60.

Sex. Some tumours show a predisposition to occur either in men or women. For example, carcinoma of the lung and stomach are more common in men and carcinoma of the breast and gall bladder are more common in women.

Race. Some people appear particularly susceptible to carcinomas while others appear immune. Many factors are at work but the distribution among different races and in different countries can be striking. For example, carcinoma of the cervix of the uterus is almost unknown amongst Jewish women; however, circumcision is universal among Jewish men and it may be that this removes a cause of malignancy. Carcinoma of the liver is common among the Bantu in South Africa, but not among the white population. Breast carcinoma is particularly common in North America and Europe, but extremely rare in Japan although the incidence is now rising.

Chemicals. Substances which evoke a malignant change in the tissues are called carcinogens. The hydrocarbons which occur in soot are carcinogenic and the first disease for which industrial compensation was granted in Great Britain was carcinoma of the scrotum in chimney sweeps. Tar and many other products of coal are also capable of inducing malignant change in the skin. The commonest cancer in men in Britain and the United States occurs in the lungs of cigarette smokers.

Hormones. Some strains of mice if injected repeatedly with oestrogens, a hormone normally secreted by the ovaries, develop breast cancer. Almost 50 per cent of human breast cancers appear to depend on oestrogens for their continued growth and this is the basis for removal of the ovaries, adrenals and pituitary in an attempt to control the spread of breast cancer in women.

Ionizing radiation. Radium, X-rays and radioactive isotopes are among the most potent causes of malignant change in man. In the early days of radiotherapy, before workers in this field knew the dangers inherent in the rays, it was not uncommon for them to receive unsafe levels of exposure. Later they developed malignant lesions of the skin of the hands, often after 20 or more years had elapsed. Exposure to X-rays or radioactive isotopes should be avoided in the foetus, children and young adults.

Chronic infection. Long-standing sepsis is occasionally complicated by malignant change and a carcinoma can very rarely occur
in a chronic leg ulcer, the result of varicose veins or chronic
osteomyelitis. Carcinoma of the tongue is more commonly seen in
those infected with syphilis.

Chronic irritation. The continued abrasion of the tongue by a
septic or rough stump of a tooth or irritation from ill-fitting
dentures can lead to the development of carcinoma.

Carcinoma and sarcoma

Malignant tumours can be classified according to the tissues in which
they arise, and they are best divided into two groups. The first is the
carcinomas, or cancers, which are malignant tumours of epithelial
tissues. They get their name from the Latin word 'cancer', meaning
a crab, probably because a crab travels sideways and illustrates the
manner in which such tumours infiltrate surrounding tissues. The
second large group is composed of the *sarcomas*, which are
malignant tumours of connective tissues. The connective tissues of
the body are made up of all the fibrous and fatty packing between
the other layers of tissues and also the bones, cartilage and muscle.

The main difference between carcinomas and sarcomas is the
manner in which they spread, apart from local infiltration.

Carcinomas usually travel by the lymphatics, first affecting the
lymph nodes, and the malignant cells are only later swept away in
the bloodstream to arrive and multiply in quite distant organs. For
the most part, however, they travel to some other part of the body
by the lymphatics.

Sarcomas, on the other hand, usually grow locally and then small
emboli of malignant cells escape into the bloodstream and *secondary
deposits* or *metastases* develop in other organs where these cells are
arrested, the commonest sites being the lungs and liver.

The diagnosis of malignancy in a tumour may be very difficult,
but the following characteristics are helpful. The tumours are *not
encapsulated*; they tend to *infiltrate* surrounding tissues, and the actual
extent often cannot be seen with the naked eye. Their spread by
lymphatics or bloodstream leads to secondary deposits in almost any
or every part of the body. The growth of these secondaries often
results in a general feeling of ill health or *malaise* and eventually
gradual loss of weight, anaemia and a rather sallow complexion.

The degree of malignancy of different growths varies enormously. Some grow so slowly that after many years they can still be

eradicated surgically, while others may destroy their host in a few months. The latter is particularly true of the sarcomas which tend to occur in younger patients and to grow rapidly. Carcinomas, on the other hand, vary greatly in their malignancy but do not usually arise in patients before middle age.

Because malignant tumours rarely give rise to pain in the early stages of their growth, they often escape diagnosis at the time when successful treatment could be carried out. For this reason, when malignancy is suspected it is customary to remove a small piece of tissue or *biopsy* from the affected area and send it to the pathologist. The latter examines sections of it under the microscope and is usually able to state whether or not the cells show invasive properties, that is, whether it is benign or malignant.

Treatment

The treatment of malignant tumours is clearly the *prevention* of their development where this is possible, and when they do arise, their early diagnosis followed by prompt *excision* or *irradiation*.

Workers in trades where there may be exposure to tar, oil, soot or other carcinogenic substances should wear suitable protective clothing and should be examined regularly by a doctor to detect the first signs. In these days radioactive materials are widely used in the diagnosis of disease and treatment of patients and also in industrial processes. It is important that everybody should know the precautions to take when dealing with them.

The early diagnosis of malignant tumours depends primarily on a good liaison between the medical practitioner and his patients so that the latter report anything unusual at the earliest possible date. In addition it is wise for people to know which organs of the body are likely to develop malignant changes and how to recognize the early signs. In the UK self-examination, e.g. of the breasts and cancer detection clinics are rare, but there are parts of the world where the population is much more cancer conscious and it is possible that this may lead to patients presenting themselves for treatment at an earlier stage of the disease. On the other hand, these advantages have to be weighed against the fact that many people become unduly anxious about developing a malignant disease when such a possibility is being constantly brought to their notice. The nurse can play a great part in encouraging the public to seek medical attention when the first signs of malignancy appear. Women frequently ask a female nurse for advice in such matters and she should be quite emphatic that any unusual lumps or swellings should be seen by a doctor and that any postmenopausal bleeding, however, slight, should never be ignored.

The treatment of malignancy is by surgery, by some form of radiotherapy, by chemical compounds which destroy malignant cells, or a combination of any or all of these. The giving of hormones such as stilboestrol and testosterone and the removal of adrenal glands and the pituitary may be employed in the treatment of advanced breast cancer.

Surgery. A tumour may be excised, e.g. mastectomy is usually performed for a carcinoma of the breast. It is known that certain tumours tend to spread in a typical way and therefore the operation is usually planned to excise the tissues which are most likely to be affected, whether or not they appear to be so on clinical examination. For example, when carcinoma of the sigmoid colon has been diagnosed and it appears possible to remove it surgically, colectomy will be performed. This includes the removal of the area of lymphatic drainage in the mesentery as well as a generous amount of apparently healthy colon since it is the adjoining tissue and the lymphatics in which the tumour spreads. In these days when great strides have been made in the maintenance of a patient after severe operations, such as replacing lost blood and giving suitable antibiotics, the kind of surgery employed for malignancy becomes more and more aggressive. This is justifiable when it is possible to remove all the malignant tissue, but it must be remembered that no operation should be so mutilating as to make life subsequently not worth living.

The guiding principle in the surgical approach to malignant disease is that the operation should be most radical when the tumour is localized, because in such circumstances a cure is more likely to result. Even when the disease is hopelessly incurable it may still be justifiable to perform a palliative operation to make life more comfortable for the patient.

Radiotherapy. Malignant disease is treated by radiotherapy in three different ways using (1) X-rays, (2) radium or cobalt and (3) radioactive isotopes.

X-rays. These are electromagnetic waves of very short wavelength and they have the property of penetrating the tissues and destroying those cells which are actively growing or in process of division. It is only the growing cells which are very sensitive to these rays so that, in a way, such treatment is specific for the malignant tissues. On the other hand, the healthy surrounding tissues are also damaged to a lesser extent by the X-rays and this damage is the limiting factor in the amount of radiation which can be given. X-ray machines are of different powers and the more powerful the machine the more penetrating the rays it produces. If very penetrating rays are used, these will do less damage to the superficial tissues and will be more lethal to the underlying tumour. In order that healthy tissues are as little damaged as possible, it is usual to irradiate a tumour from a number of different directions.

X-ray therapy may cause quite severe nausea and general upset in the patient, and it is usual to spread out the treatment over a number of weeks, giving radiation daily depending on the capacity of the machine. The cobalt machine and linear accelerator (Fig. 6.1) are the apparatus in regular use.

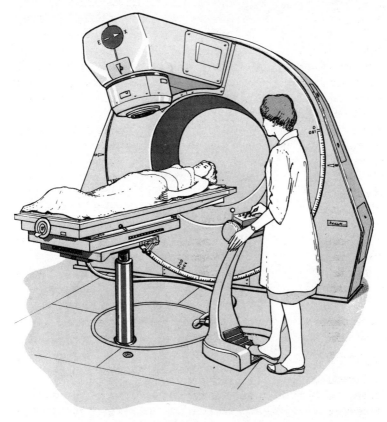

Fig. 6.1 (a) Linear accelerator. The patient lies on the table, which can be adjusted to any position.

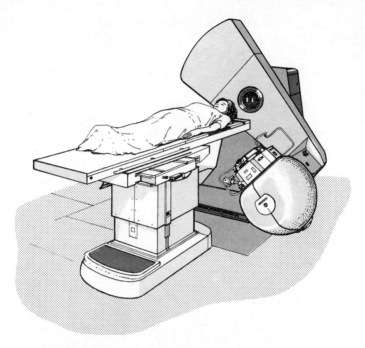

Fig. 6.1 (b) Cobalt unit.

Mental state. Each patient reacts differently to a course of radiotherapy, and the nurse must endeavour to understand individual difficulties and help in any way possible. It is usual for the patient to feel generally unwell and depressed, and it may help if the patient is encouraged to talk with the more cheerful occupants of the ward or with others who have undergone similar therapy.

The patient's will to get better is often the most important part of any treatment. This will to live can be fostered by maintaining the patient's interest in many different ways. Visitors bring stimuli from outside the sickroom while radio and television programmes can focus interest on things other than the patient's own disease. Occupational therapists are able to encourage such patients to employ themselves in creative work, which is a splendid antidote to mental depression.

Patients suffering from incurable diseases often seem to realize it yet seldom ask if they will get better, perhaps because they fear the answer. If a patient does ask the nurse about the prospect of recovering the opportunity to build morale should be seized. The team of medical nursing and ancillary staff must speak with one voice or confidence will be undermined.

Mucous membranes, especially of the mouth and throat, become dry after irradiation and call for frequent mouth washes and a little honey or paraffin, or a sweet to suck.

Anaemia often complicates both malignant disease and radiation therapy, and the administration of iron or even a blood transfusion may go far in improving the general condition and morale of the patient.

Radiation sickness. Medicine may be ordered to control nausea and vomiting. Certain of the antihistamine drugs have been found useful in controlling nausea. Promethazine (Avomine), cyclizine (Marzine) and meclozine (Ancolan), 1 tablet two or three times a day, may be given, but patients' reactions to these drugs are unpredictable.

The skin may show an initial bright red erythema, peel and later become deeply pigmented. Irradiated skin requires special care, and should be kept dry by applying aminacrine, 1 in 1000, twice daily. The moist stage may be prevented or delayed by painting with 1 per cent gentian violet, but if moist desquamation occurs, an oily dressing is most comfortable and tulle-gras may be applied.

Radiotherapy is always carried out under the direction of a doctor assisted by a physicist who is able to calculate the amount of irradiation which should be given to the tumour.

Radium and Cobalt. Radium is an element obtained from pitchblende and is a source of very powerful radiation. The rays given off by radium—alpha, beta and gamma—are of different penetrating power, the most penetrating being the gamma. In order that the overlying tissues, especially the skin, shall not be damaged, it is usual to filter off the softer alpha and beta rays by encasing the radium in a heavy metal such as lead or gold. The radium may be put in needles which can be either thrust directly into the tumour to be irradiated (*interstitial irradiation*), or arranged in an applicator which is placed on the surface of the tumour (*surface irradiation*). Radium is dangerous if not handled properly and also extremely expensive, so great care has to be taken that it does not come in contact with any healthy tissues and that it is not mislaid during the treatment of a patient. Radium should never be handled except under medical supervision. At the present time *cobalt* which has been made radioactive in an atomic pile has largely taken the place of radium because the cobalt is much less expensive to produce.

However, it is not so lasting in its properties and has to be renewed after a number of years. *The cobalt bomb* consists of a quantity of radioactive cobalt, suitably shielded with a heavy metal such as lead so that its rays can be directed at the diseased area of the patient.

Physics. All radiations are subject to the 'inverse square law', which states that their intensity varies inversely as the square of the distance from the source. Thus when external radiation is used, the skin must always receive a greater dose than the tumour deep to it. The risk of serious damage to the skin can be diminished by moving the source of radiation further away, for then, although the strength of the source of radiation must be proportionately increased, the relative excess of skin dose over tumour dose is lessened. This desire to give a greater dose to the tumour without damaging the skin has led to the building of more and more powerful sources of irradiation which can be used further away from the patient. Fast neutrons from a cyclotron are one of the most recent examples.

Radioactive isotopes. A convenient form of irradiation treatment is that obtained from the use of radioactive isotopes. Various substances can be placed in an atomic pile and rendered radioactive. These radioactive substances can then be used for implantation into a tumour, e.g. irradiated wire, or seeds of gold or tantalum, can be placed in bladder tumours. Yttrium rods are introduced via the nose into the pituitary, caesium is used for cervical cancer, and iridium wires in the breast. In addition, certain substances are selectively concentrated in different parts of the body, such as *iodine* in the *thyroid* and *phosphorus* in the bone *marrow*. If these substances are given in radioactive form they are concentrated by these tissues which are then irradiated. Thus it is possible to treat *hyperthyroidism* and some forms of cancer of the thyroid gland with radioactive iodine. The disease, *polycythaemia vera*, in which too many red cells are manufactured, can also be alleviated by giving radioactive phosphorus, which irradiates the marrow and suppresses the formation of the red cells.

Compounds made up of large molecules are not absorbed into the circulation and therefore if made radioactive can be used to irradiate body cavities since they remain localized to the area in which they are injected. *Radioactive gold* prepared in a colloidal form, which means that it is composed of very large particles, can be injected into the pleural or peritoneal cavities when these are diffusely involved by malignant disease. The malignant deposits will then be subjected to intense local irradiation of far greater intensity than could be provided by external application with X-rays or cobalt.

Precautions. When radioactive isotopes are being used the nursing staff should take care not to contaminate anything, especially their own hands, with the isotope or any radioactive excreta from the patient. The hospital physicist issues instructions depending on the type and amount of isotope used and may request observation of some of the following precautions:

1 Reducing to a minimum the time spent attending to the patient.
2 Seeing that the patient is strictly confined to the ward for a stated period of time.
3 Limiting the length of time visitors may remain near the patient.
4 The wearing of gloves and gowns when attending to dressings, handling bedpans, collecting specimens of urine.
5 Restricting the patient to the use of an individual bedpan and urinal.
6 Providing special containers for soiled linen and clothing.
7 Requiring the nurse to use a monitor (Geiger counter with loud-speaker) to detect radioactivity of excreta, bedding and dressings.
8 Devising special methods of disposal of excreta.

Finally, radiotherapy carries its own complications. It will be remembered from earlier in the chapter that exposure to radiation may itself induce in time a malignant change and therefore such therapy is not usually given to young patients unless no alternative is available.

A combination of surgery and radiotherapy is often used with advantage, for example a lobectomy for cancer of the lung is followed by X-rays to destroy any remaining cancer cells in the surrounding tissues.

Chemotherapy. A number of chemical substances have been elaborated in recent years which have a toxic effect upon dividing cells and can therefore be used to destroy malignant tumours. When cells proliferate they pass through the cell cycle which is made up of a number of phases. In the mitosis or (M) phase the cell divides into two; this is followed by a gap (G) and then a synthetic phase (S) before the whole cycle repeats. The purpose of chemotherapy is to damage or prevent cells from multiplying during their most sensitive period.

The limiting factor must always be the toxicity of the drug on the normal tissues of the body and the most vulnerable tissues are almost always those which manufacture the white and red blood cells, i.e. bone marrow.

These cytotoxic substances can be used in many ways. They may be *injected* or instilled locally as, for example, into the pleural cavity. They may be used regionally by intra-arterial *infusion*, for example a block of tissue such as the floor of mouth and tongue may be treated by infusing the external carotid artery. When a malignant lesion occurs in the head and neck region and is unsuitable for excision or further irradiation, infusion therapy may offer good palliation. Even greater amounts of cytotoxic drugs may be given if the part affected can be excluded from the general circulation, for example, by a tourniquet around the root of a limb. *Perfusion* of the limb is then done via cannulas inserted into the main artery and vein, which are connected with a pump oxygenator by which oxygenated blood is circulated through the excluded limb. Perfusions can only be performed for periods of an hour or so, whereas infusion can be maintained for days. In perfusion a larger amount of cytoxic drug can be given, whereas by infusion less can be given for a much longer time. It is possible for the patient to be normally active, with a container of cytotoxic drug, a tiny clockwork or electric pump leading to a cannula in an artery or vein. This may stay in place for many days.

Systemic treatment with cytotoxic drugs is in regular demand for treating cancer which has metastasized to other parts of the body and generalized diseases such as myeloma and leukaemia. Three or four cytotoxic drugs are usually given in combination, some orally and some intravenously. Methotrexate, vincristine, cyclophosphamide and adriamycin are common examples.

7
Pre-operative Care

Most patients approach their first operation with fear and trepidation. This is because they do not know what is going to happen to them and it is therefore an important part of a nurse's duty to try and explain any treatment given and to be prepared to answer questions about what is likely to take place. Apart from the personal anxiety that a patient may feel at this time, there is the added worry as to how those at home are managing without them. Most people dread an anaesthetic for they do not know how they will behave as they regain consciousness and in addition there is always the thought at the back of their minds that they may not recover. Not only is an operation a mental ordeal for the patient, but it is also a physical one, as there is sure to be a certain degree of pain and sometimes considerable disability, although the latter is often only temporary.

Arrival in hospital

Patients arriving in hospital should feel that they are expected, and the manner in which they are greeted is all important. First impressions of the ward and of the nursing staff should induce a feeling of confidence as this helps to create a sense of security. When a patient is admitted to the ward there are a number of formalities which must be complied with and these will vary to some extent with each particular hospital.

Routine procedures

It is always necessary to obtain the full particulars of the patient, and the name, address and telephone number of the nearest relatives. In the case of anyone under the age of 16 the parents will be interviewed and permission obtained in writing for operation. Before any operation is performed it is essential that a proper consent form be signed. In recent years, as a result of the increase in medicolegal cases, such requirements have become much more important. It is desirable to find out the religion of the patient, and, if the hospital is a large one, it is courteous to advise the chaplain as soon as possible of the patient's admission. Since patients may come from foreign countries or for religious or other reasons have particular dietary habits, these should be asked about and respected as far as possible.

It is becoming routine procedure in hospital to provide an identity bracelet for each patient newly admitted. This bears the patient's name, hospital number and ward and should not be removed until the patient is discharged.

The patient's temperature, pulse, blood pressure and respiration rate are recorded, and any abnormalities found should be reported forthwith so that appropriate action is taken. The patient is weighed and the height is recorded, as this information is necessary to calculate the correct dosage of many drugs and anaesthetic agents and it also provides a base-line for future progress. A specimen of urine is obtained and tested for its specific gravity, albumin, sugar and acetone. A blood sample is taken for grouping and cross-matching, and if necessary for sickling. The chest will be X-rayed. Any abnormalities are reported at once to the surgeon. It is wise to enquire if the patient is menstruating or obtain the date of the last period, and ask about bowel and micturition habits.

In hospital, patients may find it difficult to sleep at night, the surroundings are strange, there are many unusual noises and they are likely to lie awake worrying about their condition. For this reason sedatives are often employed and are especially necessary on the eve of an operation so that the patient may have a good night's rest, e.g. Nitrazepam (Mogadon) 5 mg.

As well as preparing the patient physically for surgery, it is equally important to prepare him mentally. Studies have shown that the patient who is relaxed and well prepared for surgery progresses much better postoperatively than the patient who is anxious and full of unanswered questions and often unnecessary fears. For this reason it is important to take the time to explain any infusions or monitoring devices that will be used postoperatively. At the same time the patient should not be frightened by too much technical jargon. It takes skill to win the patient's confidence and yet impart knowledge that the nurse feels will help.

The patient's relatives also have a need to be informed of what to expect. It can be just as frightening for them as for the patient himself.

Special procedures

Many special investigations may be called for before a major operation is undertaken. The haemoglobin has to be estimated, and if the patient is acutely ill or has been ailing for a long time further tests may be required such as estimation of the serum proteins and serum electrolytes. If the patient has been vomiting or losing fluid by other routes, it will be necessary to make good this deficit and fluid will then be given intravenously. Breathing exercises may be ordered and often supervised by a physiotherapist for patients who are likely to remain in bed for some time after the operation, so that in the postoperative period they will breathe efficiently and avoid chest complications. The physiotherapist may also, in the pre-operative period, teach the patient other exercises that they will have to do postoperatively. These may include limb exercises to prevent the development of muscle wastage, foot drop and deep vein thrombosis, complications that can occur very quickly postoperatively but can with care be avoided. If there is any suggestion that the patient has a common cold or any infection of the respiratory tract, it is usual when possible to delay admission for two weeks or to postpone operation. If this is not done there is a risk that bronchitis or pneumonia may mar the postoperative period. Certain operations require specific pre-operative tests and investigations, these will be described in the appropriate chapters.

Patients who smoke are advised to refrain from doing so for at least 24 hours before the operation.

Premedication

It is customary for the anaesthetist to visit the patient to assess suitability for anaesthesia and prescribe premedication which is administered 1 to 2 hours before operation, so that when the time comes for the patient to be taken to the theatre he is properly prepared for the anaesthetic. Premedication usually consists of two drugs; one such as atropine (injection 0.25 to 1.0 mg) or scopolamine (injection hyoscine hydrobromide 0.3 to 0.6 mg) to dry up secretions, so that the chest does not become flooded with mucus and fluid due to irritation by the inhaled gases; and the other a hypnotic such as morphia (injection morphine sulphate 8 to 20 mg) or omnopon (injection papaveretum 10 to 20 mg), so that the patient is already a little sleepy and comfortable before the induction of the anaesthetic. The drugs most commonly used at present are omnopon and scopolamine, but a combination of morphia and atropine (injection atropine sulphate 0.25 to 1.0 mg) is also often employed. The dosage of drugs for children is adjusted according to age and height. Children under two years may be given atropine alone, an older child might receive an additional short-acting barbiturate. It is preferable that the premedication is *not* injected into an arm or leg if the limb is the site for operation, due to risk of infection. Following premedication the patient should be permitted to rest quietly, and should not be allowed to get out of bed because of the drowsy effects of the premedication.

Pre-operative preparation

Because the patient is taken into the operating theatre, where an aseptic technique is to be followed, i.e. the exclusion of bacteria which might cause infection in the wound, the patient's skin and clothing must be suitably prepared. The site of the operation is shaved and the patient requested to have a bath or shower. Some surgeons request that the skin be painted with an antiseptic solution such as iodine in spirit and a sterile dressing applied. A freshly laundered open-backed cotton nightgown is put on. Dentures should be removed and placed for safekeeping in a suitable receptacle in the bedside locker. The mouth should be checked for crowned or loose teeth and the anaesthetist informed or theatre should be notified. If the patient has any prosthesis it should also be removed. Patients should be strongly discouraged from wearing make-up because lipstick, nail polish and rouge can be very misleading to the anaesthetist, who may judge the degree of oxygenation by the colour of the mucous membranes and skin.

All jewellery should be removed and kept safely. Wedding rings may not easily be taken off and can be covered with adhesive tape to prevent scratches and burns when machinery is used in the theatre.

In order to prevent the patient vomiting during the induction of the anaesthetic, solid food and fluid is withheld for 4 hours before the time of operation. Occasionally this may not be possible when the patient has to be taken to the operating theatre urgently and in such circumstances the anaesthetist must be informed. The nurse should ensure that the last meal taken before this fast is a light one. It is desirable that the patient should have a bowel action on the morning before the operation and this may be encouraged by a mild laxative or suppository. The bladder should be empty, and if the patient is unable to pass urine this should be reported to the surgeon when the patient arrives in the operating theatre. Before pelvic operations, especially in women, a catheter is passed into the bladder so that this may be emptied before the operation begins. Frequently a self-retaining or Foley type of catheter is used for this purpose. This is often performed in the operating theatre after the induction of anaesthesia.

8
The Operating Theatre

Patient care in the operating theatre

Many nurses new to theatre work often miss the patient contact which they are accustomed to having in the wards and feel that work in the operating theatre revolves around complicated equipment and instruments. The aim of this section is to illustrate the important role of the nurse in the care of the patient undergoing surgery, providing the continuity of care commenced on the ward.

In many hospitals the nursing process extends into the operating theatres. The nurses visit the patients pre-operatively to introduce themselves and identify any special needs of the patient relevant to his care in the operating theatre. Such needs may include skeletal deformities making positioning of the patient on the operating table difficult for certain operations; or skin lesions which require additional protection. Awareness of such needs allows the theatre nurse to be prepared and give the best care possible.

Receiving the patient in the anaesthetic room

It is usual and desirable for a ward nurse to accompany the patient to theatre and remain in the anaesthetic room until induction of anaesthesia is complete and the patient is unconscious. The admission of the ward nurse to the anaesthetic room is governed partly by the policy of the hospital and partly by the design of the operating suite. Newly designed theatre suites often have a system of transfer or a holding bay. The identity of the patient is confirmed by the theatre nurse, who greets the patient by name and checks his wristband.

The consent form is checked for correct completion and signature by the patient, or relative if the patient is aged under 16 years.
The site and nature of the operation is confirmed.
The time, dosage and effect of premedication are noted.
The patient's notes and X-rays are checked to be present and complete and any known allergies registered.
The theatre nurse checks for removal of all jewellery, dentures, prosthesis, etc.

Prior to receiving any patient in the anaesthetic room, the nurse will have prepared the necessary equipment and checked that it is in good working order. She will also know if blood has been made available for the patient and where it is located. At no time is a patient left alone in the anaesthetic room and duties should be performed with quiet efficiency and a reassuring manner. The rôle of the ward nurse is ostensibly a social one, providing friendly support.

Anaesthesia

Anaesthesia means 'without sensation'. In general anaesthesia the patient is rendered unconscious, whereas under local anaesthetic consciousness is retained.

General anaesthesia may be administered by inhalation of gas or vapour, by intravenous injection of a barbiturate, or by intramuscular injection, usually with Ketamine.

Inhalation agents. *Halothane* is a very potent anaesthetic agent which gives rapid induction and recovery with little postanaesthetic nausea and vomiting. It is non-inflammable, non-explosive and non-irritant. It provides little analgesia but good relaxation and is very widely used.

Ethane provides rapid induction and recovery, good muscle relaxation and is non-inflammable.

Cyclopropane is a potent anaesthetic agent, non-irritant, highly explosive and very expensive. It has largely been superseded by Halothane although it is still used for children.

Nitrous oxide produces rapid induction of a light anaesthesia suitable only for minor surgery such as dental extractions. It is usually used in combination with oxygen and Halothane for maintenance of anaesthesia.

Ether gives off an inflammable and explosive vapour which is highly dangerous in the theatre where diathermy and electrical apparatus are employed. Its vapour is also irritating and quite often causes postanaesthetic nausea and vomiting. It is, however, a safe anaesthetic agent.

Intravenous drugs. *Thiopentone sodium* is a commonly used barbiturate producing rapid induction of anaesthesia. It provides no analgesia. If introduced outside the vein into either the tissues or an artery, its action is both painful and serious.

Methohexitone is a short-acting barbiturate suitable for quick procedures. Recovery is quick.

Once induction has been achieved, anaesthesia is maintained with a combination of drugs, used with maximum safety to produce the best conditions for surgery. Muscle relaxants like suxamethonium, curare and flaxedil are administered to produce complete relaxation. With the muscle paralysis resulting from the use of such drugs, artificial ventilation will be necessary and is achieved by the introduction of a cuffed endotracheal tube, which is usually attached to a ventilator. Intravenous analgesics like pethidine or neurolep-tanalgesics like fentanyl or phenoperidine are often used.

Local anaesthesia. *Procaine, Lignocaine and cinchocaine* are the three most commonly employed injections for producing local analgesia. By means of a hypodermic needle a small weal is raised in the skin and then a longer fine needle is used to reach the tissues it is desired to anaesthetise. This method is best suited to small operations on the skin and subcutaneous tissues, e.g. removal of sebaceous cysts and operations on mucous 'membranes such as the eye and mouth.

Nerve blocks may be used where it is proposed to operate on a wider area. The best example is a block of the brachial plexus which allows surgery to be performed on the arm.

Epidural anaesthesia, which may be used in childbirth consists of introducing the anaesthetic solution in the space between the dura mater and the bony and fibrous walls of the vertebral canal. A fine catheter may be threaded through the needle if the anaesthetic effect is needed for some hours, so that further solution can be injected. The anaesthetic usually requires 15 to 30 minutes before taking full effect.

Spinal analgesia. This is much less frequently employed in Britain today than formerly. It is carried out by having the patient sit up or lie on his side and then introducing a long thin needle into the spinal theca between the spines of the fourth and fifth lumbar vertebrae. An analgesic, such as Lignocaine or cinchocaine is then injected. These drugs may cause a profound fall in the blood pressure and therefore injections of vasopressor substances such as noradrenaline or pholedrine should be at hand. Spinal anaesthesia is particularly useful for perineal operations. It should never be used in the very young or very old nor in the presence of shock or neurological disease.

During surgery the patient is constantly observed by the anaesthetist, who regularly records blood pressure, pulse and respirations. The anaesthetist is also responsible for maintenance of the circulatory volume and appropriate intravenous infusions will be given. If the surgery is to be complex and of long duration, additional monitoring equipment is required such as an ECG machine and a CVP line.

Positioning and handling of the anaesthetised person is a skilful task and vitally important in the prevention of trauma to the patient. The aim in positioning a patient is to provide good access for both the surgeon and anaesthetist without placing the patient at risk. There should always be an adequate number of people available to transfer the patient on and off the operating table safely, and to position the patient appropriately. Since the anaesthetist is responsible for maintaining the respiratory and circulatory functions of the patient, his assent should always be sought before the patient or any part of the patient is moved. Special care of the limbs is essential; the arms should be neither over-extended, nor allowed to fall off the operating table, either of which may cause damage to the brachial plexus. The legs, if left straight, should be supported under the heels to relieve calf pressure and prevent deep vein thrombosis. If the legs are to be raised, as in the lithotomy position, they should be handled simultaneously by two people and supported securely. Adequate padding should be used as required to alleviate pressure and prevent any contact between the skin and metal objects, a contact which could result in diathermy burns. There are few positions used in the operating theatre that a conscious patient would naturally adopt, hence the importance of stressing the care needed to prevent trauma. Some operations are unavoidably of long duration, and the prevention of pressure sores developing can be achieved by the use of a well-padded mattress and water blankets. A water blanket of the ripple variety is used and assists in maintaining body temperature.

The application of the diathermy plate requires mention. Diathermy is the use of an electrical current to achieve haemostasis. The diathermy plate is essential to complete the circuit of the electrical current which passes from a machine through the body tissues and is returned to the machine via the indifferent electrode (diathermy plate). If no plate were in position, the electrical current would return to earth at the nearest point of contact between the patient and any metal object. The upper thigh is most commonly used for this purpose; alternatively the buttocks can be used. In either instance, the skin should be dry and free of excessive hair to give good safe contact. The electrode plates used today are generally disposable and are made in suitable sizes for adults, infants and the newborn.

The technique of antisepsis

Less than a hundred years ago any surgical operation was regarded as carrying a real threat to life and if the wound did not become infected it was considered unusual. Surgery as we know it today really dates from Lister, who introduced the technique of *antisepsis* as a direct outcome of Pasteur's work on micro-organisms. Lister discovered that if the surgeon's hands, instruments and dressings were made as clean as possible and if infection was kept under control by means of carbolic acid in the form of a spray (Fig. 8.1) and a lotion, then clean tissues could be opened and closed with every chance of their healing by first intention. It was an easy step from this to evolve a technique whereby micro-organisms were entirely excluded from the operation field, so that antiseptics were no longer necessary. The great advantage of the *aseptic technique* over the antiseptic one was that antiseptics not only destroyed micro-organisms but also the tissues themselves and thus healing was of necessity delayed. With asepsis the tissues are left healthy and undamaged and with the exclusion of organisms are able to heal normally.

Asepsis is a commonly used term throughout hospitals, but probably nowhere so much as in the operating department. All instruments, drapes, sutures, drains, dressings, gowns, gloves and solutions used during surgery must be sterile, and it is the 'scrub' nurse's responsibility to ensure the strictest of aseptic conditions and techniques. Many hospitals today are provided with sterile instrument sets and drapes etc. from a central sterile supply department (CSSD). Others are not and provision for sterilizing equipment is made in the theatres. Where an autoclave or any other method is

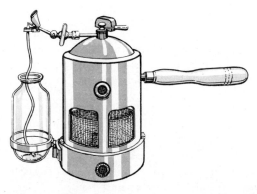

Fig. 8.1 Lister's carbolic spray.

used to achieve sterility the staff should be fully versed as to their appropriate uses and methods of functioning.

The scrub nurse has many duties pertinent to the care of the patient, including the counting and checking of the instruments, sutures, needles, and swabs used during an operation. These checks are made prior to starting the operation, on the closure of any cavity, such as the peritoneal cavity, and at the end of the operation before the skin sutures are inserted. Provisions are made in every operating theatre for the recording of such checks, and the theatre nurse should know the policy of the hospital for this procedure.

Personnel working in the operating theatre have a responsibility to prevent the spread of infection. Any member of staff with a cold, sore throat, open wound or any other source of infection should refrain from work and seek treatment. Patients can be a source of cross-infection, and staff should be informed of the correct procedures for operating on infectious patients. There are usually local policies for dealing with people who have tuberculosis or positive Australia antigen, etc. Likewise, there should be a routine for the reporting, recording and treating of any accidents occurring to either staff or patients.

Apart from the aforementioned, there are many other aspects of theatres and the work performed there which are centred around providing a safe environment for the patients. Maintenance of the correct temperature and humidity in the theatre with good ventilation providing adequate air changes is necessary. Equipment requires regular checking, overhaul and maintenance by the appropriately trained people. Good lighting for the surgeon and anaesthetist must be provided.

Supervision and teaching of learners in the department is the responsibility of the trained staff. Correct usage of equipment and the following of procedures and local policies is essential.

Preparation for operation

The patient. It is necessary that the patient should not bring infection into the operating theatre and for this reason he has a shower or bath, so that the usual contaminating organisms on the skin are removed. A freshly laundered gown is put on, the hair is covered with a light cap and the legs are usually left uncovered. The site of operation is cleansed by shaving off any hairs and washing with soap. If the surgeon requests it, the skin is prepared using spirit soap, and when completely dry is painted with an antiseptic solution over a wider area than that in which the surgeon is expected to operate. By such means, the field in which the surgeon makes his incision is freed from bacteria, but as an added precaution the skin surface is always painted with an antiseptic after the patient has been placed on the operating table.

Surgeon and nurse. Those who are to take part in the surgical operation must, in like manner, prepare themselves so that they will not introduce infection into the wound. The outdoor clothing is first changed for a freshly laundered dress or suit which is light, since the temperature in the operating theatre will be higher than that outside. An impervious mask is put over the face and a cap over the head. The hands and forearms are washed under running water for 5 minutes. The hands and fingernails are scrubbed with a sterile nail brush; it is unlikely that scrubbing for longer confers any benefit and may be harmful. Some surgeons prefer a soap or fluid containing hexochlorophene but this is occasionally irritant to the skin and ordinary bland white Castile soap is excellent. When the scrubbing-up process is complete, an assistant produces a sterile towel upon which the hands and forearms are dried. A sterile gown is then donned and an assistant ties it up at the back. Finally, a pair of sterile rubber gloves is pulled on; these are usually thin and supple in texture. Rubber gloves greatly improve asepsis since when the hand perspires infection may be pushed out from the sweat pores and so contaminate the wound. It is important that the gloves should be free from punctures and tears and they should fit well. It is not advisable for a surgeon or nurse to 'scrub-up' if they have open cuts or infections on their hands.

CSSD *and* TSSU

These abbreviations refer to the Central Sterile Supply Department and Theatre Sterile Supply Unit, which may be housed in one department and which have become essential for the efficient supply of sterile dressings and instruments in hospital. Superheated steam under pressure followed by a vacuum ensures that all bacteria and their spores are destroyed and that the contents of the packs when removed are dry. These packs wrapped in cloth and/or paper contain everything required for an operation, gowns for the operating team, or dressings for a patient's wound. They are stored in a central unit to be delivered to theatre or ward as required.

All the instruments used in a surgical operation must be suitably sterilized.

9
Postoperative Care

The recovery room

Many operating suites today have the facility of an adjoining recovery room where patients are cared for in the immediate postoperative period, until consciousness is regained and their respiratory and cardiovascular systems are stable.

The recovery room is equipped with piped suction and oxygen to each bed, facilities for cardiac monitoring and the relevant equipment for assisted ventilation. In addition, the recovery room should have all the necessary equipment for recording blood pressure, changing dressings, emptying and changing drainage bags, and maintaining intravenous infusions and irrigation systems. Above all, trained nursing staff with experience in monitoring the recovering patient and knowledge of postanaesthetic and postoperative complications is essential.

Where the facilities of a recovery room are not available a suitably trained and experienced nurse will collect the patient from theatre and escort him back to the ward. In the handover of the patient, the ward nurse should check for herself the condition of the patient, that respirations, colour, pulse rate and wound site are all satisfactory. She should have the patient's notes and X-rays and be informed of the operation performed and the names of the surgeon and anaesthetist together with instructions for intravenous therapy and analgesia and any further special nursing care ordered by the surgeon or anaesthetist. The patient is transferred back to the ward by two people on a special trolley, or the bed in some instances, the nurse walking by the patient's head in order to ensure a clear airway. The nursing care on the ward is the same as that carried out in the recovery room.

Nursing care in the immediate postoperative period

The immediate priority in caring for the unconscious patient is the maintenance of a clear airway with or without an artificial airway. To achieve this, the jaw should be held well forward and supported at the angle of the mandible, thus preventing the tongue falling back and causing an obstruction (Fig. 9.1). The nurse should not be lulled

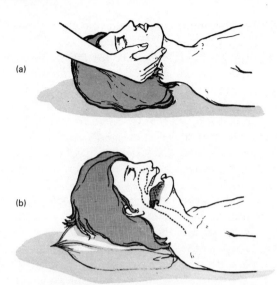

Fig. 9.1 (a) Holding the jaw well forward at its angle to maintain a clear airway.
(b) Obstruction of the airway by allowing the tongue to fall back.

into a false sense of security in thinking that an artificial airway will prevent obstruction occurring. The airway can also become obstructed by a plug of mucus or a foreign body obstructing the larynx, or by spasm of the larynx as the reflexes return. An acute obstructed airway is an emergency and medical help should be obtained since the possibility of cardiac arrest may follow. If the airway is partially obstructed the patient's breathing will be noisy and the patient restless. This must be investigated immediately.

Until consciousness is regained, the patient should be nursed in the semiprone position unless this is contra-indicated, as for example in the patient following thoracotomy, when lying on the unoperated side may embarrass respiration.

The pulse, blood pressure and respirations are monitored and recorded at 15 minute intervals. Regular observations of these signs help early recognition of the onset of postoperative shock, reactionary haemorrhage or respiratory depression.

Oxygen is given by a Hudson-type mask or nasal cannula at a rate of 4–6 litres/minute. In the case of bronchitic patients a Venturi mask is used giving an oxygen concentration of 28 per cent at a rate of 4 litres/minute. Care should be taken to place the mask comfortably over the patient's mouth and nose, away from the eyes.

Intravenous infusions should be secured and maintained at the prescribed rate. The importance of fluid and electrolyte balance has been stressed previously. A chart should be available to record all intake and output of fluid. Intake may be intravenous or by some other method, for example bladder irrigation following prostatectomy. Output may be by vomit, urine or wound drainage. Each form of intake and output should be carefully measured and individually recorded to effect a correct and adequate fluid balance.

Wound dressings should be secure and dry and they should be observed for oozing. Additional packing may be necessary if blood loss is great. Excessive loss from the wound should be reported to the surgeon.

Drainage tubes should be secure. A variety of drainage apparatus is in use today and the nurse should be familiar with each type, its usage and how to change the bottles or bags which accompany certain drains, such as the 'Redivac' or under-water seal bottles.

The level of consciousness of the patient should be closely observed. The first reflexes to return following anaesthesia are the tracheal, laryngeal and cough reflexes. These have usually returned before the patient is removed to the recovery room. The reflex activity which the nurse should be alert to is that of swallowing and vomiting. Close attention is required during this stage. If an artificial airway is *in situ* at this stage it is advisable to withdraw it an inch or so to prevent contact with the back of the throat, an irritation which may provoke retching. Soon after the return of swallowing reflexes, response to painful stimuli becomes evident but overstimulation is to be avoided, since it may induce the patient to reject his airway prematurely. It is preferable and safer that the patient removes his own airway. When the patient can respond to the spoken word return to consciousness is complete.

The need for pain relief in the recovery period will depend largely on whether opiates have been administered in the premedication or during anaesthesia and on the nature of the surgery. Analgesia should not be withheld in the postoperative period, and once it has been administered as prescribed, the patient should be retained in the recovery room under observation for at least another half an hour, during which time any effects on blood pressure or respirations will have become evident.

Following the return of consciousness the patient may be raised to the semi-recumbent position and made more comfortable by the addition of pillows, a change of linen if required and a light wash of hands and face. The patient should be kept warm at all times and the atmosphere in the recovery room should be quiet and calm, with the nurses performing their duties gently and efficiently. Regular attention is given to pressure areas and gentle breathing and limb exercises are encouraged for those patients who may remain for a long period in the recovery room.

Following complete recovery, the patient is collected from the recovery room by a ward nurse, preferably the same one who escorted the patient to theatre. A complete report of the operation, infusions, irrigations, anaesthetic techniques, analgesia, drainage apparatus, recovery-room care and observations is given together with any further nursing care ordered. It is usual for a vomit bowl and a postanaesthetic pack to accompany the patient back to the ward. This consists of a mouth gag of the Ferguson type, a wooden spatula, tongue forceps, absorbent gauze to wipe away mucus and a Guedel-type airway. The trolley should have facilities to support any infusions, an oxygen cylinder and face-mask. If the journey back to the ward is a long one, portable suction apparatus should be made available.

Epidural and spinal anaesthesia

Techniques in anaesthesia permit surgery to be undertaken on the patient who is at risk from a general anaesthetic. Patients with cardiac or respiratory diseases may fall into this category. Operations on the body below the lower abdominal region may be performed under spinal anaesthesia. Epidural anaesthesia is widely used in obstetrics. Contra-indications to spinal anaesthesia are shock, low blood volume, cardiac failure and severe anaemia; it is also unsuitable for children and when there are spinal deformities or infections of the back.

Patients who have had spinal anaesthesia require special nursing care until the effects of the anaesthesia have worn off. Until sensation and muscle activity return, particular attention should be given to the limbs, with regular observation of colour and sensation of the lower limbs. Comfortable positioning without undue pressure is important. Hypotension is common following spinal anaesthesia and the patient is nursed flat or with the head of the bed lowered, until the systolic blood pressure shows a return to normal. Nursing the patient flat also helps to prevent the headache that often accompanies spinal anaesthesia. Remembering that there is temporary loss of sensation, the urinary bladder may become very distended and an observant nurse can take action to alleviate this.

Ketamine hydrochloride (Ketalar). Injection of Ketalar produces a state of dissociative anaesthesia where the patient experiences a

changed state of consciousness accompanied by analgesia. It is used
mainly as an induction agent for paediatric anaesthesia, especially
where repeated administration is likely. However, its use is
restricted because of the associated incidence of hallucinations and
other psychotic sequelae that may follow. In adults this occurs to a
much greater extent that in children and the incidence is unac-
ceptably high. Consequently recovery from such a form of
anaesthesia should be allowed to take its own course with as little
disturbance as possible.

General postoperative care

The authors can only offer general principles in postoperative care
together with guidelines by which a patient-care plan may be
formulated by the nurse according to her assessment of the patient's
needs. As no two patients will make the same rate of progress on the
road to recovery, the nursing-care plan needs to be flexible,
permitting change as the patient's condition and progress alter.

Personal hygiene and comfort. Thoughtful and skilful execution
of the fundamental nursing duties which promote cleanliness and
comfort can do much to generate a feeling of well-being and increase
morale in a patient. In the early stages following surgery, a patient
will require blanket bathing and assistance with toilet facilities. As he
becomes more ambulant, the patient will be able to perform these
tasks for himself, but for those patients confined to bed for any
length of time, it is the attention given to details such as hair care,
oral hygiene, eye care, skin care and personal freshness that become
important. An attentive nurse can, with initiative and imagination,
employ any of several methods to promote comfort, ensure warmth
and relieve pressure and pain.

Fluid balance. A postoperative record of fluid intake, orally or by
any other means, and of urinary or any other output will be
maintained for all patients for different lengths of time according to
the type of surgery performed. In some cases this may be 24 hours,
in others, a period of days, or even weeks. Intravenous therapy may
be used following surgery, to maintain a correct electrolyte balance
and prevent underhydration. Irrigation systems are used after
certain operations, and careful balance of intake and output is
required. Other points to remember include wound drainage,
vomit, nasogastric and other aspirate.

Wound care. Wound healing is dependent on a good food supply, adequate protein intake and vitamin C. The latter may be given
supplementary to the patient's diet, in either tablet or injection form.
Wound dressings are applied to protect from contamination, to give
pressure and support and to maintain apposition of the skin edges.
Wounds should be kept as dry as possible, since bacteria thrive in
warm moist conditions. Wound dressings should be changed only
when necessary: when they become moist, when sutures are to be
removed or drains shortened, if discomfort is felt by the patient, or if
there is an unexplained rise in temperature. Strict aseptic techniques
should be employed when dressings require changing.

Wound drains are inserted at operation to enable the escape of
pus, blood or tissue fluid, which ensures wound healing from the
bottom upwards. If drainage is not employed, fluid is likely to
collect and cause breakdown of the wound. Drains may be attached
to bottles or bags with gentle suction applied, or they may be left
open into a dressing. Invariably they are secured to the skin by a
suture, and some have a safety pin inserted through them to prevent
the drain slipping back into the wound once the stitch has been
removed. Often, shortening of a drainage tube in stages prior to
complete removal is necessary and is performed with the aseptic
precautions employed for any wound dressing. Any abnormality in
appearance, odour or exudate from a wound should be reported to
the person in charge of the ward.

The removal of sutures is undertaken at the time appointed by the
surgeon, usually 7–10 days after operation. Those on the face and
neck are removed much earlier, 3–5 days, because the blood supply
is good and minimal scar tissue is desirable. Sutures on the back may
be left longer, as the blood supply is less good. Deep tension sutures
may be removed before or after the skin sutures, as the surgeon
prefers. Some wounds may not have skin sutures to remove due to
the use of absorbable subcuticular suture material. Clips of the
Michel or Kifa variety may be used for skin approximation and
require special clip removers.

Analgesia. Pain is often considerable during the first 12–24 hours
and should be relieved by the administration of the drugs ordered by
the surgeon. Usually, one of the controlled drugs like Omnopon
may be prescribed for pain relief in the first 24 hours, with an
alternative such as Pentazocine or Panadol to alleviate less severe
pain in the later stages of recovery. Analgesia should not be
withheld, but drugs with addictive properties are to be administered

with care to prevent a recurring need being developed by the patient.

Pain causes restlessness and irritability in a patient and can retard recovery. Analgesia may be necessary prior to certain treatments, such as breathing or limb exercises supervised by a physiotherapist. Abdominal wound incisions can be painful enough to discourage a patient from deep breathing, which is undesirable because of the complications this may produce.

Administration of the appropriate analgesia and sedation will provide for adequate rest and sleep, necessary to promote healing.

Diet. Adequate nourishment and hydration incorporating essential proteins, vitamins, particularly vitamin C, and carbohydrates is vital for recovery and wound healing. Except in gastric and intestinal operations, fluids may be given by mouth as soon as the patient recovers from the anaesthetic and any postanaesthetic vomiting has been relieved. A light diet is usually offered until the bowels have been opened and a gradual return to a normal diet can then be encouraged. Any special dietary requirements or preferences should be noted and followed where possible.

In some instances nutrition may need to be administered by methods other than the oral route, such as by nasogastric tube, gastrostomy tube or by an intravenous feeding line. In these cases, a carefully planned diet providing all essential nutrients is required. Advice on the preparation and composition of special dietary needs can be sought from the hospital dietician.

Elimination. Alteration in bowel habit can occur due to hospitalization alone and is distressing for many patients. If a bowel action has not occurred by the third postoperative day the administration of glycerine suppositories may be required to prevent constipation developing. Defaecation may also be encouraged by allowing the patient to adopt as normal a posture as possible, by the use of a commode or by taking the patient to the toilet in a wheelchair. After operations involving the anal region, such as haemorrhoidectomy or perineal resection, special nursing care is required. Elimination of waste products also includes the passing of urine. This can sometimes be delayed following surgery, and nursing attention should be directed at noting and recording the first act of micturition or its absence.

Exercise and ambulation. As soon as the patient's condition permits he should be allowed to adopt the position most comfortable. Early ambulation is encouraged to prevent all the possible complications that occur from remaining immobile, such as deep vein thrombosis, chest infections, and pressure sores. Active exercises including breathing exercises are to be encouraged and passive limb movements performed where applicable. Since it is to the patient's benefit for him to be mobilized as soon as possible, the nurse needs to be firm in her handling of the patient and offer an explanation for what the patient usually sees as bullying tactics in order to make life easier for the nursing staff. Patients who understand their treatment and its necessity are usually co-operative.

Complete recovery leading to discharge from hospital can be lengthy after major surgery; it can also, in the later stages, be boring. An occupied patient is usually a more contented patient. Relatives and visitors can help by providing books and magazines and some form of light occupation to while away the time. The assistance of an occupational therapist can also be sought, especially if there is a need for rehabilitation to home life such as in the case of an amputee.

On the other hand there are an increasing number of patients who are discharged home early after surgery. These patients are referred to the care of the community nurse, who will visit them and check on progress, change wound dressings, remove sutures and so on.

Some patients may require help and support from specialist sources. In this category may be included patients with stomas, mastectomy patients and others with similar long-term conditions who may need to seek advice or just moral support. The community services can be arranged by the ward sister before discharge of the patient.

Communication. A patient who suddenly finds himself in hospital encounters a strange environment amongst a large number of different people and he becomes a victim of the ministrations of all who work therein. This can be, and often is, a frightening experience and the individual's reaction to this can vary from being withdrawn and retiring to being aggressive and demanding. People admitted to hospital have a need to maintain their dignity and independence, and the recognition and respect of this by hospital staff is vital. All too often nursing and medical staff forget that the well-intentioned treatment that they administer is totally new to a patient and is frequently performed with a clinical air and a certain lack of sensitivity. Time spent in talking to, explaining and above all listening to a patient is invaluable in developing a trusting and relaxed relationship.

Postoperative complications

Vomiting. Modern anaesthetic agents cause much less vomiting than those which were used formerly, but patients still feel nauseated after operations and occasionally vomit. If vomiting is profuse, a Ryle's or Levine's tube may be introduced into the stomach through the nose. The gastric contents are then aspirated at regular intervals or the tube is connected to a continuous-suction pump. It is often a great advantage to insert the tube pre-operatively. Sips of cold water or soda water or pieces of ice to suck often tide the patient over this period.

Pain. This is often worse in the early hours after an operation, and when a drug has been ordered on the patient's prescription sheet there should be no delay in administering it. Frequently a small dose of morphia is given and not repeated thereafter, but at night-time some other sedative may also be prescribed. Pethidine (Inj. Pethidine or Tab. Pethidine 25 to 100 mg) is given with good effect for colicky pain.

Urine. Retention of urine may complicate the postoperative period for two reasons. The abdomen may be painful because of an incision, thus making it difficult for the patient to pass water, or the patient may find it difficult to micturate while lying in bed. Simple measures to remedy this should be tried first. The patient is encouraged to pass urine in a changed position, or a tap may be left running near the bedside since the sound of running water is often helpful. A drink of water and a hot-water bottle placed over the patient's abdomen sometimes produce the desired result. Finally a drug such as carbachol, e.g. 0.25 to 0.5 mg, may be ordered and is given by injection. The latter can only be used when the operation does not involve the urinary tract. If all these measures have failed, it is necessary to pass a catheter and this must be done with strict aseptic precautions, as infection at this time is more easily introduced than when the patient is in good health.

Bronchitis and pneumonia. After an operation when the incision reaches near to the costal margin, or actually involves the chest wall, it is difficult for the patient to breathe deeply because of pain. If a lung is not fully aerated, the fluid within tends to stagnate and becomes infected, and if the patient is prone to recurrent respiratory diseases these are likely to be lighted up by an anaesthetic. Bronchitis may occur with a painful dry cough which later becomes productive. Alternatively, a tough plug of mucus may obstruct a bronchus so that the lung distal to this will not be aerated and if X-rayed will be seen as a fairly solid area. Such an event causes a rapid increase in the pulse rate, out of proportion to the rise of temperature which accompanies it and vigorous physiotherapy is required to relieve it. If this treatment is not successful it may be necessary for the patient to have a bronchoscope passed, when the offending bronchus is cleared by aspiration. Administration of oxygen is of value when the patient shows any signs of cyanosis.

Pneumonia, which in the postoperative period is usually bron-chopneumonia, is a serious complication of any operation. It is treated by breathing exercises, the encouragement of expectoration of the mucopus which has formed and by the administration of suitable antibiotics to control the infection. If the breathing is laboured and difficult, steam inhalations may be helpful, or a tent may be placed about the patient's bed with a steam kettle to ensure that the air inspired is warm, moist and soothing.

Haemorrhage. Bleeding is not a common complication of operations, but may occur within the first hours after the patient returns from the operating theatre. If it is serious the patient will become pale, the pulse rate will rise rapidly and all the signs of shock appear. The blood may be seen externally in the dressings, but since the haemorrhage may be internal it is important that the closest watch be kept on the patient's pulse rate. It will be necessary to return the patient to the operating theatre so that the bleeding point, or points, can be controlled and blood administered intravenously to make up for that which is lost. Secondary haemorrhage is an extremely rare complication in these days and is due to the erosion of a blood vessel by sepsis. It occurs about ten days after an operation, since it takes this time for infection to destroy the vessel wall. When it does happen the loss of blood may be very severe, but fortunately is often heralded by tiny losses a few hours before.

Paralytic ileus. Paralysis of the bowel following an operation is usually caused by peritonitis. The treatment is to aspirate the contents of the bowel by a Ryle's or Miller Abbott's tube and to replace the fluids which the patient loses by giving intravenous saline and glucose. The aspiration is best carried out continuously by means of an electric pump, and this treatment may have to be continued for some days.

Pulmonary embolus. In this condition a clot becomes detached from a vein and is swept back in the bloodstream to the heart and then held up in the pulmonary circulation. The largest of such clots will be arrested at the bifurcation of the pulmonary artery and this is associated with intense pain in the chest, distress, an urge to defaecate and sudden death. Where smaller emboli occur, the block may be in a vessel supplying only one segment of the lung. In such circumstances the administration of heparin to prevent further clotting and oxygen administered by a mask will be required. Morphine will be administered for relief of pain.

Wound infection. Infection in the wound of a clean operation should never occur for it means that there has been some fault in the surgical technique. However, many operations are carried out when infection is already present and then such a complication may be expected. If the wound has been close-stitched the stitches will have to be removed in order to let the pus escape. Anaerobic infection may complicate an abdominal wound and the resulting pus is foul smelling. Antibiotics may be given should the causative organisms be known. Occasionally an abdominal wound bursts open even though no obvious sepsis is present. This is more likely to happen where increased intra-abdominal pressure occurs, as in coughing or vomiting, or when the patient's healing processes are faulty due to previous ill health and malnutrition. With such a *burst abdomen* it is a matter of great urgency that it be covered with a large, sterile, moist pack of gauze or a sterile towel and the patient returned to the operating theatre for immediate surgery. Only by this means can peritonitis and all its sequelae be avoided.

Other complications. There are many other complications which can cause trouble in the postoperative period. The patient may have difficulty in having a bowel action and it may be necessary to insert a suppository or give a small enema. Distension may be relieved by introduction of a flatus tube.

A wound may break down and a faecal fistula appear. If this occurs a few days after the operation, it is not necessarily of serious import and very often it will close spontaneously without further treatment.

Many other conditions, usually treated by a physician, may complicate this postoperative phase because patients with heart disease, or previous chest disease, are likely to have an exacerbation of their troubles due to the added stress of an anaesthetic and a surgical operation.

When the patient has to spend a long time in hospital, as in the postoperative stages of chest surgery, the nurse needs to show much sympathy and understanding. Often during each stage of the illness, new demands are made as patients adjust themselves to changing circumstances. A good nurse derives great satisfaction from this relationship, but it is advisable to remain emotionally detached.

The intensive care unit (ICU)

The Intensive Care Unit is best described as an area where seriously ill patients can be treated and cared for by highly qualified staff, in the best possible conditions with the most modern equipment available.

Intensive care implies continuous observation. To achieve this, specially trained and qualified staff with a high nurse to patient ratio, giving a 24-hour service, are needed. In addition, a unit furnished with appropriate equipment for cardiac monitoring, assisted ventilation, emergency cardiopulmonary resuscitation and so on, is essential.

The selection of patients for admission to an ICU should be decided upon by agreed criteria. Inevitably, the patient turnover and mortality rate in such a unit is high, because of the very nature of its work. To compound this by inappropriate patient selection can only be detrimental to staff and patient morale. As a general principle, the patients' illnesses should be judged to be reversible and those in the terminal stage of chronic diseases do not fall into this category.

The decisions on patient care in an ICU are often under the control of an experienced anaesthetist, who collaborates with the relevant physician or surgeon about the patients' management. This is a desirable situation for nursing staff, whose instructions for care need to be clear and not constantly changed by different doctors. However, this is an arguable point and often an issue of conflict.

Patients who have undergone major thoracic, arterial or neurological surgery may be transferred direct to ICU from the operating theatre. This is usually determined prior to surgery and a bed is reserved. Occasionally, circumstances arise during surgery, when continuous observation postoperatively is decided to be in the patient's best interests and arrangements are made for transfer to ICU. This decision is usually taken by the anaesthetist whose responsibility it is to monitor and maintain circulatory volume, respiratory function and electrolyte balance. The decision is obviously taken in consultation with the surgeon.

In addition to the highly specialized nursing procedures performed in the ICU the fundamental patient care must not be forgotten. Included here is the regular and meticulous recording of vital signs and fluid balance. Many ICU's have their own specially designed charts on which all observations, medication, nursing care and any other treatment given in each 24 hours are recorded. This provides an overall picture of the patient's progress at a single glance.

There are both advantages and disadvantages in establishing an ICU, but it is recognised that the former outweigh the latter inasmuch as the concentration of expensive and complex equipment together with highly skilled staff makes economic and practical sense. However, it does mean that nurses in training do not gain the experience of nursing critically ill patients on the general wards, and they should spend some time in an ICU, preferably during their final year.

10

Head and Neck

Many congenital defects occur in the head and neck, and because they are so conspicuous they require early treatment. An account of cleft lip and cleft palate will be found in the chapter on paediatric conditions, but there are also a number of congenital lesions which may not produce symptoms until many years after birth.

Branchial cysts and fistulas

During the early stages of development, the foetus goes through a period in which it resembles a fish rather than a mammal. There are branchial (gill) clefts along each side of the upper end of the embryo (Fig. 10.1); occasionally these do not completely fuse together, leaving an opening. A small space can be shut off, or sequestrated, between them and when this happens a *branchial cyst* (Fig. 10.2) is produced. This is usually oval and lies obliquely deep to the upper third of the sternomastoid muscle. It may increase in size quite rapidly and, if seen in an older patient, may mimic malignant disease. More commonly it is seen in a child or young adult when it attracts attention because of its size, or because it has become infected. The treatment of a branchial cyst is excision and often the correct diagnosis is not made until an operation for removal of the swelling is performed. A *branchial fistula* or, as it is often called, a

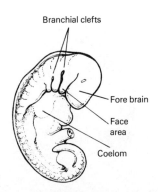

Fig. 10.1 Side view of an early embryo showing branchial clefts.

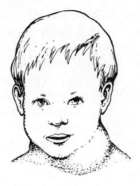

Fig. 10.2 Branchial cyst in a child.

cervical sinus presents as a tiny opening in the skin of the neck at the inner border of the lower third of the sternomastoid muscle and usually discharges some clear sticky fluid. The track passes upwards and backwards between the internal and external carotid arteries and occasionally opens just above the tonsil. The opening in the neck may have a protuberance beside it which, of course, makes it more unsightly. The sinus may become infected and progress to abscess formation. Such an abscess recurs at intervals and since it arises in a track lined with epithelium it is not able to heal. Treatment is by complete excision of the whole track. Cervical sinus is often familial, i.e. occurs in a number of members of the same family.

Tongue

On rare occasions the fraenum beneath the tongue (Fig. 10.3) is so short that the tongue cannot be protruded, with the result that

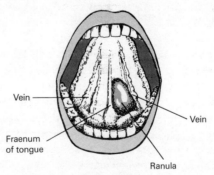

Fig. 10.3 Under-surface of the normal tongue.

speech is impaired. The condition is called *tongue-tie* and is readily cured by incising the fraenum or performing a small plastic operation beneath the tongue. Many parents blame a short fraenum or tongue-tie when the baby is slow to talk, but this is rarely the cause. Another rare condition is an unduly mobile tongue which falls back and obstructs the airway in the newborn baby. This is an extremely dangerous situation and a stitch has to be put through the tip of the tongue in order to secure it to the chin lest the baby suffocate. It is unfortunately often associated with underdevelopment of the lower jaw and mental retardation. A cyst beneath the tongue is called a *ranula*.

Glossitis. This is a word used to describe many conditions in which the surface of the tongue is altered by pathological processes. It does not necessarily infer that the condition is inflammatory. Any kind of redness, soreness or unusual appearance of the tongue is referred to as glossitis, but the most important of these is *leukoplakia*. In this condition there is an overgrowth of the superficial layer so that white patches appear, looking rather like splashes of milk. Leukoplakia is often the result of chronic irritation such as that produced by smoking or ill-fitting dentures. The importance of the condition is that it is prone to undergo a malignant change and the tumour which then most commonly develops in the tongue is a *squamous carcinoma*.

Ulcers of the tongue. These may be simple or malignant. Simple ulcers include the painful ones which accompany dyspepsia and those which follow any kind of trauma such as that due to biting the tongue or the abrasion caused by a roughened denture. In addition, a malignant change can make its first appearance as an ulcer, usually on one edge of the tongue in its anterior two thirds. If the ulcer is malignant it is often painless, firm or indurated to the touch, and with edges which tend to be rolled outwards or everted.

Carcinoma of the tongue. This is seen much more frequently in men than women and in those who are heavy smokers. It is also more common in those patients who have had syphilis and its incidence in different countries varies markedly. It typically presents as an ulcer on the edge of the tongue but may also appear as a heaped-up tumour on its surface. It can be treated by radiation or by surgical excision. When cancer occurs in the anterior two-thirds of the tongue, it is treated by the insertion of *radium needles* in such a way as to expose the tumour to an evenly distributed crossfire from the radium rays. Such an arrangement of radium needles is referred to as a volume implant.

The treatment of carcinoma of the tongue should always be preceded by proper attention to oral hygiene. The mouth is cleaned using hot mouthwashes at two hourly intervals. Carious teeth are extracted and metal fillings removed. In the case of male patients the moustache is shaved and the external skin cleaned using hot soapy water.

After excision of a carcinoma the remaining portion of the tongue is sutured and painted with Whitehead's varnish. It should not be allowed to fall back and block the airway, therefore a ligature is passed through it and a forceps attached so that it can be pulled forward. When the patient is able to swallow, fluids may be given using a spouted feeding-cup with a rubber tube attached. The mouth should be cleaned at frequent and regular intervals. The patient is usually most comfortable in the sitting position.

When radium needles are applied there is considerable swelling followed by the formation of sloughs. The mouth should be irrigated frequently and the fluid used tested with a monitor for radioactivity before being thrown away, in case one of the needles has come adrift. The radium needles are usually attached to sutures which are fastened externally to the patient's cheek; in order to ensure that the needles are still in position the nurse should check the number of these strings three times daily. The patient is instructed not to talk while the radium is *in situ*, which is usually for 7 to 10 days. Early ambulation prevents chest complications.

When a tumour has spread to the lymph nodes underneath the chin (submental), behind the angle of the jaw (submandibular) or beside the jugular vein, it is necessary to excise these nodes. The operation of excising all the lymph nodes and adjoining tissues in the posterior triangle of the neck is called a *block dissection*.

When a carcinoma occurs in the posterior third of the tongue, it is not usually amenable to surgical excision and must be treated by some form of *radiotherapy*. Radium needles can rarely be inserted but it is often more convenient to use the beam of a cobalt machine or linear accelerator.

Alternative treatment for carcinoma in the posterior third of the tongue or for a carcinoma which has recurred after excision is the intra-arterial infusion of a cytotoxic drug (see Chapter 6).

Nursing care

The care of a patient who has had an operation on the neck, face or mouth needs special mention here. This form of surgery is invariably carried out under general anaesthesia, and after the operation the patient is gently laid on the side opposite the wound, to prevent soiling of the dressing should vomiting occur. The patient should be supported with pillows in the lateral position with one knee flexed and the upper arm flexed over the body. The foot of the bed should be raised so that the head is lower than the body in order to encourage drainage of mucus and vomit. Care must be taken to support the head when moving the patient to a comfortable position and the pillows should be arranged to give adequate support. When consciousness returns the patient is sat up in bed. As soon as possible he is encouraged to walk a little to prevent thrombosis in the leg veins. It is important that the patient breathes deeply and breathing exercises are best supervised by a physiotherapist.

Oral hygiene is essential and the mouth should be kept clean by the use of a toothbrush and frequent mouthwashes, e.g. 1 in 4 solution of glycerine thymol compound (glycer. thymol co.). If the patient is unable to manipulate the toothbrush the nurse may be required to do this. Using the moistened brush and dentifrice she brushes the teeth in an up and down direction, cleaning the molar and premolar teeth before the incisors. The mouth is then rinsed with a mouthwash.

Sometimes it is necessary to use cotton-wool swabs held in forceps, the ends of which should be well protected. The swabs are dipped in a solution, e.g. 1 in 4 glycer. thymol co., or 1 per cent sodium bicarbonate, and the vestibule of the mouth cleaned first. Using fresh moistened swabs the tongue is then cleaned in a similar manner; the mouth is then rinsed. Soda water with a little lemon juice may be used as an alternative mouthwash. Dissecting forceps should be used to remove the soiled cotton-wool swabs from the artery forceps to a paper bag for disposal by incineration.

The teeth

The care of the teeth is primarily the duty of the dental surgeon, but it is necessary for the nurse to know about normal and abnormal findings in the mouth.

Most dental surgery is carried out using local analgesia, the dentist injecting the solution either directly beside the tooth or into the main nerves supplying the upper and lower jaws. Occasionally it is necessary for the patient to have a general anaesthetic and a mouth gag is employed to keep the jaws separated. Sponges are often used and should have tapes attached to them so that they are not lost sight of; they are taken out of the mouth immediately the operation is finished. It is also most important to retain all the teeth or portions of teeth after removal, so that they are not inhaled or swallowed and can be inspected by the dental surgeon at the end of the operation.

After operation, it is the nurse's duty to maintain a clear airway until the patient returns to consciousness. Local applications may be ordered to prevent swelling, e.g. compresses of a double fold of lint cut to the required size and wrung out in iced water—these should be changed frequently. Small ice-bags (special half-moon shaped ones are sometimes available) may be used. The ice is broken into small pieces and the sharp edges removed by the addition of a little salt, this also reduces the temperature of the mixture. The ice-bag is half filled by means of a teaspoon, the air is expelled and the cap screwed on firmly. The ice bag is covered with a flannel bag and applied to the particular part. The area of skin is carefully observed and the bag removed if there are any signs of changes in the circulation, such as mottling. It is important that these patients have frequent antiseptic mouthwashes, e.g. 1 in 4 solution of glycer. thymol co.

There are 20 first or *milk teeth* and these start erupting at between six to nine months of age, all being present by the third year. There are, however, many exceptions to these dates. There are 32 second, or *permanent teeth* and these start appearing after the fifth year. Occasionally the third molars or wisdom teeth, do not erupt and if tilted at such an angle that they press on the second molars, may cause severe pain and lock-jaw; they are then described as *impacted molars* (Fig. 10.4).

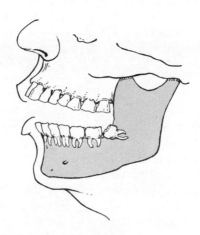

Fig. 10.4 Impacted wisdom tooth or molar.

It is usual to name the milk teeth with the letters A to E, starting from the central incisors and working laterally, as shown in Fig. 10.5.

$$\frac{E\,D\,C\,B\,A \quad A\,B\,C\,D\,E}{E\,D\,C\,B\,A \quad A\,B\,C\,D\,E}$$

Fig. 10.5 Lettering used for milk teeth.

The permanent teeth are numbered from 1 to 8 in both the upper and lower jaws, as is shown in Fig. 10.6. It is useful for the nurse to understand these formulae and be able to check the patients' teeth.

$$\frac{8\,7\,6\,5\,4\,3\,2\,1 \quad 1\,2\,3\,4\,5\,6\,7\,8}{8\,7\,6\,5\,4\,3\,2\,1 \quad 1\,2\,3\,4\,5\,6\,7\,8}$$

Fig. 10.6 Numbering used for permanent teeth.

The commonest disease of teeth is caries. This is considered to be due to the presence of micro-organisms, the growth of which is favoured by sugar, hence the need to limit the consumption of confectionery by children. Fluoride is also necessary for good tooth development.

The gums

The gums, which are formed by the mucous membranes surrounding the teeth, are often the site of disease. Infection of the gums is referred to as *gingivitis* and may be the result of the entry of organisms such as the spirillae of Vincent's Angina, or of a deficiency disease such as scurvy, which is caused by lack of vitamin C. The gums may also recede from the borders of the teeth when the latter, due to exposure, become more liable to decay or caries. Occasionally the gums are greatly hypertrophied and this may be due to a congenital condition or a mild infection. Hypertrophied gums require excision. Certain metallic poisons like lead and mercury leave a telltale black line round the teeth and thus examination of the gums may sometimes be a useful diagnostic measure.

The lips

The lips may be the site of fissures, which can be chronic. The lower lip in man is a common site for malignant disease, the lesion being a squamous carcinoma.

The jaws

There are two jaws, the upper and the lower. The upper jaw or *maxilla* contains the maxillary antrum and this is dealt with in the next chapter. The lower jaw, or *mandible*, is particularly mobile and is often the subject of trauma. It may be fractured by a direct blow, as in boxing or as the result of a road accident. The fracture is almost always an open one because much of the inner surface of the mandible is covered only by a single layer of mucous membrane. A fractured jaw, when not grossly displaced, can be treated by a simple bandage around the head, this brings the lower and upper teeth together and thus employs the upper jaw as a splint for the lower. Feeding is then carried out by means of a tube passed via a gap between the teeth. It is necessary to irrigate the mouth frequently and this may be carried out using a rubber catheter and a syringe. A solution of glycer. thymol co. 1 part to 4 parts of warm water is efficient but if the mouth becomes infected a solution such as peroxide of hydrogen 1 in 100 is more effective. This is best followed by rinsing with a pleasant-tasting fluid to remove any septic material which has been loosened.

When the fracture is more severe, and especially if it is necessary for the patient to lead a more normal life, a fractured mandible can be held firmly in place by a *cap-splint* (Fig. 10.7) made of plastic

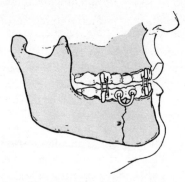

Fig. 10.7 Cap-splint for a fractured jaw.

material or by a metal plate applied to the crowns of the teeth on each side of the fracture line.

When the fracture occurs posterior to the tooth-bearing part of the jaw, it is necessary to adopt other methods such as the introduction of small metal pins. These are driven into the fractured fragment and also into the jaw anterior to the fracture; fixation is then provided by connecting the pins with an external bar (Fig. 10.8). Because these fractures are usually open, the nursing care must aim to prevent oral sepsis, which might infect the underlying bone and cause osteomyelitis of the mandible.

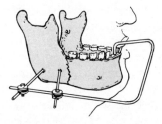

Fig. 10.8 Fixation used for fracture of the posterior part of the mandible.

Fractures of the upper jaw are not as common as those of the lower. When the higher part of the cheek bone, i.e. the zygoma, is fractured, it is often *depressed* and requires elevating by an operation so as not to leave an unsightly deformity and the possibility of double vision. If the nose is broken this requires immediate care. Finally, the whole central part of the body structure of the face may be driven inwards and will then require elevation under general anaesthesia.

The joint between the lower and upper jaw is called the *temporomandibular joint*. It is occasionally dislocated, usually during a yawn, and the best method of reduction is to reproduce the original movement. Arthritis may cause painful limitation of movement at the temporomandibular joint. Sometimes it clicks loudly and causes the patient much discomfort, especially when eating. If the clicking becomes troublesome it may help to excise the small intra-articular cartilage, which can be compared to one of the semilunar cartilages in the knee joint.

Salivary glands

These are the paired parotid and submandibular glands. There are numerous other small ones in the floor of the mouth which are not of great importance. The commonest cause of swelling of the parotid glands is mumps, but this never progresses to suppuration and does not call for surgical intervention. The salivary glands may also be infected by organisms from the mouth, especially in children, and the swelling is made worse by eating because this causes a flow of saliva which cannot freely escape so that the gland becomes distended and painful. Recurrent parotid swelling may arise from allergy. The duct from the parotid gland opens inside the cheek and if it becomes narrowed it will be necessary to dilate it. The submandibular gland may become the site of infection, but this occurs less frequently than in the parotid.

A stone or *calculus* may form in a salivary duct and is found more often in that of the submandibular gland, i.e. Wharton's duct. The stone is composed of almost pure calcium carbonate and therefore shows up well when X-rayed. It may sometimes be seen peeping out of the duct in the floor of the mouth. In a typical case the patient complains of swelling of the gland when food is eaten and occasionally the pain is quite severe because saliva cannot escape past the obstruction. A stone occurring in the duct is removed under local analgesia and the patient is afterwards told to use mouthwashes such as a solution of 1 in 4 glycer. thymol co. until the wound is healed. When a stone occurs within the substance of the gland it is necessary to excise the whole gland, usually the submandibular since stones rarely form in the parotid gland.

Tumours occasionally arise in the salivary glands but are much more common in the parotid than the submandibular. The most usual type of tumour is one which is called a *mixed salivary tumour* and represents a very bizarre appearance under the microscope. Although not at first malignant it increases in size locally, producing for itself a false capsule as it presses on the surrounding gland tissue. After many years it may undergo a malignant change. Treatment consists of excision of the tumour, which must be meticulous and complete for otherwise it is liable to recur. Recurrences, if they occur, are usually multiple and therefore much more difficult to excise.

Excision is a difficult operation because the facial nerve passes through the substance of the gland, breaking up into its main branches therein. Injury to the nerve, causes paralysis of the face resulting in a most unsightly deformity. If facial paralysis is already present when the patient is first seen, this is good evidence that the tumour is a malignant one. Such tumours can be sensitive to *radiation* and since they are frequently unsuitable for excision are treated in the radiotherapy department.

Lymph nodes

In the neck there are many lymph nodes which follow a certain general distribution although it is quite common for them to occur in sites which do not follow an orderly anatomical plan. The main lymph nodes are situated immediately underneath the front of the chin in the submental area, behind the angle of the jaw where they drain from the tonsils, and along the line of the jugular vein where they drain most of the structures in the mouth and neck. Others are found in the occipital region and above the clavicles. Certain small groups lie in relation to definite structures, such as those found above the isthmus of the thyroid gland. Lymph is one of the routes by which infection spreads, it is also of importance in combatting infection. The lymph travels to a lymph node, where it is filtered and this is often the site where the organisms are arrested; if they multiply the node becomes swollen, painful and frequently warm to the touch. Pyogenic organisms usually lead to suppuration. Where lymph nodes are enlarged, tender and warm as a result of infection, relief of pain can be obtained by the application of warmth in the form of fomentations or antiphlogistine. In addition, splinting the neck by means of a collar padded with cotton wool may also help to relieve pain and assist resolution.

When the organisms are tuberculous, there is no warmth and the typical cheesy or caseous pus which forms is referred to as a *cold abscess*. Frequently the abscess is shaped like a collar stud with a small collection of pus under the skin and a much larger one below the deep fascia, the two areas communicating with one another through a small opening.

The lymph nodes of the neck are frequently involved in malignant disease. Certain malignant conditions affect the lymph nodes primarily while other malignant processes involve them secondarily, as for example carcinoma of the tongue, which spreads to the lymph nodes in the posterior triangle.

Hodgkin's disease, or *lymphadenoma*, is a condition which primarily affects the lymph nodes, especially in the neck and upper part of the chest of young adults (Fig. 10.9). The nodes become discretely enlarged, of firm consistence and rubbery. The condition is diagnosed under the microscope after biopsy of an affected node. There are many other types of lymphoma, all of which are malignant and progressive. They are treated by radiotherapy and the injection of cytotoxic chemicals. By means of wide-field irradiation and, when necessary, cytotoxics, patients have remained free from recurrence of Hodgkin's disease for more than 10 years and are presumed cured.

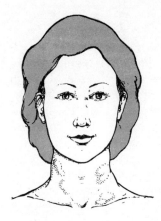

Fig. 10.9 Enlarged lymph nodes in the neck in lymphadenoma (Hodgkin's disease).

Lymphosarcoma is another malignant disease affecting lymphoid tissue which is usually treated by radiotherapy. *Leukaemia* is often a fatal disease in which the white blood cells are produced in ever-increasing numbers, eventually destroying the patient. The lymph nodes are usually enlarged and soft. Cytotoxic drugs are used to induce a remission, which in childhood may last for years.

When lymph nodes are enlarged, those in the neck are so readily palpable and accessible that one of them is often removed for *biopsy*. The pathologist inspects it under the microscope and can usually tell the surgeon what the disease is that has caused the enlargement.

There are a great many other important conditions in the head and neck which have not been mentioned in this chapter, but they will be found under their respective headings in other parts of the book. For example, the thyroid gland is described in the chapter on the endocrine system, basal cell carcinoma (rodent ulcer) and squamous carcinoma of the skin, both of which are commonly seen on the face, are dealt with in the chapter on the skin.

11
Ear, Nose and Throat

The ear, nose and throat, ENT, or otorhinolaryngology department is a highly specialized one and relatively more outpatients than inpatients are dealt with than in other parts of the hospital. The investigations which have to be carried out require special equipment and it is necessary to be able to darken the room. Such a clinic is therefore housed where possible in a department of its own.

Investigations

Because inspection of the inside of the ear, nose and throat requires a bright light and special instruments, the room is darkened and a powerful spotlight placed behind and to one side of the patient's head. The surgeon wears a mirror with a central aperture over his eye. He looks through this mirror at the patient and the light is reflected along the line of sight, thus enabling him to see parts which would not otherwise be visible, while leaving both his hands free to handle the instruments. The care of the electrical equipment and the cleansing of the mirrors used in the department is the responsibility of the nurse in charge. X-rays are frequently required and special viewing-boxes have to be provided so that the films can be seen in the darkened department if necessary.

In addition to the actual inspection and investigation of the ear, nose and throat, it is often necessary to carry out audiometry or hearing tests and these require a soundproof room with apparatus capable of producing sounds of known pitch and loudness. Finally, patients may require instruction in how to speak, either when they have not previously been able to do so properly or when they have had operations upon the larynx. Therefore a speech therapy department is run in conjunction with the ENT department.

The ear

Congenital lesions

There are many congenital abnormalities of the ear. The outer ear is developed from six small tubercles and if these do not fuse together correctly they produce a crumpled ear. Very rarely the outer ear is absent and then there is an associated maldevelopment of the inner ear and complete deafness. An artificial ear of plastic may be provided to improve the patient's appearance. Some children have prominent or bat ears which stand out at right angles to the side of the head. These need to be corrected early in life or otherwise the child is tormented by the other children at school. Much more commonly an *accessory auricle* is present and this takes the form of one or more little nodules of cartilage covered with skin situated just in front of the normal ear. An abnormality which may give rise to chronic sepsis is an *ear-pit* or *pre-auricular fistula*. In this condition a blind pit is situated a centimetre or so in front of the ear and is usually surrounded with rather scaly skin. This fistula may become infected, and when it does it will never heal completely, because there is an epithelial lining to the track. Often the track is associated with cartilage and a cure is obtained only by complete surgical excision.

Earache

Pain in the ear is a common symptom and is not necessarily due to disease of the ear itself. Pain is often referred from lesions in the tongue, jaw (e.g. impacted wisdom tooth), the thyroid or enlarged lymph nodes in the neck. Thus the patient who presents with pain in the ear may require an extensive clinical examination, apart from the examination of the ear itself. The commonest cause, however, of earache is inflammation of the middle ear or *otitis media*. The pain is throbbing, the eardrum bulges and treatment is immediate intramuscular injection of penicillin or other antibiotic. Further treatment is described below.

The normal ear produces a certain amount of *wax* or *cerumen*, which certainly in hot dusty climates has a protective function. Occasionally an excess of wax is produced, or it becomes swollen and impacted causing deafness and pain. The removal of the wax may be done with instruments, but is more commonly carried out by syringing. This task often falls to the nurse, and it requires skill, patience and gentleness in order to remove wax from the ear without causing pain or damaging the sensitive eardrum (tympanic membrane). Drops, e.g. castor oil or sodium bicarbonate solution, may be instilled in the ear at night two or three times before the ear is syringed, to loosen the wax. For syringing, a warm solution of sodium bicarbonate is used and the stream is gently directed along the roof of the meatus while the ear is pulled upwards and backwards. The patient holds a dish snugly against the neck to catch the water and should be shown any wax that is removed.

The outer ear, which includes the pinna and the skin-lined tube leading to the drum, is often the site of infection, *otitis externa*. The organisms responsible for this are frequently staphylococci and may be difficult to eradicate. The outer ear and drum are inspected by means of an aural speculum (Fig. 11.1).

The middle ear (Fig. 11.2) extends inwards from the tympanic membrane and contains the small bones, or ossicles, which transmit sounds from the drum to the cochlea or organ of hearing. This part of the ear communicates with the back of the throat via the *Eustachian tube*. Infection may enter the middle ear via this tube and results in *otitis media*. The patient suffers acute throbbing pain in the ear with some deafness, and if pus forms it may rupture through the tympanic membrane and discharge into the outer ear. Acute otitis

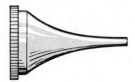

Fig. 11.1 Aural speculum.

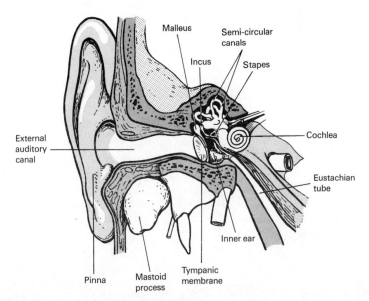

Fig. 11.2 The anatomy of the middle ear.

media is treated with penicillin by intramuscular injection, or other suitable antibiotic, and incision of the bulging inflamed tympanic membrane to let out the pus. A specimen of the pus is sent to the laboratory for identification and to discover its sensitivity to antibiotics. The operation is done under brief general anaesthesia (e.g. nitrous oxide) and is called a *myringotomy* (Fig. 11.3). After this treatment the patient should be told to lie on the affected side to encourage drainage of the pus. A gauze dressing with a large pad of cotton wool may be bandaged in position, but it is important that drainage be maintained. When the discharge stops the patient should be warned not to swim or bathe until the surgeon considers it safe to do so. *Myringoplasty* is the operation in which a skin graft is used to repair or reconstruct the eardrum after simple perforation.

Middle ear infection can spread to three important sites (Fig. 11.4):

1   It may involve the *mastoid air cells*, which are found within the mastoid process, the bony protuberance just behind the ear. In this site, pain and tenderness occur and the infection, if it does not respond to antibiotics such as penicillin, will require surgical

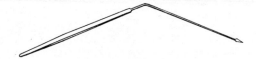

Fig. 11.3 Myringotome.

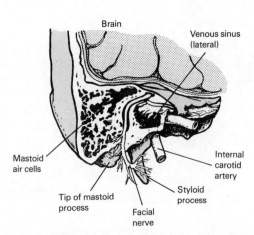

Fig. 11.4 Mastoid air cells and adjoining structures which may be involved by infection.

drainage. If the drainage is only of the adjoining air cells for an acute infection in the mastoid area, it is referred to as a *cortical or Schwartze mastoidectomy*. If the infection is allowed to become chronic, it may have to be dealt with by excising not only these air cells but also the ossicles and some of the adjacent bone. Such an operation is called a *radical mastoidectomy* and carries with it limitation of hearing in that ear. The modern operation of *tympanoplasty* attempts to reconstruct the eardrum by skin grafts and so to ameliorate the deafness after mastoidectomy.

2   The infection can spread upwards from the mastoid area to the meninges causing *meningitis* and *cerebral abscess*, the latter being an abscess within the brain substance. This complication is a serious one and requires adequate dosage with antibiotics and also surgical drainage of the infected area, which is usually performed by the neurosurgeon.

3   The *lateral venous sinus*, which runs just within the skull at this site, can be *thrombosed* by the infection and will require exploration by making a burr hole in the skull, nibbling away the surrounding bone with rongeurs and then removal of the blood clot.

The commonest complication of *otitis media* is continuing low-grade suppuration of the middle ear with perforation of the eardrum and a chronic discharging ear. Many patients with this condition are treated in the ENT Outpatient Department, but far less than in pre-penicillin days. They require careful aural toilet, and when the condition does not clear up, surgical treatment as described above may be necessary. These patients should always be warned not to swim or bathe for fear of stirring up the infection.

Nursing care for tympanoplasty and myringoplasty. The skin is prepared as for mastoidectomy. Tympanoplasty consists of reconstructing the middle ear after its destruction by sepsis. De-natured bone or small plastic prostheses are commonly employed. Myringoplasty is the formation of a flexible eardrum after it has been perforated by infection; thin cartilage is commonly employed. The patient usually returns to the operating theatre for the first dressing, when a wisp of cotton wool will be left in the ear, to be replaced as necessary.

Deafness

The organ of hearing, or cochlea, is situated within the inner ear and when this is involved by inflammation, deafness results.

Another common cause of deafness is *otosclerosis*; in this disease, the membranous covering of the oval window (fenestra ovalis), to which the stapes transmits the vibrations from the eardrum, becomes the site of bony deposits and thickening. As a result the sound waves are not conducted to the middle ear and the patient has *conduction deafness*. The operation of stapedectomy is usually performed, the technique varying from surgeon to surgeon. Hearing may be excellent immediately after operation, but improvement may be delayed and in any case lessens in time.

Nursing care after operations on the middle ear. Giddiness or vertigo often complicates operations on the middle ear, so a drug such as promethazine chlorotheophylinate (Avomine) 25 to 50 mg is given the night before operation and three times a day thereafter if required. Vomiting may also be a complication and chlorpromazine 25 to 50 mg is usually prescribed to control it. The hair is shaved as for mastoidectomy. As infection would mar the result, an antibiotic is given. After operation the patient is laid on the operated side and is kept lying down for the first 24 hours, as he is usually giddy and drowsy. Thereafter the patient is encouraged to raise the head, which is supported by pillows, and on the second day sits out of bed for a short while. From the third day the patient is encouraged to be up as much as possible and the physiotherapist supervises head exercises to improve the patient's balance. The first dressing is often done in the operating theatre on about the fifth day and a wisp of cotton wool is left in the ear.

Associated with the cochlea is the organ of balance made up of three semicircular canals which, together with the vestibule, is called the labyrinth. When the labyrinth is diseased, the patient suffers attacks of *vertigo* or giddiness and when these attacks are associated with tinnitus, or noises in the ears, and *vomiting*, the condition is referred to as *Menière's syndrome*. Treatment is by medical measures as long as possible. If the hearing is good vestibulectomy is performed but when deafness occurs the surgical treatment is to destroy the labyrinth, i.e. labyrinthectomy.

The nose

Examination of the nose is usually carried out using a Thudicum's speculum (Fig. 11.5) and a head mirror with a bright light, e.g. bull's-eye lamp, over the patient's head. The nose is the organ of

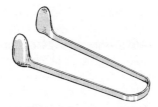

Fig. 11.5 Thudicum's speculum.

smell and the olfactory nerve supplies the upper part of its mucous membrane. It is divided centrally by a septum, which may become deviated to one side and require straightening, an operation called *submucous resection.*

Nursing care. After submucous resection a nasal bolster or pad is applied under the nose to prevent the patient from touching the area and introducing infection. The patient is nursed sitting up to encourage the drainage of serum and discharge and is told not to blow his nose or smoke. Steam inhalations and nasal drops are ordered if there is congestion.

There are three turbinates projecting inwards from each lateral wall. They may become engorged, making breathing difficult and require a spray or drops of normal saline containing 1 per cent ephedrine to shrink them. Chronic infection of the nasal cavity can lead to the formation of *polyps*, these gradually increase in size and obstruct the airway (Fig. 11.6). They are removed by a wire snare

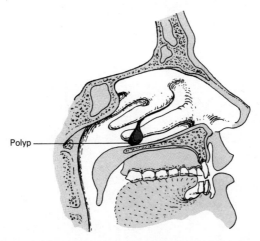

Polyp

Fig. 11.6 Section through the nose; the polyp shaded black hangs below the middle turbinate.

after the interior of the nose has been rendered insensitive with cocaine.

Epistaxis, or nose bleed, is one of the commoner symptoms of nasal disease, but may also occur in otherwise healthy individuals due to excitement. Infection, high blood pressure, foreign bodies and tumours can all cause severe bleeding from the nose. The patient should sit up leaning forward and be instructed to pinch the nostrils between the thumb and forefinger for 15 minutes. The pressure encourages the formation of a clot. The patient should breathe through the mouth and this can be encouraged by giving him a roll of bandage to hold between the teeth and so keep the mouth open. If the blood only escapes in drops it will probably stop spontaneously, but if the bleeding is more copious the nose is irrigated and lightly packed with ribbon gauze soaked in hydrogen peroxide, or adrenalin 1 in 1000 solution, or special gauze such as Calgitex. If a bleeding point is seen, the surgeon cauterizes it with a hot wire or a bead of chromic acid.

The sinuses

The important structures surrounding the nose are the *paranasal sinuses* (Fig. 11.7). The two large box-like ones on each side of the nose are the *maxillary antra* and these are often the site of infection. In acute *sinusitis*, antibiotic therapy is ordered and congestion is

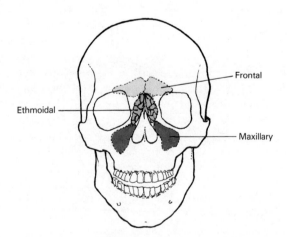

Fig. 11.7 Frontal, ethmoidal and maxillary sinuses (from above, downwards) have been indicated on each side by shading.

relieved by the use of nasal drops or a spray of normal saline containing 1 per cent ephedrine to shrink the engorged mucous membrane. The antra drain into the nose by small openings, or ostia, but since these are not at the lowest level of the antra, fluid such as pus may accumulate. When this happens it is usual to puncture and wash out the antrum. This is commonly done under local analgesia in the outpatient department, a small swab soaked in 25 per cent cocaine being placed in the nose preparatory to making the puncture. In children, fine polythene tubing may be introduced into the antra, the tubing being left in place and the ends fixed to the cheeks with adhesive strapping. The nurse is instructed to irrigate the antra through the tubing at regular intervals using a syringe. The child is instructed to lean forward over a receiver and breathe through the mouth while the irrigation is in progress so that the fluid flows out of the nostrils. It is very important to empty any air out of the syringe before attaching it to the tubing or a bursting sensation is produced. If infection recurs, a permanent opening may be made in the nose to drain the antrum. After such an operation, when infection occurs a cannula can be slid into the antrum and the contents washed out with a syringe. When an antrum is chronically infected, a *Caldwell Luc* operation may be necessary to make a new opening and remove the diseased lining membrane. The antrum is approached by an incision through the gum over the canine teeth and it is cleaned out under direct vision.

Situated in the upper part of the nose are the *ethmoidal sinuses* and these, when infected, produce polypoid projections which require excision by an operation called *ethmoidectomy*. The most inaccessible of the sinuses is the *sphenoid*, which lies above and behind the nasal cavity and forms part of the base of the skull. It is rarely infected and can be drained via the nose by puncture.

Children often push small beads or buttons into their noses and this leads to a persistent nasal discharge until the object has been removed with forceps. Other causes of nasal discharge are infection in the sinuses and, less commonly, malignant disease. Atrophy of the mucous membrane which lines the nose, if associated with excessive dryness and crusting, is called *atrophic rhinitis* and requires treatment with nasal drops and irrigation.

For nasal irrigation the patient should lean forward over a receiver. A rubber catheter attached to a syringe is filled with the irrigating fluid, e.g. normal saline, gently inserted about 2 inches along the floor of the nostril and the fluid introduced so that it flows back into the receiver. This treatment is continued until the fluid returns clear.

The throat

Tonsils and adenoids

The tonsils are collections of lymphoid tissue on each side at the back of the throat; in children there is also a pad of lymphoid tissue on the roof of the nasopharynx, called the adenoids. It is quite common for the tonsils and adenoids to be large in infancy and early childhood, but with the passage of time they generally shrink in size. When they are the site of recurrent infection they may require removal and this is carried out under a general anaesthetic. The indications for T's and A's, as the operation is called, are not clear since tonsils always shrink with age and mere size is not significant. If recurrent acute attacks of infection cause serious loss of schooling or if deafness develops there is little doubt that an operation will help, but the final decision may be difficult. The tonsils are removed by dissection and a wire snare is often employed to complete the operation. Tonsils can also be removed with a guillotine, but this is much less satisfactory. The adenoids are curetted away with a sharp spoon or adenotome.

Nursing care. It is very important that the airway be kept free during recovery from the anaesthetic and the patient should be lying in a semiprone position with the uppermost leg flexed and the lower arm brought well forward. The head is kept low so that blood will not be inhaled into the lungs. The nurse must repeatedly note the rate and volume of the pulse, reporting any change, so that the throat may be examined for reactionary haemorrhage. If the patient is seen to be swallowing it may indicate haemorrhage. A portable electric sucker with soft rubber catheter attached is useful for keeping the airway free of blood and mucus. As soon as consciousness returns, sips of water are given as it is important not to allow the throat muscles to become stiff. The patient ought to take breakfast such as porridge and a boiled egg the day after the operation and often cold fluids and ice cream are soothing. Acetylsalicylic acid (aspirin) 0.75 g to 40 ml of water should be gargled and swallowed about 20 minutes before a meal. An analgesic and antiseptic lozenge such as trocha benzocaine co. is sucked after eating.

Patients get up on the second day following tonsillectomy and seldom need an aperient; however, if a lot of blood has been swallowed it may be advisable to give one, e.g. liquid paraffin 15 ml with an equal amount of magnesium hydroxide. Children are often allowed home on the third or fourth day following operation, but the parents are warned to send for the doctor should any signs of bleeding occur. Adults usually stay in hospital until the sixth or seventh day following operation as they take longer to regain normal health.

When infection strikes at a tonsil and leads to the formation of an abscess between the tonsil and the wall of the pharynx, it is referred to as a quinsy and requires surgical drainage. Local analgesia is preferred for this operation since if a general anaesthetic is given there is always a risk of inhalation of pus. The fauces are sprayed with lignocaine 1 per cent. Occasionally an abscess from the tonsil tracks behind the pharynx and causes the posterior wall to bulge forward obstructing the airway.

Larynx

The larynx or voice-box (Fig. 11.8) is made up of a series of cartilages connected by membranes, the whole enclosing within them the vocal cords. Above is the *hyoid bone* with, just behind it, the *epiglottis*. The thyrohyoid membrane stretches down from the hyoid bone to the *thyroid cartilage*, the largest cartilage of the three. Below this the *cricoid cartilage*, shaped like a signet ring, is situated, connected by the rather short cricothyroid membrane to the thyroid cartilage above. Posteriorly, two small *arytenoid cartilages* are situated on the upper border of the cricoid cartilage and the vocal cords stretch forward from these two arytenoids to be attached to the thyroid cartilage anteriorly.

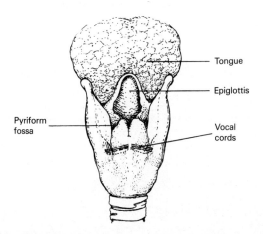

Tongue

Epiglottis

Pyriform fossa

Vocal cords

Fig. 11.8 Tongue, epiglottis and larynx seen from behind.

The epiglottis deflects swallowed food and liquid so that it is passed back into the oesophagus instead of entering the larynx. Rarely this mechanism breaks down and a bolus of food becomes impacted in the larynx causing suffocation if it is not removed. Treatment is urgent, a slap on the back and a finger thrust down to hook the bolus out. If unsuccessful, tracheostomy must be carried out at once.

The innervation of the vocal cords is primarily through the recurrent laryngeal nerves, which cause abduction of the cords. If one of these nerves is damaged the cord lies near the midline and hoarseness and loss of voice result. If both nerves are injured the two paralysed vocal cords almost meet in the midline, and if the patient undergoes exertion he is unable to obtain enough air through the narrow slit which remains. At rest breathing is usually very noisy, especially during sleep, and a tracheostomy will be necessary if any distress is present on exertion.

Infection may also cause obstruction of the larynx, as may the oedema caused by inhaling steam or hot fumes.

The relief of laryngeal obstruction is by *tracheotomy*, or, more correctly, *tracheostomy*, which means making an opening or stoma into the trachea below the cricoid cartilage (Fig. 11.9). A tracheostomy tube is then inserted (Figs. 11.10, 11.11 and 11.12) and it is kept clear of mucus by sucking this out with a fine rubber tube attached to a suction apparatus, preferably a powerful electrical one. Tracheostomy is used to help patients who have difficulty in breathing, as in poliomyelitis, severe injuries of the face, head and neck, and burns. Breathing may be assisted by connecting the tracheostomy tube to an electronically controlled respirator such as

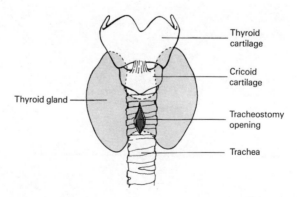

Fig. 11.9 Site for tracheostomy.

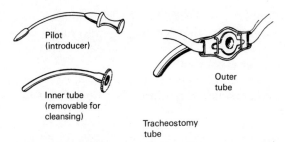

Fig. 11.10 Component parts of a metal tracheostomy tube; (a) pilot (introducer), (b) outer tube, (c) inner tube (removable for cleansing).

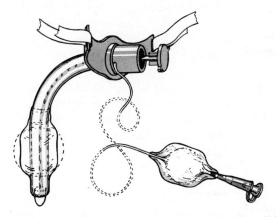

Fig. 11.11 Tracheostomy tube made of plastic with an inflatable cuff for positive pressure respiration using a mechanical respirator.

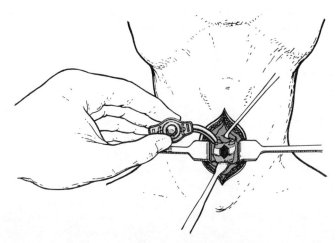

Fig. 11.12 Operation of tracheostomy; tube about to be inserted.

the Blease, which rhythmically inflates the lungs. Thus tracheostomy may be an elective or emergency operation.

Indications for tracheostomy.

1 Obstruction of the respiratory passages due to
   (a) external compression due to tumour or oedema,
   (b) trauma,
   (c) paralysis,
   (d) spasm,
   (e) foreign bodies.
2 The need to assist respiration, e.g. after thoracic surgery when the patient is too ill or weak to cough up secretions.
3 Cessation of normal respirations, e.g. due to failure of the respiratory centre in the medulla because of head injury or narcotic poisoning.

Pre-operative care. When a tracheostomy is to be performed as an elective operation, the psychological preparation of both patient and relatives is important. It is advisable to explain simply that the operation will alleviate the respiratory problems and that although speech will not be possible immediately following surgery, the patient will be taught how to speak with a tube *in situ*.

Postoperative care. A trolley is prepared by the bedside of the patient prior to receiving the patient back from the operating theatre. On this trolley should be facilities for sterile wound dressings, a spare tracheostomy tube of the same size and kind as the one used, sterile tracheal dilators, suction catheters and equipment for oral hygiene. Other equipment includes a suction machine, a mechanical humidifier and, for the patient's own benefit, a bell, note-pad and pencil. If assisted ventilation is required the patient will be transferred direct to ICU from theatre.

The patient will usually be conscious on return to the ward and may be nursed sitting up if his condition permits this. The inhaled air will require moistening and filtering since it no longer passes through the nasal passages. The humidifier required has been mentioned. For filtration, a gauze 'veil' dampened in warm distilled water can be hung over the opened end of the tracheostomy tube.

Suction through the tracheostomy tube is an exhausting procedure for an ill patient and speed and skill are essential. The procedure is performed with aseptic precautions. Suction should only be applied on *withdrawing* the suction tube from the trachea.

If a metal tube has been used, the inner segment will require removal for cleansing two or three times daily. The outer tube should be made secure with tapes tied comfortably around the patient's neck. If the outer tube should fall out, it must be replaced instantly to prevent the opening contracting. Immediate insertion of the tracheal dilators will assist at this point.

Speech is not impossible following tracheostomy but is to be discouraged for the first few days after the operation, since covering the end of the tube during expiration forces air into the surrounding soft tissues causing surgical emphysema.

A Negus-type tracheostomy tube may be used for the long-term patient since it has a 'speaking valve'.

Tumours of the larynx. Simple tumours may occur in the larynx and the commonest is a *papilloma* of the vocal cord. This occurs in childhood and causes partial obstruction to breathing and hoarseness, it usually disappears spontaneously. In singers or those who use their voices a great deal, a nodule may arise requiring surgical removal.

Malignant tumours of the larynx can arise on the vocal cords themselves, *intrinsic tumours*, or in the structures surrounding the larynx, *extrinsic tumours*. Malignant disease affecting a vocal cord often grows slowly and may be excised endoscopically. When the tumour is more extensive *total laryngectomy* is undertaken. This consists of excising the whole of the larynx and the surrounding tissues and leaving the patient with a permanent tracheostomy. The operation is a severe one and causes considerable mental as well as physical upset to the patient. However, in well-selected individuals the result can be satisfactory and a patient can be taught not only to speak but also to sing by swallowing air and ejecting forcibly. In the case of more extensive growths and those lying posteriorly, part of the pharynx and upper oesophagus has to be sacrificed with the larynx, an operation called *pharyngolaryngectomy*. An oesophagostomy is necessary and the patient is fed by tube for the first 4 to 6 weeks. Subsequently skin grafts or transplanted bowel are used to reconstruct the pharynx and allow the patient to swallow normally. Whenever possible these patients are treated by radiotherapy, which plays an important part in the treatment of malignant disease of the larynx. After treatment the services of a speech therapist may be required. When the larynx has been removed the patient is taught to speak by regurgitating swallowed air, so-called oesophageal speech.

Nursing care. A patient who has a surgical operation upon, or radiation therapy to, the larynx is best nursed supported in a sitting position in a bed with a tent. A sucker is kept ready beside the bed, preferably of the powerful electrical type, so that the tracheostomy tube can be kept free of mucus. These patients are fed through an oesophageal feeding tube which is left in position until the patient has learnt to swallow, usually about the seventh to tenth day. The feeds should be increased gradually from small amounts of water at first, until an adequate fluid diet is introduced at 2 hourly intervals. Milk, cream, eggs, salt, honey and glucose should be given together with vitamin C in the form of orange juice. Some of the drinks may be flavoured with Marmite, which contains the vitamin B complex, and proprietary foods containing dried milk solids are useful to maintain nutrition. Oral hygiene must be attended to and frequent mouthwashes given.

An account of cleft lip and cleft palate will be found in the chapter dealing with paediatric surgery.

12
The Thorax

The surgery of the thorax, that is of the lungs and pleura, oesophagus, heart, great vessels and structures in the mediastinum, has evolved relatively recently but in order to obtain better access the chest is often opened by surgeons operating on the stomach, liver and kidneys. The nursing of a patient who has had a chest operation makes considerable demands on the staff; supervision of drainage tubes, intravenous fluid administration and the use of suction apparatus are all of vital importance. Moreover, emergencies may arise in which the time factor is critical if the patient's life is to be saved.

In making a patient ready for a chest operation, the following are required in addition to the usual preparation for surgery. Respiratory function is estimated by clinical measurement of vital capacity and forced expiratory volume. General observation of the patients' breathing is valuable also. Breathing exercises are taught, usually in conjunction with a physiotherapist, and can improve respiratory efficiency. Instructions as to the importance of being mobile postoperatively in order to prevent circulatory disorders are also given.

Lungs and pleura

Each lung is covered by a smooth, shining membrane called the pleura; this is reflected at the root of the lung onto the mediastinum and lines the inner wall of the chest cavity and the dome of the diaphragm. A small amount of fluid is found between these two layers of pleura, the visceral layer covering the lung and the parietal layer lining the inner wall of the chest. During inspiration the pleural layers move over each other with a minimum of friction. Inspiration is carried out by an upwards and outwards movement of the ribs and a downward movement of the diaphragm. This muscular action increases the negative pressure within the thorax and air is drawn down the trachea and main bronchi to expand the lungs.

Pleural effusion

When infection reaches the pleural cavity there is an outpouring of the fluid which separates the two layers of the pleura. Such a collection of fluid is called a pleural effusion (Fig. 12.1) and if it progresses to form pus, it is termed an *empyema*. Fluid in the pleural cavity causes compression of the underlying lung, so that lung capacity is diminished and dullness occurs over the chest wall due to the underlying fluid. The fluid may be aspirated by inserting a needle through one of the intercostal spaces between two of the ribs, usually using local analgesia (Fig. 12.2). It is most important that air is not introduced into the pleural cavity, since it diminishes the

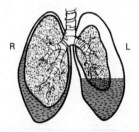

Fig. 12.1 Pleural effusion on the right side. Hydropneumothorax on the left (note the collapsed lung).

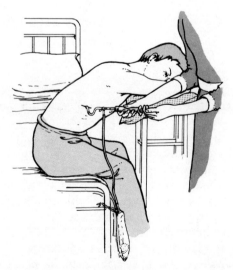

Fig. 12.2 Two-way syringe used for the removal of pleural fluid.

negative pressure necessary for the act of inspiration. If much air is allowed to enter it will collapse the lung. Therefore, a two-way tap on the syringe is used so that fluid can be aspirated from the chest and expelled into a receptacle without having to remove the syringe from the needle. An explanation is given to the patient as to what is about to happen and the nurse helps him into the correct position. This will be either leaning over a bed table, or lying on the unaffected side supported by pillows with the arm of the affected side raised above the head. Such a position will widen the intercostal spaces and facilitate insertion of the needle.

Nursing care. During aspiration of fluid from the pleural cavity the nurse should observe the patient carefully for signs of shock, which might result from the sudden withdrawal of fluid from a body cavity. The patient is asked to remain still and to give warning of any desire to cough so that the aspiration can be temporarily stopped and so avoid puncturing the visceral pleura with the needle. When the fluid has been removed some antibiotic may be injected into the pleural cavity. When the procedure is completed the patient should rest for half an hour. Any reaction to the aspiration should be reported immediately, as it might indicate bleeding. Specimens of pleural fluid should be carefully labelled and sent immediately to the clinical laboratory for culture and determination of sensitivity of organisms and for cytology. The character and amount of fluid withdrawn should be noted in the patient's records.

Empyema

The importance of not draining an empyema too soon was first realized during the pandemic of influenza during 1918–20. At that time streptococcal empyema very commonly accompanied the disease and when intercostal drainage was instituted, collapse of the lung followed, proving too great a burden for an already sick patient. When the empyema was aspirated through a needle and inspected from day to day, it was possible to ascertain by the thickness of the pus when adhesions had formed between the two layers of pleura. Thus drainage of the empyema was safe when the pus contained about seven-eighths of its volume as solid matter. This test is still a useful one when deciding to drain an empyema, an operation rarely called for today. Staphylococcal infections usually produce very thick pus whereas in streptococcal infections the pus is often thin and watery and adhesions between the pleura do not form until considerably later. Occasionally a collection of pus forms between two lobes of the lung and is then called an interlobar empyema.

Treatment. Drainage of an empyema is carried out in the operating theatre under local analgesia or general anaesthesia. A short length of rib is bared of periosteum and excised. A wide-bore drainage tube is inserted after the loculations and adhesions have been broken down within the pleural cavity by an exploring finger. The drainage tube is secured to the skin with a 'purse string' suture and is connected to an underwater seal; this consists of a sterile bottle with a rubber stopper and two tubes passing through it. The drainage tube in the chest is connected to the longer glass tube which dips under the surface of a measured quantity of sterile water in the bottle. The shorter tube passing through the cork is open to the air via a filter. By this means pus can drain freely from the chest into the bottle, but air cannot enter the chest because there is a column of fluid in the tube, drainage of fluid is assisted by frequent 'milking' of the tube. When the patient coughs, bubbles of pus and occasionally gas can be seen escaping from the longer tube. Some empyema tubes have a fine catheter incorporated in the wall so that the abscess cavity can be irrigated.

Nursing care. The patient is nursed in the sitting position supported by pillows, and the rubber tubing should be arranged so that it is not compressed and allows free drainage. The fluid level in the long glass tube should be carefully observed to see that it is 'swinging'; the level varies as the pressure in the pleural cavity changes during respiration. The amount and type of drainage from the patient's chest should be carefully noted and when the bottle is changed great care should be exercised to clamp the rubber tubing in two places to prevent air entering the pleural cavity. The aperture of the tubing may be closed temporarily with a sterile spigot or gauze swab. Great care should be taken not to lift the bottle above the level of the patient's chest or there is a danger of fluid being aspirated into the chest cavity. If the bottle should be accidentally broken, two clamps should immediately be applied to the drain.

The tube is retained until the pus stops draining. Drainage may be assisted by the instillation of a solution of streptokinase and streptodornase, substances prepared from streptococci, which are capable of dissolving the solid matter in pus and making it liquid enough to run out of the tube. Occasionally this causes a severe reaction with hyperpyrexia. The expansion of the lung to fill the chest cavity is encouraged by vigorous breathing exercises, which are best superintended by a physiotherapist. With children, games are devised to encourage the patient to breathe deeply and expire actively. A large mirror placed at the foot of the bed will often help the individual to breathe more effectively and show how well the chest moves.

The introduction of antibiotics has made the incidence of empyema much less common and has also simplified treatment.

Chest injuries

If the chest wall is crushed or pierced, air will enter the pleural cavity and the lung will collapse; such a condition is described as a *pneumothorax*. The effect will be not only to deny the patient the use of that lung but by pushing the mediastinum over to the opposite side to compress and make the remaining lung less efficient. The treatment of pneumothorax is to aspirate the air as soon as possible and to continue aspirating it if necessary. It may be necessary to connect the drain to an underwater seal and a small suction apparatus such as a Roberts pump.

Occasionally the patient may rupture a bulla or cyst on the lung and then the air continues to enter the. pleural cavity with each breath. Sometimes a valve-like effect is produced by injury and a high positive pressure is built up in the pleural cavity; this is called a *tension pneumothorax*. If the pressure is not released, the patient becomes cyanosed because of the inability of the opposite lung to expand. Treatment is by the insertion of a tube through the intercostal space. The tube is provided with a small valve so that air can be forced out of the pleural cavity but no longer drawn in, or it is connected to an underwater seal.

Chest injuries may also be accompanied by bleeding within the pleural cavity, a condition called *haemothorax*. Haemothorax may also result from bleeding due to injury to the intercostal vessels or the lung parenchyma, and it may be complicated by a pneumo-thorax. Blood within the pleural cavity does not clot at first because the movement of the lung removes the fibrin from the blood so that it remains fluid. Thus it is possible to aspirate a haemothorax for some days after the original injury. In time, however, the fibrin organizes and covers the lung surface and this layer of fibrin, being tough and inelastic, prevents proper lung movement. This may be circumvented, however, by the injection of streptokinase and streptodornase into the pleural cavity to dissolve the exudate. If, however, the fibrin has been allowed to form over the lung and 'freeze' it, then the chest has to be opened widely and this layer stripped off the lung, an operation called *decortication*.

Bronchiectasis

This condition, which may be congenital or acquired and is a complication of cystic fibrosis of the pancreas, is one in which the bronchi and bronchioles are dilated and the dilations almost always contain pus. The lung is incapable of proper respiration and foul, stinking sputum is expectorated in large amounts. The patient becomes toxic and if a child, does not thrive or grow properly. He is an embarrassment to himself and those around him because of the offensiveness of the sputum.

Bronchiectasis is much improved by *postural drainage*, which consists of the patient lying steeply tilted, head down, each day and coughing up the sputum as it drains out of the cavities. This drainage is assisted by active breathing exercises carried out under the guidance of a physiotherapist. If the disease is localized to one lobe, the diseased part may be excised. If the disease is bilateral, excision carries a poor prognosis.

Nursing care. The nursing of a patient who has had part or all of one lung removed needs great care, the main aim being to restore normal respiration, full aeration of the lung and full mobility of the chest wall and to prevent atelectasis or collapse of the lung. The patient requires oxygen if cyanosed and this is given by oxygen tent or light polythene face-mask (Fig. 12.3).

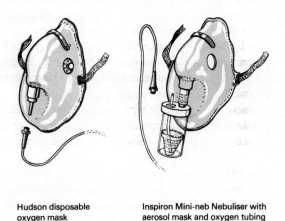

Hudson disposable
oxygen mask

Inspiron Mini-neb Nebuliser with
aerosol mask and oxygen tubing

Fig. 12.3 Oxygen face-masks.

The pleural cavity may be drained in two places, one drain being inserted into the apex of the pleural cavity to permit air to escape, the other into the base to allow drainage of blood or serum. These drains are of the underwater seal type and require the previously mentioned care. When the drainage is no longer required, X-rays are taken before the drains are removed to make sure re-expansion of the lungs is satisfactory. When the tubes are removed it is important to apply tulle-gras or petroleum jelly gauze dressing immediately, so that no air enters the pleural cavity. Frequently a stitch with long ends is left in position for tying as the tube is withdrawn.

When consciousness is regained the patient is well supported with pillows in the appropriate position; usually the patient should sit upright, but instructions about this should be obtained from the surgeon. It may be required to nurse the patient leaning towards the affected side in order to help the remaining lung tissue to expand. Good posture is most important if disfigurement is to be avoided, and the patient should be constantly encouraged to maintain a correct position. A large mirror may again be helpful. A strong bandage fixed to the foot of the bed for the patient to pull on may also aid recovery. Breathing exercises are carried out with the assistance of somebody to support the chest wall, and the patient is encouraged to cough, for it is of the utmost importance that the bronchi be cleared of sputum. Only by this means is it possible to prevent collapse of a segment or lobe and allow complete re-expansion of the remaining lung tissue. Nurse and physiotherapist must collaborate in this vital part of the patient's care. Changing the patient's position at frequent intervals will encourage coughing and an expectorant may be given before these exercises.

Drugs may be ordered for the relief of pain, e.g. pethidine 50 to 100 mg intramuscularly. It is usual not to give drugs such as morphine and codeine, which depress the respiratory system, until the patient's condition is much improved.

The diet is increased gradually but progressively. In order that the patient shall take sufficient nourishment during what is of necessity a long convalescence, the meals should be served attractively and punctually.

Pulmonary tuberculosis is no longer a severe problem in developed countries owing to the introduction of streptomycin, isoniazid, PAS (para-amino-salicylic acid) and rifampicin, since these drugs are effective in controlling the infection. Most patients with a tuberculous lung infection are cured by a course of suitable chemotherapy.

Lung tumours

Cancer of the lung is one of the commonest malignant diseases, being found much more frequently in men than in women and being more often seen in heavy cigarette smokers. The early signs and symptoms are haemoptysis, i.e. spitting up blood, pain in the chest, loss of weight and shortness of breath. The disease often runs a rapid course and the tumour may spread by the bloodstream, frequently producing metastases in the skeleton and brain. The successful treatment of lung cancer depends on its early diagnosis and this is aided by mass radiography, which enables it to be recognized before the patient has any obvious clinical signs.

Bronchoscopy. This procedure, in which a straight, illuminated tube is introduced through the mouth and down the trachea into the right or left main bronchus, is of considerable value in diagnosis. Bronchoscopy is usually performed under a general anaesthetic but in skilled hands may be done under a local. The fibreoptic endoscope gives excellent visibility. If a local analgesic is used the nurse should withhold anything by mouth until the effect of the analgesic has passed off. Since the tumour usually arises in one of the bronchi, it may be seen and a small portion removed with biopsy forceps for microscopic examination. When the tumour occurs in the periphery of the lung, the symptoms may not be so obvious, haemoptysis is less likely and the tumour cannot be seen at bronchoscopy, but the prognosis following resection is better.

Lung cancer is treated by the removal of a lobe (*lobectomy*) or the whole lung (*pneumonectomy*) on the affected side. Alternatively radiotherapy may be used alone or in combination with surgery.

Pneumonectomy. At operation the chest is opened widely and the pulmonary artery and veins at the hilum of the lung are first isolated and divided between ligatures. In like manner the bronchus is closed, often with strong nonabsorbable sutures such as silk. Any affected lymph nodes are dissected out. The chest wall is then closed with suction drainage. Although a large dead space is left behind, the heart and mediastinum move across and the organization of blood clot eventually fills much of the cavity. Occasionally the surgeon decides not to use a drainage tube. If there is no drainage tube the nurse must watch the patient very carefully for signs of internal haemorrhage and respiratory distress due to the cavity filling too rapidly with blood. Should such a situation arise, immediate steps will be taken to aspirate the fluid and a blood transfusion must be set up.

Oesophagus

Congenital abnormalities

Developmental abnormalities of the oesophagus are not uncommon, but they are often overlooked. The lesion most often seen is *atresia of the oesophagus* (tracheo-oesophageal fistula). In this condition the upper part of the oesophagus ends in a blind sac and the lower part communicates with the trachea, usually at the bifurcation. As a result of this, fluid swallowed by the baby quickly fills the small pouch, spills over into the trachea or larynx and causes a choking, cyanotic attack. This syndrome of vomiting and cyanosis at birth is characteristic of the lesion and it is often the midwife who first makes the correct diagnosis. This is one reason for the first feed given to a newborn baby being sterile water.

The presence of the lesion is confirmed by passing a fine rubber catheter through the nose into the upper pouch, instilling a few drops of lipoidol and taking an X-ray picture. The blind pouch is then easily seen and the fact that the lower end of the oesophagus communicates with the trachea is demonstrated by the presence of gas in the bowel. The treatment is by operation, which is usually carried out through the right side of the chest. The two ends of the oesophagus are reunited or anastomosed after detaching the lower one from the trachea. Such babies offer many problems in nursing.

Nursing care. Before operation the baby is nursed with the head of the cot lowered in order to minimize inhalation of mucus. Penicillin is given and the baby is turned at least every half-hour so that all parts of the chest have the opportunity to move and so aerate the lungs. The mucus at the back of the throat is sucked out with a small catheter and syringe, and should they be required, fluids are given by subcutaneous or intravenous infusion. After operation, the baby is nursed with the feet lower than the head and an oxygen tent is often necessary. A drainage tube will be connected to the right pleural cavity and passed to an underwater seal. The baby again needs turning from side to side at intervals to help expansion of the lungs and feeding is not started for some days. A gastrostomy may have been performed and this allows a slow continuous milk feed. A fine polythene tube may be passed by the nose through the anastomosis into the stomach during the operation. Milk can then be given by this route.

Short oesophagus

This condition is one in which the oesophagus ends well above the diaphragm and thus part of the stomach lies in the mediastinum. It is associated with regurgitation of feeds and may be seen in babies or adults. It is often the end result of a diaphragmatic or *hiatus hernia* (p. 144) and is complicated by bleeding from the oesophagus, ulceration and stricture formation.

Foreign bodies

Foreign bodies are sometimes swallowed by children and, if large enough, will stick in the oesophagus. Adults occasionally swallow dentures or sharp objects such as chicken or rabbit bones, which may become impaled upon the oesophageal wall and thus obstruct the lumen. An X-ray picture can confirm the diagnosis and if the foreign body is not opaque to X-rays, a small amount of radio-opaque fluid is given by mouth and the site at which it is held up can be seen on the fluoroscopic screen. If the foreign body shows no inclination to move on, then the patient is anaesthetized and an oesophagoscope passed. Forceps are passed through the oesophagoscope in order to remove the foreign body or, on rare occasions, it may be pushed into the stomach so that it passes on through the gastro-intestinal tract.

Cardiospasm or achalasia

This is a condition in which food does not pass from the oesophagus into the stomach. The onset of the condition may be sudden or insidious and it is seen more commonly in young women. The cause is unknown but appears to be related to some abnormality of the nerves supplying the lower end of the oesophagus.

When a barium examination is made the oesophagus is found to be dilated and sometimes tortuous. It narrows at the level of the diaphragm and it is with great difficulty that small amounts of food pass through into the stomach. As a result of this disability the patient slowly loses weight and often vomits rather offensive, stale food.

Treatment. The treatment of cardiospasm is determined by the severity of the condition. In mild cases the lower end of the oesophagus may be dilated with bougies. In severe cases, *cardiomyotomy* or *Heller's operation* is performed in which an incision is made from the stomach to the oesophagus, dividing the muscle coats for about 10 cm but leaving the mucosa intact. This operation, which resembles that of Ramstedt for pyloric stenosis, gives a high proportion of cures. It may be performed by either the abdominal or thoracic route.

Stricture

Stricture of the oesophagus usually follows the swallowing of some corrosive fluid such as an acid or strong alkali. It is a condition not often seen in the UK. The mucosal lining of the oesophagus is destroyed and replaced by fibrous tissue which makes it extremely difficult for anything but fluids to get into the stomach, eventually there may be complete obstruction.

Treatment. The treatment is to keep the lumen open by the regular *passage of bougies*. The patient is taught to do this and he usually becomes quite skilful at it.

Where complete obstruction has occurred a *gastrostomy* has to be performed in order to feed the patient. The abdomen is opened and a small pouch of the stomach is brought up to the surface and sutured in position. A tube is passed through the opening or stoma while the patient is still on the operating table and some water is run in by means of a funnel in order to test the patency of the gastrostomy. The patient is then fed through this opening until the general health has improved. It may be possible to pass a bougie from the stomach upwards through the oesophagus then, if a thread is attached to the bougie, this can be left in position and subsequently used to guide dilators through the oesophagus. When all attempts to find a lumen in the damaged oesophagus fail, it is necessary to reconstruct another and this may be done by bringing up a loop of small or large bowel deep to the skin and anastomosing it to the pharynx or stump of oesophagus in the neck.

Dysphagia associated with anaemia

This is a condition which occurs in women in whom an iron deficiency hypochromic anaemia is associated with glossitis, achlorhydria and an atrophic condition of the pharyngeal mucosa. There is, in addition, spasm of the muscle surrounding the junction of the pharynx and oesophagus which makes swallowing difficult. The difficulty in swallowing, or dysphagia, can be relieved by passing bougies, but the most important matter is the treatment of the anaemia. This condition has a sinister reputation because it predisposes to carcinoma of the upper end of the oesophagus. The syndrome is referred to in this country as the Paterson Brown — Kelly, and in America as the Plummer—Vinson.

Varices

Oesophageal varices consist of dilated, tortuous, thin-walled veins at the lower end of the oesophagus where it opens into the stomach. They result from *portal hypertension* and are associated with *cirrhosis* of the liver or some block in the portal venous system.

Treatment. The varices may rupture causing severe haematemesis and the treatment is replacement of the blood lost, followed by an operation to relieve the portal hypertension. This consists of anastomosing the portal vein to the inferior vena cava or occasionally anastomosing the left renal and splenic veins. In an emergency a Sengstaken tube is used to control the bleeding. This is a triple-lumen tube which is passed into the stomach and the terminal balloon inflated. The tube is then withdrawn until the balloon is held up at the cardia when the proximal balloon is inflated. This is sausage-shaped and exerts pressure on the lower oesophagus, so occluding the veins: meanwhile the contents of the stomach are aspirated through the third lumen.

Hiatus hernia

The opening in the diaphragm through which the oesophagus passes to join the stomach is called a hiatus. It is a muscular ring and the fibres of the right crus of the diaphragm divide to enclose it. It is this junction between the oesophagus and stomach which is so critical in preventing regurgitation of the gastric contents. It appears that one of the most important things about this junction is the angle at which the oesophagus meets the stomach. In the very young and in the old, there occasionally develops a weakening of the muscles guarding this opening so that part of the stomach herniates into the chest. The herniation may occur acutely with a knuckle of stomach rolling up beside the oesophagus and causing pain, sickness and perhaps bleeding. More commonly the whole circumference of the stomach slides or telescopes up into the chest directly through the hiatus, the oesophagus appearing to become shorter.

The result of this herniation is that the lower oesophagus now becomes exposed to the hydrochloric acid and pepsin from the stomach and this leads to inflammation, or oesophagitis. The mucosa of the lower end of the oesophagus becomes swollen and red and may ulcerate. Haemorrhage may occur in the form of a haematemesis, or the continued loss of small amount of blood may lead to anaemia, especially in infants.

Treatment. The condition described as a hiatus hernia is treated in a variety of ways. The patient, if an adult, is encouraged to sleep with the head of the bed raised; for an infant a small padded chair is constructed, nicknamed a sentry box, so that he can spend both day and night in the vertical position. Alkalis by mouth assist in neutralizing the acid and various operations have been devised to repair the hernia or to fix the stomach back in its proper place in the abdominal cavity, the most popular is *fundoplication*. In obese patients, strict dieting often leads to improvement.

Carcinoma

Carcinoma of the oesophagus in Western countries is typically a disease of men over the age of seventy; in the Middle and Far East it is often seen in younger patients. There is a steadily increasing dysphagia, at first for solids and later for liquids, which results in great loss of weight and lack of energy. The patient can often point to the site of the obstruction by saying where the food seems to stick. As the disease progresses other structures in the chest may become involved. The trachea may be invaded and a fistula may develop between it and the oesophagus. The recurrent laryngeal nerve may be involved producing hoarseness; more rarely the tumour spreads distantly by the bloodstream and produces metastases in other parts of the body. The tumour is common in Malaysia and Japan.

The diagnosis is made by taking X-ray pictures of a barium swallow which show the tell-tale, irregular, rat-tail narrowing of the oesophagus.

Treatment. The treatment of carcinoma of the oesophagus is rarely satisfactory, especially when the patients are old; also they are often very wasted when they present themselves for treatment. If the tumour can be excised, a thoracic approach is used and the two ends of the oesophagus sutured together. If the tumour is at the lower end of the oesophagus a thoraco-abdominal operation is carried out and the stomach brought up into the chest cavity to bridge the gap. When the patient is too ill, or the tumour is too extensive for these manoeuvres, an oesophagoscope is passed and a Mousseau – Barbin

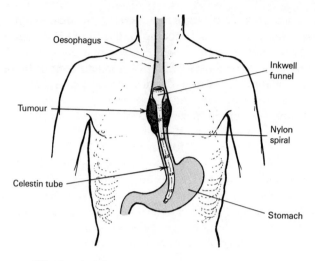

Fig. 12.4 Celestin tube after insertion through an oesophageal carcinoma.

or Celestin tube (Fig. 12.4) inserted. These are funnel-shaped plastic tubes with a long 'tail', which is threaded through the growth into the stomach. The abdomen is opened and a small incision made in the stomach wall through which the 'tail' is threaded and then pulled. The funnel of the tube then fits snugly into the growth and the 'tail' is trimmed and stitched to the stomach wall to keep it there. Fluids are then able to pass through the tube and the patient gains nourishment. The diet has to consist of fortified skimmed milk with added vitamins, or a normal diet may be made fluid in a liquidiser. The meal should be completed by a drink of water to try and clear anything adherent to the sides of the tube. The toilet of the mouth needs particular attention.

If the oesophagus becomes completely obstructed a gastrostomy is performed so that the patient can be fed. The diet then has to be a fluid one, being introduced with a tube and funnel into the gastrostomy. The nurse should remember that the appetite is aroused by the sight, smell and anticipation of food, and she should try to give the patient pleasure at meal-times, at the same time stimulating the secretion of saliva to keep the mouth fresh. Paper handkerchiefs and a receiver may be required if the patient cannot swallow saliva.

X-ray therapy is also used for those patients unsuitable for surgical treatment, and supervoltage therapy is the most suitable for this type of tumour.

Heart and great vessels

The treatment of abnormalities and diseases of the heart and great vessels has made great strides due to improvements in anaesthesia but perhaps most of all due to an increased knowledge of the anatomy, physiology and pathology of the heart and therefore an understanding of how treatment may be undertaken.

Trauma

The heart and the great vessels may be damaged by bullets, shrapnel, or direct injury as in a road accident, and such lesions are naturally more frequent in war time. The immediate problem in such a patient is to staunch the haemorrhage, replace the blood which is lost and take the patient as soon as possible to a hospital where operation can be undertaken immediately.

Many foreign bodies have been removed from the walls and within the chambers of the heart. The heart muscle withstands incisions and stitches extremely well and the heart continues to beat even when severely damaged, which allows many quite complicated manoeuvres to be undertaken. If the pericardial sac, which is the fibrous bag in which the heart is contained, becomes filled with blood it will press on the heart and stop it beating; a condition referred to as *cardiac tamponade*.

Congenital heart disease

Patent ductus arteriosus. In this condition the communication between the aorta and the pulmonary artery which normally exists in foetal life persists after birth (Fig. 12.5). In the foetus the lungs do not expand and therefore the pulmonary circulation is not properly functioning. The blood pumped into the pulmonary artery is bypassed into the aorta and the lungs remain airless and relatively bloodless. At birth the pulmonary circulation opens up for the first time and the ductus arteriosus contracts down and is obliterated.

If the ductus remains patent, blood passes from the aorta into the pulmonary artery at each contraction of the left ventricle and the circulation is, therefore, much less efficient. There is no cyanosis. The ductus not only puts a strain on the heart, but it may also become infected with bacterial endocarditis. For this reason the ductus is double ligatured or divided at an early age, usually between two and six years.

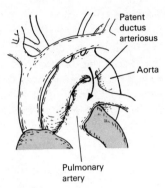

Fig. 12.5 Patent ductus arteriosus.

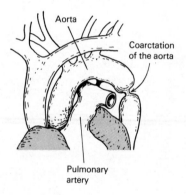

Fig. 12.6 Coarctation of the aorta.

Coarctation of the aorta. In this condition the aorta or main blood vessel leaving the heart is narrowed, usually in the arch or its descending part (Fig. 12.6). As a result, the patient has a high blood pressure in the upper half of the body and a low one in the legs. If left untreated the increased pressure in the upper half of the body leads to such complications as rupture of the aorta or cerebral haemorrhage. X-ray pictures may be taken after the injection of a radio-opaque substance into one of the veins near the heart, and the pictures (angiocardiographs) will show dye leaving the heart and outlining the narrowed aorta. Operation consists of excising the narrow portion and joining the two ends of the aorta by fine sutures. Where the gap is too long for the ends to be approximated, a woven teflon tube may be inserted.

Pulmonary stenosis. A baby may be born with a narrowing of the pulmonary artery, which takes the blood to the lungs. The narrowing may consist of a segment of vessel which is improperly developed or the valves may be fused together leaving only a tiny aperture. This operation requires the use of a cardio-pulmonary bypass while the heart is opened and the abnormalities corrected.

Fallot's tetralogy. This is a more complicated cardiac lesion which includes pulmonary stenosis, a patent interventricular septum, hypertrophy of the right ventricle and an aorta which overrides the septum. Such children are cyanosed and short of breath, they are often referred to as 'blue babies'. Treatment may consist of anastomosing the right subclavian artery to the pulmonary artery so that blood passes through the lungs and is thus oxygenated. When the child is older and fitter the circulation is put on to bypass and the heart is opened to allow full correction of the defects.

Atrial septal defects. Occasionally the septum between the right and left atrium does not develop normally and a hole remains between the two sides of the heart. This can be closed, and in order to do so various techniques have been evolved. To enable the heart to be opened and the septum closed, the patient can be cooled by placing iced water bags around the body after anaesthesia has been induced and circulating the blood through a cooling system to achieve hypothermia. This technique makes the requirements for oxygen and therefore the blood flow much less. Alternatively the cardio-pulmonary bypass is used and the hole closed with sutures or a patch fixed in place with the heart stopped and free of blood.

Ventricular septal defects. These defects can only be closed by employing a heart–lung machine.

Acquired heart disease

Pericarditis. The only form of pericarditis which requires surgical treatment is that following tuberculous disease. This leads to a chronic fibrous constriction of the pericardium and prevents the heart from beating properly. As a result, fluid accumulates in the tissues and the patient becomes breathless and oedematous. Operative treatment consists of excising as much of the diseased pericardium as practicable. Such patients are required to lose as much fluid as possible before the operation and their drinking is therefore strictly curtailed and they are given diuretics.

Mitral stenosis. As a result of acute rheumatism in childhood the valves of the heart may become fibrosed and narrowed in later life.

The commonest valve to be involved is the mitral. Mitral stenosis causes the patient to become increasingly breathless and lacking in energy. The condition can be relieved by splitting open the valve at its commissures by means of a finger introduced through the left atrial appendage, an operation called valvotomy. A dilator may be introduced simultaneously through the left ventricle and guided into position by the finger in the atrium. When the valve is so damaged by fibrosis and calcification that it cannot be improved by simple valvotomy it has to be replaced by an artificial mitral valve. While the circulation is maintained by a heart–lung machine, the diseased valve is cut out and a prosthesis inserted.

Aortic stenosis can be produced in exactly the same way by rheumatism, but is rarer. The aortic valve, which is made up of three small leaflets, is less accessible and less easily mobilized in order to make it function properly. The aortic valve can also be excised and an artificial valve inserted in its place. The Starr valve consisting of a ball in a cage, is commonly used. Both the mitral and the aortic valves may be involved by the same process and it then becomes necessary to replace both valves, usually at the same time.

Nursing care

Patients who have undergone operations on the heart or great vessels require skilful nursing with most careful attention to detail. They usually go to the intensive care unit first (Chapter 9) where they are mechanically ventilated for the first 24–48 hours.

Oxygen. This is required on most occasions and is given by a mask covering the nose and mouth. If a mask is not well tolerated, an oxygen tent must be used and when this is expected it is a good plan to give the patients a trial run in one before the day of operation. Infants can be nursed in an 'incubator' in which oxygen saturation, humidity and temperature are all readily controlled. When there is great difficulty in breathing a tracheostomy is performed at the time of operation and the patient can then be maintained on a respirator.

Blood. Transfusion of blood is necessary both during and after the operation and the speed of flow which has been ordered must be maintained.

Position. As soon as the patient recovers from the anaesthetic he is lifted into a semirecumbent position or sat up, according to the doctor's instructions. Such patients are always the joint responsibility of both physician and surgeon and both are concerned in the management of the postoperative period. It is usual to nurse such patients in special recovery wards until they are fit enough to return to their own ward.

Drugs. These may be ordered for the relief of pain as frequently as every 4 hours during the first 24 hours.

Breathing exercises. The patient's position is changed at frequent intervals, and breathing exercises are superintended by a physiotherapist from the first day and, if ordered, also at night. If they exhaust the patient unduly, they may have to be restricted until the patient has recovered more strength. Sputum must be coughed up and the nurse should support the wound with the flat of one hand, using the other for counterpressure on the opposite side of the chest while the patient coughs. When a tracheostomy has been made the secretions have to be sucked out at frequent intervals.

Diet. Fluids may have to be restricted if the patient develops oedema, but he should be encouraged to take as full a diet as possible. The salt content of the diet may have to be restricted in order to help diminish the oedema.

Drainage. The drainage tube is attached to an underwater seal bottle (Figs. 12.7 and 12.8) or an electric suction apparatus may be used. A careful watch must be kept that the fluid is swinging freely

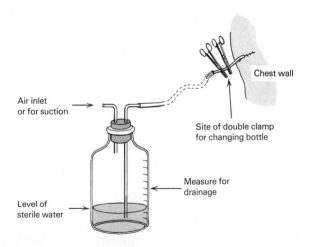

Fig. 12.7 Closed chest (underwater seal) drainage.

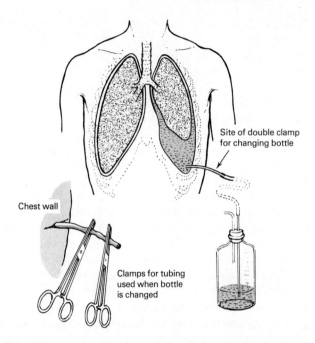

Site of double clamp
for changing bottle

Chest wall

Clamps for tubing
used when bottle
is changed

Fig. 12.8 Drainage of the pleural cavity into an underwater seal bottle.

in the drainage bottle and the amount of drainage and its nature is recorded regularly. The drainage tube is removed when the discharge ceases and the wound immediately covered with a sterile dressing and adhesive strapping. The sutures are removed on the sixth to tenth day following operation.

Observations. Pulse rate, respiration, temperature and blood pressure will be recorded at frequent intervals and charted, any sudden change in any one of them being reported immediately to the medical officer in charge. The patient's heart rate is usually monitored on an ECG machine.

As the general condition of the patient improves, the amount of activity permitted is increased, the patient being allowed to sit out of bed and eventually walk with assistance. The length of time for which the patient is nursed at rest varies greatly with the type of operation and the age of the patient; for example, a small child after ligation of a patent ductus will probably be running about the ward on the third postoperative day whereas the adult who has had extensive open-heart surgery may well have to stay in bed for 2 or 3 weeks.

13
The Breast

Operations upon the breast form a large part of the work in surgical wards because carcinoma of the breast is the commonest malignant tumour in women, 8000 dying from this disease every year in England and Wales alone.

Anatomy

The female breast develops rapidly at puberty to extend from the second rib above to the sixth below and from the edge of the sternum medially to the axillary fold laterally. On the nipple will be found the openings of fifteen to twenty lactiferous ducts, each one of which has a small dilatation called an ampulla draining a single lobe of the gland. The whole of the breast is embedded in fat which makes precise determination of its limits difficult, it frequently sends an extension, called the axillary tail upwards and laterally into the axilla.

The nipples

Cracked or fissured nipples are a complication of lactation and produce an extremely painful condition. This often results in a reduction of the milk flow, since the mother finds it too painful to allow the baby to suck. In addition the crack allows the entry of organisms which may multiply and so produce a breast abscess.

Mastitis

The term mastitis includes not only inflammation of the breast but also other conditions, often of hormonal origin, in which the function of the breast is upset.

Mastitis neonatorum. This condition occurs in about 50 per cent of infants towards the end of the first week of life and consists of swelling of the breasts and the secretion of fluid resembling colostrum. It results from the infant obtaining from the mother before birth some of the hormone which stimulates her own breasts to secrete. It is equally common in male and female babies and disappears spontaneously in the course of a few days unless it becomes infected, when a small abscess may form.

Puberty mastitis. This condition occurs in children of both sexes when one or both breasts become firm and tender for a brief period at puberty but it resolves without treatment in the male while in the female the breast continues to enlarge.

Gynaecomastia

Young male adults may develop enlargement of the breasts and become acutely embarrassed at exposing the torso. The cause is rarely discovered but treatment is by excising the breast tissue through an incision at the junction of the areola and normal skin, the scar is thus invisible and the normal nipple is retained. In older men who are treated with stilboestrol for prostatic cancer the nipple darkens and the breast swells.

Breast abscess

A breast abscess forms almost always as a complication of lactation. At this time the breast is extremely vascular and may be engorged with milk, as a result infection enters either along the dilated ducts or via a crack in one of the nipples. The organism is usually *Staphylococcus pyogenes*, or occasionally the streptococcus. The breast becomes painful, red and swollen and often throbs; the temperature is raised and the patient feels unwell. If treatment with

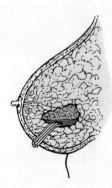

Fig. 13.1 Breast abscess with a drainage tube in position.

large doses of penicillin is given, resolution usually takes place and the inflammation subsides without pus formation.

When pus forms, an abscess may develop in any quadrant of the breast, or behind the breast lifting it forwards; it requires incision and drainage. Since the abscess is usually made up of a number of small cavities, the divisions between these are broken down at the same time so that all the cavities drain through the one opening in the skin (Fig. 13.1)

Nursing care. The penicillin ordered will be given by intramuscular injection or an antibiotic will be taken by mouth every six hours.

Congestion of the breast may be relieved by expressing the milk with firm manual pressure or removing it with a breast pump. The baby is not allowed to suck at the infected breast. A firm breast bandage or brassiere should be applied to give support.

After incision of an abscess the wound will be dressed daily and the drainage tube shortened as the discharge lessens. If the abscess is slow to heal the surgeon may order irrigations of a 1 per cent solution of hypochlorite to be given using a fine catheter. After irrigation, a penicillin solution may be instilled into the cavity.

Galactocele

This is a milk cyst and results from the blockage of one of the main ducts of the breast during lactation. The importance of a galactocoele is that a correct diagnosis should be made as it may be mistaken for a carcinoma. The cyst requires aspiration with a syringe and needle or, rarely, excision.

Fibroadenoma

There are two kinds of fibroadenoma; both of them are simple tumours occurring usually in the breasts of younger women. A hard fibroadenoma is slow growing, very firm on palpation and mobile within the breast tissue. It is treated by local excision. A soft fibroadenoma may be seen in somewhat older patients, grows more quickly and is bulkier in size. Again the treatment is local excision.

Duct papilloma

A papilloma may develop in one of the ducts of the breast. It gives rise to different signs. There may be a bloody discharge from the nipple due to erosions on the surface of the papilloma and there may also be a cystic swelling in the breast due to blockage of a duct and retention of products proximal to it. Such a papilloma requires excision, together with that segment of the breast in which it occurs, as it is known that the condition when left may undergo a malignant change.

Mammary dysplasia or chronic mastitis

This condition, which goes under a variety of other names such as fibro-adenosis or Schimmelbusch's disease, is not an inflammatory condition as the name implies but is probably due to the interplay of various hormones on the breast tissue. Before each menstrual period it is not uncommon for the breast to be a little engorged and possibly more active. These constantly repeated phases of hyperplasia and involution of the breast appear to lead, especially in women who have not been pregnant, to changes which take place partly within the ducts and partly outside them. The lining of the ducts becomes heaped up and may go on to block some of them completely. This in turn leads to cyst formation. Outside the ducts a reaction takes place with the production of much fibrous tissue which is not uniformly distributed and this results in a characteristic lumpy feeling when the breast is palpated with the tips of the fingers, but which cannot be detected with the flat of the hand. The signs of mammary dysplasia are lumpiness of the breast, which may be painful and is not usually associated with discharge from the nipple or enlargement of the axillary lymph nodes. The condition is benign and the patient should be reassured and instructed to wear a firm support in the form of a suitable brassiere. When there is any doubt concerning the diagnosis, the breast is explored at operation and the affected segment removed. If a carcinoma is found, a more extensive operation is done, as described below. If any doubt about the diagnosis still remains after the affected area has been laid open in the operating theatre, a piece is examined immediately by the pathologist using a frozen section technique. Depending on the pathologist's report as to whether the lesion is benign or malignant, the appropriate operation is carried out.

Carcinoma

Since the breast is such a common site for malignant disease, the early diagnosis of carcinoma is all important and therefore any lump in the breast is considered to be malignant until proved otherwise.

Carcinoma of the breast often consists more of fibrous tissue than tumour cells and such a hard growth is known as a scirrhous carcinoma.

The tumour may become attached to the skin causing it to be indrawn and puckered. It may spread to involve the muscles of the chest wall. It also spreads by the lymphatics to the lymph nodes, most commonly involving those in the axillary and the intercostal spaces (Fig. 13.2). Later the supraclavicular nodes are involved and the disease may spread widely into the chest or abdomen. When the carcinoma is disseminated by the bloodstream, metastases are found anywhere in the body but especially commonly in the bones.

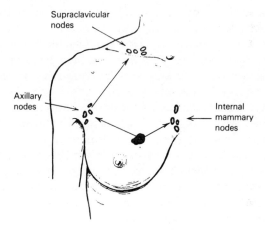

Fig. 13.2 Spread of carcinoma to the axillary, internal mammary and supraclavicular nodes.

The international classification is T for primary tumour, N for nodes and M for metastases. Breast cancer may also be divided into four *stages* according to the extent of the spread. The *first stage* is one in which the growth is confined to the breast. In the *second stage* there are, in addition, palpable but mobile nodes in the axilla. The *third stage* includes involvement of the skin over a wide area or fixation to the underlying muscles; if there are nodes palpable in the axilla they must still be mobile if the disease is to be included in this stage. The *fourth* and last *stage* is one in which the growth has extended beyond the breast, as shown by fixation of nodes in the axilla and the presence of involved nodes more distally, such as those above the clavicle, and spread to bone, lung or other organs.

Diagnosis. The diagnosis of carcinoma of the breast is of such importance that it is customary to obtain histological proof before proceeding to a planned operation. There are three main techniques available for this. The first is by fine needle aspiration biopsy, in which a needle is passed into the tissue without the need for local anaesthetic and with a syringe exerting suction. A small sample of cells is obtained, which are smeared on a microscope slide, fixed, stained and immediately examined by a pathologist who is a cytologist and can give a diagnosis. Alternatively under local anaesthesia a high speed drill or cutting (Trucut) needle is used to obtain a cylinder of tissue which is then fixed and stained. In about two days a histological diagnosis can be given. The third method is to prepare the patient for mastectomy, excise the palpable lump and have an immediate frozen-tissue report. If positive for carcinoma, mastectomy is done. If the lesion is benign, the wound is closed. A further technique is mammography, in which the breast is X-rayed using a special soft-tissue technique; carcinoma produces minute areas of calcification which are considered diagnostic of malignancy.

Treatment. The treatment of breast carcinoma depends on the stage of the disease. Stage one is treated by mastectomy, which consists of the removal of the affected breast, an area of skin, the underlying muscles and a block of tissue which includes the lymph nodes in the axilla. Many surgeons prefer to leave the underlying pectoral muscles untouched if they are not invaded by the carcinoma, an operation called a modified radical mastectomy.

The operation is first explained to the patient and she is assured that the loss of the breast can be completely disguised by an artificial breast made of sponge rubber or plastic.

Pre-operative care. In addition to the routine preparations for surgery, supervision of breathing exercises by a physiotherapist is recommended, since respiration in the postoperative period can be painful and, if not performed adequately, can lead to lung complications. Of prime importance prior to breast surgery, and with mastectomy in particular, is the mental preparation of the patient. The psychological repercussions following such surgery can be great and much support from nursing staff will be needed. The involvement of the husband during this period can also be a real help.

Post-operative care. After operation the patient may be suffering from shock and the nurse will then be required to maintain an infusion of blood or saline. Careful observation of the patient's pulse rate and colour will be necessary.

The axilla is usually drained using a suction apparatus and a tube is left in place for at least 4 days or until the serous discharge stops. The drainage tube is connected to a low-power suction pump to encourage the escape of serum. Sometimes an evacuated bottle or rubber bulb is used which, as it expands, sucks out the serum.

On regaining consciousness the patient is supported in the sitting position and for the first 24 hours it is usual to rest the arm by the side. After this time movements are encouraged and the physiotherapist teaches the patient how to lift the arm and eventually touch both the back of the head and the small of the back. The nurse should urge the patient to make these efforts at intervals during the day. Brushing the hair is excellent practice for regaining return of movement. The dressings are often soaked due to oozing from the wound and need changing after 24 or 48 hours. The wound needs special care as the incision is a long one and may be under tension. The sutures should be kept dry and if there are signs of haematoma formation, it should at once be reported to the surgeon. Stitches are usually left in until the eighth or tenth day, but if tension stitches have been used they should be removed earlier. Early mobilization should be encouraged.

After the wound has healed it is essential to supervise the patient's convalescence. Continuing support during and after convalescence may be required by those patients who are having difficulty in accepting the partial or total removal of a breast. Assistance and counselling may be sought through the Mastectomy Associations.

When it is considered that all the malignant disease has not been excised, a course of radiotherapy may be prescribed for the patient, this usually takes about 3 weeks to complete. In some clinics a course of chemotherapy is given. When a tumour is unsuitable for surgical excision, i.e. in stages three and four, radiotherapy may offer excellent palliative treatment. The X-rays given may be of supervoltage, such as those provided by a linear accelerator or cobalt machine. Often an immediate regression of the tumour is obtained.

When the disease has spread widely in the body or when following good initial results after mastectomy there has been a recurrence, further measures are employed. The ovaries can be removed and this occasionally leads to regression of the tumour tissue. Stilboestrol may be given by mouth to a woman past the menopause, or testosterone to a younger woman by implant or injection. It is likely that both these hormone preparations act by suppressing pituitary activity. There may, however, be many undesirable side effects.

Total adrenalectomy performed in conjunction with öophorectomy has been followed by good results in some patients. For this operation see the chapter on the endocrine system. Hypophysectomy, or removal of the pituitary, or its destruction by implanted radon or yttrium seeds may be beneficial. After such treatment the patient requires replacement of the hormones which are no longer produced in sufficient amount, and this will mean taking cortisone and thyroid extract by mouth for the rest of her life. Relatives should have the seriousness of the condition carefully explained to them so that they may be able to help the patient.

Prognosis. Patients who have breast carcinoma in stage one have a good prospect of cure, and between 80 to 90 per cent of such patients survive for 5 years or more. In stage two, when the axillary lymph nodes are involved, mastectomy combined with X-ray therapy gives a 50 to 60 per cent survival rate for 5 years. Finally, in stages three and four the outlook is poor although there are occasional exceptions. Comparable statistics of survival from different forms of treatment are difficult to assess because so many variable factors are working in individual cases.

14
Hernia

A hernia, or rupture, is a swelling formed by the protrusion of part of an organ through a breach in the wall of the containing cavity. It occurs most commonly in the abdomen, but the term is applied to other parts of the body. For example, if there is an opening in the diaphragm through which bowel passes into chest, it is described as a diaphragmatic hernia. The treatment of hernias forms a large part of the surgical service of a hospital and a good understanding of the different varieties which may occur, the complications to which they may give rise and their appropriate treatment is important.

Types of hernia

The most common forms of hernia are associated with the abdominal wall, and in order of frequency they are: inguinal, femoral and umbilical (Fig. 14.1). There are others, such as ventral, or incisional and diaphragmatic, which will be described later.

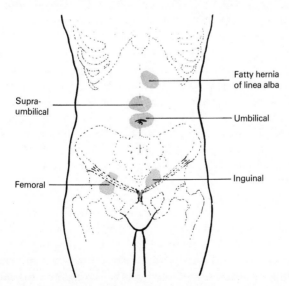

Fig. 14.1 Common sites of hernia.

Inguinal hernia. This condition may be congenital or acquired. The congenital variety is usually indirect, that is, the hernia pushes its way down the normal inguinal canal before appearing at the surface, where it may pass on to enter the scrotum or, in the female, the labium. When it is an acquired lesion it is frequently a direct hernia, that is, it pushes its way straight out through the abdominal wall and does not traverse the length of the inguinal canal. The sac of a hernia is made of peritoneum, and the swelling therefore increases in size when the patient coughs or cries because the increased tension in the abdominal cavity is transmitted to the hernia. Anything which increases the pressure in the abdomen, such as heavy lifting, coughing or straining at defaecation, will similarly increase the size of the hernia.

The treatment of an inguinal hernia depends on the type of hernia and the age of the patient. In infants the hernia can be controlled by a small rubber horseshoe truss. Operation is performed when it is convenient to admit the baby to hospital, which is usually after weaning has taken place. In some centres the baby is allowed home on the day of operation, returning later to have the stitches removed, or subcuticular closure may be used. In older patients a choice is made between the wearing of a truss or a radical operation which will aim at removing the sac and repairing the weakness in the abdominal wall. In old patients, especially those who suffer from chronic cough or diseases which increase intra-abdominal pressure, a truss is prescribed; in younger patients who have to lead a more active life the treatment of choice is an operation.

Femoral hernia. In this type of hernia the abdominal contents, typically bowel, omentum or bladder, protrude along the femoral canal into the thigh. It is relatively more common in women than men and is especially likely to become irreducible. This is because the femoral canal has a narrow neck and the sac turns back on itself as it passes through the opening into the thigh. Because the swelling lies in this awkward position just below the inguinal ligament, it is unsuitable for any form of truss and a surgical operation is the only satisfactory treatment.

Umbilical hernia. This is the commonest hernia seen in babies, but it is usually unnecessary to operate because the condition disappears spontaneously, often in the first year of life. It occurs particularly in coloured babies, in whom the umbilical opening may not close until about three years of age. If the hernia is large and especially if its presence worries the mother, it is usual to control it with a little rubber belt and pad or by means of adhesive strapping. The natural closure which eventually takes place does not seem to be either accelerated or delayed by such treatment.

In patients past middle age, especially the obese who suffer from bronchitis, an umbilical hernia may develop due to a weakness in the abdominal wall immediately above the umbilicus. The sac enlarges forwards and downwards and the contents of the hernia are very prone to strangulation. Such patients always require surgical treatment. The repair operation carried out is one associated with the name of Mayo, in which the layers of the abdominal wall are dissected clear and then overlapped. The principle of the operation is similar to the buttoning of a double-breasted jacket.

Incisional hernia. This type of hernia occurs as a result of an operation in which an incision has been made in the abdominal wall. The scar weakens and stretches, allowing the contents to bulge. An incisional hernia is usually the result of complications in the original wound, such as infection or haematoma formation. It may also result from the patient having raised abdominal pressure due to severe cough or distended bowel or bladder, all of which serve to force the edges of the wound apart. The repair of such a hernia may therefore be very difficult because the same conditions which occurred at the time of the first operation probably still apply at the second. For this reason treatment by operation is sometimes contra-indicated and a belt is prescribed to support the abdominal wall.

Other hernias. When the stomach prolapses through the oesophageal hiatus or opening in the diaphragm and enters the thoracic cavity it is described as a hiatus hernia. Rupture of the diaphragm by injury, or the presence of a congenital opening in it, results in diaphragmatic hernia. Protrusion of the brain through the skull following an injury or an operation for decompression is called a cerebral hernia.

Complications

A hernia is described as reducible if the contents can be manipulated back into the cavity from which they came. Sometimes, as a result of attacks of inflammation, adhesions occur between the intestine or omentum and the sac wall so that the hernia becomes irreducible.

The neck of the sac may be so narrow that the hernial contents cannot return and occasionally in a femoral hernia the sac closes off completely and becomes filled with fluid.

When a hernia is *irreducible* there may be pressure at the neck of the sac on the veins draining the bowel or omentum inside. As a result the contents swell up due to oedema and the hernia is said to be *incarcerated*. Should the swelling progress to such an extent that the arteries supplying the incarcerated bowel or gut are completely occluded, gangrene of the hernial contents must eventually result and the condition is referred to as a *strangulated hernia*. Many strangulated hernias are operated upon before gangrene sets in and fortunately the small bowel has great powers of recovery. For this reason a strangulated hernia is always treated surgically and as soon as possible.

It is possible to reduce some inguinal hernias by manipulation, and this treatment is usually attempted first if it is considered that the contents of the sac are viable. The patient is placed in a bed, the foot of which is raised on blocks. An ice bag is suspended over the swelling and then with the patient's hip abducted and slightly flexed the surgeon tries with gentle pressure to milk the contents back into the abdomen. If this proves impossible or if there are signs of bowel obstruction, immediate operation is advised.

Treatment

The treatment of hernia and its complications has been briefly mentioned under the various types, but the general care of such patients is outlined here.

Pre-operative preparation. It is important that patients who are to undergo an operation for a hernia should be as free as possible from infection of the upper respiratory tract. For this reason if there is any evidence of a cold, the operation should be deferred for 2 weeks. The patient should be persuaded to give up smoking for a few weeks before the operation. Elderly patients are particularly prone to constipation, so a mild laxative may be prescribed for the evening before the operation. Other preparation is the same as for any abdominal operation.

Postoperative care. The operation performed for hernia may be either the removal of the sac, that is *herniotomy*, or the removal of the sac followed by a repair, that is *herniorrhaphy* or hernioplasty. In the case of herniotomy the patient is usually able to sit out of bed the day after operation and start walking soon after. When a herniorrhaphy has been performed the patient may have to stay in bed for 2 or 3 days. Whenver possible the policy is to get patients out of bed and *home* after hernia repair, encouraging them to walk but not indulge in strenuous exercise. Thus many patients, especially children, undergoing herniotomy are returned home the same day and are never admitted to the hospital. Even after herniorrhaphy patients may be sent home in three or four days. The advantages are the lessened incidence of complications such as leg vein thrombosis and embolus, the rapid return to full health and the lightening of the load on hospital beds.

Nursing care. The patient is nursed in the semirecumbent position or in whatever position is most comfortable. In male patients if the scrotum swells it is supported by cotton wool or a suspensory bandage in order to relieve the discomfort and reduce the oedema. Leg exercises, which are repeated hourly throughout the day, form an important part of the postoperative regime by preventing thrombosis of the leg veins and maintaining good muscle tone. At the same time the patient will be instructed in carrying out special abdominal exercises to strengthen the muscles, without putting undue strain on the areas which have been sutured. This is especially the case if the patient has had an incisional hernia repaired.

It is important that the patient should pass water soon after operation and that the bowels work regularly and normally. If he has difficulty in doing the former he may be assisted to stand as this often helps micturition. If this fails he will have to be catheterized. The patient is encouraged to eat a full diet as soon as he is able. Chest complications such as bronchitis and bronchopneumonia are common after hernia operations and for this reason active breathing exercises are encouraged from the first postoperative day. Where a physiotherapist is available her supervision of this part of the treatment is invaluable.

Finally, the postoperative care of the patient does not end when he leaves hospital. If he has had a herniorrhaphy he must be carefully instructed not to carry out heavy straining or lifting for three months after operation in order that the repair may be given a proper opportunity to heal soundly. The cooperation of the medical social worker at this juncture is most helpful. They can, for example, contact the employers and arrange that the return to heavy work shall be gradual. In addition in older patients it may be possible to plan convalescence, if this should be considered necessary.

A strangulated hernia

A hernia which has strangulated presents special problems since the bowel is obstructed. It is imperative under these circumstances to admit the patient to hospital as an emergency and as soon as possible the nurse is instructed to pass a nasogastric tube into the stomach and aspirate the contents. At the same time, since there will have been fluid loss due to vomiting, it will be necessary to give intravenous therapy to replace the water and electrolytes. As soon as the patient is fit enough he is taken to the operating theatre for surgical treatment. The subsequent care will include aspiration of the stomach contents by nasogastric tube and replacement of fluid intravenously until normal bowel movements return, when adequate fluids can be taken by mouth. The technique of 'suck and drip' is life-saving in such circumstances. When the patient does not come for treatment at an early date, the strangulated bowel may be gangrenous, in which case it will have to be resected. The management of such a patient will be the same as for one who has had an operation on the small bowel, which is outlined in the next chapter.

15
Stomach, Duodenum and Small Intestine

Stomach and duodenum

The stomach acts as a receptacle into which the food passes after being chewed and swallowed. It extends from the oesophageal hiatus in the diaphragm to end at the pylorus, or gateway, which leads into the duodenum (Fig. 15.1). The normal stomach has a capacity of about 1 litre and is the most dilated part of the alimentary tract. It lies high up on the left side of the abdomen beneath the ribs. The duodenum is in the shape of the letter 'C'. Starting at the pylorus it passes round the head of the pancreas and ends by becoming the jejunum (Fig. 15.2). It is about 25 cm long.

When food enters the stomach it becomes mixed with gastric juices, the most important constituents of which are hydrochloric acid and pepsin, which are secreted mainly from the upper, or cardiac, end of the stomach. The food becomes intimately mixed with these juices by the peristaltic waves which pass along the stomach walls and after a while some of the food is passed on into the duodenum, where it meets the pancreatic secretion. Unlike that of the stomach, the pancreatic secretion is alkaline and contains three main ferments which are capable of breaking down protein, fat and carbohydrate. The secretions of the stomach and the pancreas are

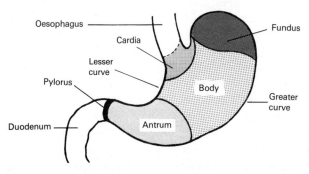

Fig. 15.1 Parts of the stomach.

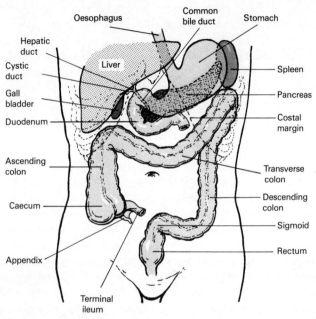

Fig. 15.2 The gastrointestinal tract.

under very delicate and rather complicated control. In part they are governed by impulses passing along the vagus nerves and in part they are under hormonal control, i.e. control due to substances like gastrin present in the bloodstream. An upset of this balance may lead to the secretion of too much acid in the stomach or too little and the duodenal secretions may be similarly affected. Any upset in the normal digestive processes is usually referred to as *dyspepsia* and when an ulcer forms in the stomach or duodenum it is referred to as a *peptic ulcer*. The importance of dyspepsia and peptic ulcer cannot be overestimated; they constitute two of the commonest afflictions of mankind today and lead to an enormous amount of ill health and loss of working hours. The great increase in the incidence of peptic ulcer in recent years has been attributed to the stresses and strains of modern life. Some confirmation of this is afforded by the fact, which anyone can observe, that an upset of the individual's nervous system, due to worry or overwork is often reflected by a disorder of the digestion.

Special investigations

Barium meal. One of the most useful investigations of stomach and duodenum is by means of a barium meal. The patient stands in front of an X-ray viewing screen and swallows a thick cream of barium emulsion which is opaque to X-rays. The meal is observed as it passes into the stomach and in addition the radiologist palpates the abdominal wall to locate any tender areas or the filling of an ulcer niche. Delay in emptying or too rapid emptying may be seen and the barium is followed through the pylorus into the duodenum and small bowel. Some hours later the patient usually returns to the X-ray department so that the passage of barium through the large bowel can also be studied.

The nurse should see that patients for X-ray examination are dressed in cotton or woollen upper garments and wear pyjama trousers free from buttons, pins and metallic fastenings. A laxative may be ordered and it should be given not later than 24 hours prior to the examination. Any medicine which might be opaque to X-rays (e.g. bismuth, iron, calcium) is avoided for a similar period.

Test meals. These tests of gastric function are carried out by fasting the patient overnight and then aspirating the gastric juice with a nasogastric tube at quarter hour intervals. In addition, after the first 4 samples, which measure basal secretion, have been collected an injection of pentagastrin (according to body weight) is given. Six further quarter-hour specimens are aspirated and represent the maximal acid secretion of the stomach. All ten specimens are carefully labelled and sent to the laboratory for measurement. The normal basal secretion is less than 5 mmol/hour and after pentagastrin secretion is about 20 mmol in a man and 10 mmol in a woman. Patients with duodenal ulcer usually secrete much higher amounts. Another method is the *all night secretion* test, in which gastric juice is aspirated overnight. Patients with duodenal ulcer secrete large volumes and high concentrations of both acid and pepsin.

Gastroscopy. In this investigation a long flexible tube or fiberscope, made of many fine glass fibres which transmit light and allow vision, is passed into the stomach. Gastroscopy is often performed under Diazepam (Valium) sedation and the back of the throat sprayed with a local anaesthetic. The patient then lies on his side while the tube is passed down the back of the throat and gently moved on through the oesophagus until the tip enters the stomach. Since the instrument is flexible, it is possible to look round inside the stomach inspecting the mucosa for an ulcer if one is suspected and noting any other abnormalities. The fiberscope may also be passed on into the duodenum to inspect it in the same way and see if an ulcer is present. The investigation is not without danger as on occasion the oesophagus may be injured or even ruptured. It is also important that for about 3 hours after the investigation patients should not be allowed to drink any hot or cold liquids since the back of the throat is still insensitive due to the anaesthetic spray and they may damage themselves without being aware of it. The fiberscope by its flexibility and transmission of light allows the stomach and duodenum to be not only seen but also photographed.

Peptic ulcer

Peptic ulcer may be gastric or duodenal and the two conditions are fairly distinct in the different symptoms they present. Gastric ulcer is almost as common in women as in men and the pain which it produces may be unrelated to the taking of food or may be aggravated by eating. Duodenal ulcer produces a pain which has been likened to that of severe hunger and it does not usually appear until an hour or more after the food has been eaten. It is often relieved by the taking of a further meal. Gastric ulcer may be accompanied by an increased secretion of hydrochloric acid, but this is not by any means the rule. Duodenal ulcer is almost invariably accompanied by hypersecretion of acid.

Patients with peptic ulcer lose weight, have nausea or vomiting and find that they have to be very careful what they eat because many indigestible foods, such as those that are fried, give them pain. When the diagnosis of an ulcer has been confirmed, the patient is usually given instructions as to diet and the regularity with which meals should be taken. If there is over-secretion of acid, an alkaline mixture is prescribed. A sedative, such as phenobarbitone 30 mg, may be ordered to allay worry or anxiety.

When the simple measures described above do not lead to a relief of symptoms and healing of the ulcer, it is necessary to institute a more thorough form of medical treatment.

Nursing care. The patient is admitted to hospital and nursed in bed. At first a very strict regime of frequent small drinks of milk or milky foods are given together with regular doses of an antacid such as magnesium trisilicate or colloidal aluminium hydroxide. Sedatives are usually prescribed freely. The diet is gradually augmented to contain easily digested solids such as a lightly boiled egg, jellies and junkets until a full light diet is taken. Pain often disappears after the first few days, but healing of the ulcer may take many weeks. The patient is discharged after being told the importance of following a careful regime and given written instructions. The drug, Cimetidine, may be ordered, which reduces the acidity so long as it is given, but its long-term effects have yet to be assessed.

When the ulcer fails to heal or rapidly recurs, an operation is performed, vagotomy and pyloroplasty, as described later in this chapter.

Complications of peptic ulcer

The complications of a peptic ulcer are haemorrhage, perforation, pyloric stenosis and carcinoma. Since they almost always require surgical treatment they are described individually.

Haemorrhage. When a peptic ulcer bleeds, the blood may pass down into the bowel and when appearing in the stool gives it a distinctive blackish colour which is referred to as *melaena*. If the blood is vomited it is referred to as a *haematemesis*. When haemorrhage from a peptic ulcer is diagnosed, the patient is immediately put to bed and usually only allowed ice to suck until there are signs that the bleeding has stopped. A nasogastric tube is passed into the stomach and half-hourly aspiration carried out. This shows if the bleeding is continuing or has stopped and may give a guide to the amount of blood lost. An intravenous infusion of saline is set up and blood is cross-matched so that it can be transfused if bleeding continues. An injection of morphia relieves the patient of anxiety and pain and helps in combating shock. If the loss of blood is severe, the foot of the bed is raised and blood transfusion started immediately. If the bleeding continues, an emergency operation is performed which ideally consists of the removal of that part of the stomach containing the bleeding ulcer.

Perforation. A peptic ulcer, especially a duodenal one which has been present for a long time, may replace the bowel wall with scar tissue and finally perforate. Flooding of the peritoneal cavity with the acid stomach contents causes intense pain, the patient is severely shocked and the abdominal wall is rigid. Such a patient is first treated for shock and then a laparotomy is performed at which the perforation is sewn up or, if it is considered desirable, a gastrectomy is performed, i.e. part of the stomach and duodenum is removed with re-establishment of bowel continuity. In very special circumstances and particularly when the perforation is small, it may be possible to aspirate the stomach contents through a large stomach tube and maintain the fluid intake by intravenous infusion until the perforation has sealed off.

Pyloric stenosis. If an ulcer occurs close to the pylorus, either on the gastric or duodenal side, when it heals, the fibrosis may almost close the pylorus with scar tissue and it is with difficulty that the stomach contents pass on. Such a condition is called pyloric stenosis and leads to a great increase in the size of the stomach, vomiting, loss of weight and dehydration. The patient is admitted, an intravenous infusion of saline is given to combat the dehydration and blood is sent to the laboratory. A large-bore stomach tube is passed and the stomach washed with normal saline since the contents are usually offensive. The treatment is always surgical and consists of either gastrectomy or a gastro-enterostomy. In the latter operation a loop of the jejunum is brought up and anastomosed to the stomach so that its contents can pass directly into the small bowel. In addition to the gastro-enterostomy a vagotomy is performed, that is division of the vagal nerves which innervate the acid-secreting glands of the stomach. The result is to reduce the secretion of acid by the stomach.

Carcinoma. A peptic ulcer may, after the passage of many years, undergo a malignant change resulting in a gastric carcinoma. However, carcinoma of the stomach arises much more commonly in patients who have no history of ulcer. The main symptom is pain which is constant (unlike that of a simple ulcer), but it may be slight or even absent. There is anorexia, which means complete loss of interest in food, and the body weight steadily falls. The diagnosis is usually made by barium meal and the treatment is gastrectomy, which may need to be total. Unfortunately such patients often have a recurrence of the growth and indeed many have inoperable tumours when first seen.

Treatment. The treatment of peptic ulcer has been outlined above and is always, primarily, a careful medical regime, but when this fails to heal the ulcer, surgical treatment is advised. For gastric ulcer a partial gastrectomy is recommended and for duodenal ulcer it is usual to perform vagotomy and pyloroplasty, although under certain circumstances partial gastrectomy may be preferred.

Pre-operative care. Before operation the patient's general health is carefully assessed and he is made as fit as possible. Adequate nourishment should be given up to the day of the operation. It is important that protein is included in the diet and this may be taken in the form of milk, eggs, fish or meat. The taking of fresh fruit drinks should be encouraged and the diet made as palatable as possible.

The haemoglobin level is estimated and corrected if low. The patient's blood is grouped so that a transfusion may be given in the operating theatre if necessary. Breathing exercises are taught pre-operatively so that the patient can more readily carry them out in the postoperative period.

Nursing care. The skin of the abdomen, lower chest and thighs are shaved and washed, ideally the patient takes a bath or a shower. The nurse will be required to pass a nasogastric tube through the nose into the stomach attaching the free end to the patient's cheek with adhesive plaster. The end should be closed with a spigot. Between 1 and 2 hours before going to the operating theatre the patient passes urine and is then given premedication, usually in the form of a subcutaneous injection of papaveretum (omnopon) 20 mg and scopolamine 0.4 mg.

Operation. In the operation of *vagotomy* and *pyloroplasty* (Fig. 15.3) the abdomen is opened and the stomach, duodenum and viscera inspected and palpated. The vagi are defined at the oesophageal hiatus in the diaphragm, doubly ligated and divided. The pylorus is incised longitudinally and sutured transversely so as to increase the size of the opening and aid drainage from the stomach, which is slowed up by vagotomy. In some clinics only the branches of the

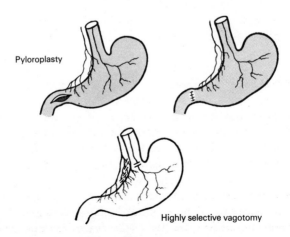

Fig. 15.3 Vagotomy and pyloroplasty.

vagus supplying the stomach are divided: *highly selective vagotomy.*
This reduces acid secretion but does not slow gastric emptying so
that pyloroplasty is not required.

In the operation of *partial gastrectomy* the abdomen is opened and
some three-quarters of the stomach removed. If the ulcer was in the
stomach, the duodenum may now be joined up to the remaining
portion of the stomach, which is partially closed to accommodate it:
this is a Billroth I operation (Fig. 15.4). If the ulcer was in the
duodenum, then the duodenal stump is closed and a loop of jejunum
is brought up and anastomosed to the remaining part of the
stomach: the Polya operation (Fig. 15.4).

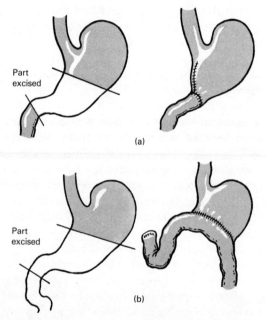

Fig. 15.4 (a) Billroth I gastrectomy. (b) Polya gastrectomy.

Postoperative nursing care. Routine care of a patient immediately following surgery is carried out. On regaining consciousness, the patient is made comfortable in the semirecumbent position,
providing the blood pressure has become stable.

Blood transfusion may be continued after surgery, if not, certain
other intravenous fluids will be administered and continued until
sufficient fluid can be taken and absorbed orally. The volume and
type of fluids will depend on the patient's levels of hydration and
serum electrolytes.

The Ryle's tube will require either hourly aspiration or continuous suction and is retained until the aspirate is minimal and there are good bowel sounds and flatus has been passed.

Once the aspirate is clear, sips of water following aspiration are permitted and gradually increased to 60 ml hourly. The Ryle's tube can then be removed, oral fluids increased and a semisolid diet introduced. Maintenance of a strict fluid balance chart is essential during this time and care of oral hygiene is necessary. Eventually a full diet will be tolerated, but stomach capacity has been reduced or it will empty less well and so meals of small quantity provided frequently are preferable.

Observance of the general care of the patient is required and carried out according to the principles of postoperative care in Chapter 8.

Gastric carcinoma

Carcinoma of the stomach is common, but of the duodenum extremely uncommon. A malignant tumour occurring in the stomach is seen more often in men than women and usually occurs after the age of forty. Occasionally it follows a chronic peptic ulcer, but more usually it arises 'out of the blue'. The first indication may be the patient feeling a lump in his upper abdomen or there may be loss of appetite, sickness and loss of weight. In time the patient develops cachexia, which is typical of malignant disease; it is due to failure to absorb nourishment, with a corresponding loss of flesh. The diagnosis of gastric carcinoma is usually confirmed by a barium meal and the treatment is total gastrectomy, if by this means the whole of the tumour can be excised. In this operation the whole stomach is removed from its junction with the oesophagus to that with the duodenum. A loop of jejunum is then brought up and anastomosed to the oesophagus. Many other operations have been devised using isolated loops of small bowel and they may be successful where it is possible to excise all the tumour. The naked eye and microscopical appearance of a gastric carcinoma are not good guides to the prognosis, which in any case is usually poor.

Many patients are found at operation to have a tumour which has already extended so far that it cannot be completely excised. In this event some kind of palliative operation may be done, for example a gastro-enterostomy to relieve the obstruction. Before operation these patients require very careful preparation. The nurse gives a daily stomach washout because there is usually a lot of foul residue due to the inability of the stomach to empty properly. There may be anaemia and this will require correction by iron or by transfusion. If the patient is cachectic this will be an indication for giving a high calorie, fluid or semisolid diet containing added vitamins. Intravenous alimentation with glucose, amino acids and emulsified fat will often make a very sick patient fit enough to undergo major surgery.

Other gastric operations

Gastrotomy. Some individuals swallow foreign bodies. Children frequently do this by accident because they like putting toys, buttons, etc. in their mouths and these may then be swallowed. Usually they pass on successfully and cause nothing but alarm to the parents, but occasionally the object is so big that it cannot leave the stomach and it has to be removed surgically, an operation called gastrotomy.

Certain individuals have a habit of swallowing hairs. Often they pull these out of their own scalp and the hairs slowly accumulate in the stomach to form a hair ball or *trichobezoar*, which may in time form almost a complete cast of the stomach. This leads to dyspepsia and loss of weight and the treatment is its removal by gastrotomy. It is also necessary to teach the individual not to continue swallowing hair. Many patients with trichobezoar are young women who need psychiatric treatment in addition to removal of the hair ball.

Gastrostomy. When a patient cannot get adequate nourishment because of obstruction to the oesophagus, as by a carcinoma, a gastrostomy may be required. At this operation an opening is made in the stomach, which is then sutured to the abdominal wall so that food can be introduced directly into the stomach. It is important that at operation the patency of the gastrostomy is confirmed by running in a little saline through a funnel and rubber tube. The tube is usually spigotted and fixed with a safety pin to a many-tailed bandage. In some cases, when the wound has healed, the tube is reintroduced before each feed and the opening maintained by inserting a specially fitted rubber bung when the tube is withdrawn. Food should be introduced at frequent intervals and a convenient mixture consists of milk to which may be added eggs, butter, soups, yeast extract and orange juice so that a well-balanced diet is given. It is also possible by means of a syringe to introduce what is virtually a normal diet if all the food is first put into a liquidiser or kitchen blender. The nurse can teach the patient how to pass the tube into the gastrostomy so that he can feed himself when he leaves hospital.

Small intestine

The small intestine, which consists of duodenum, jejunum and ileum, is the longest length of the alimentary tract and at postmortem is shown to be some 7 metres (20 feet) in all. However, in life, owing to the tone of the muscle wall, it is often less than half this length in the adult and considerably less in the baby. It is attached to the posterior abdominal wall by a mesentery which consists of two layers of peritoneum between which pass the blood vessels, nerves and lymphatics. The length of this mesentery, from its attachment to the posterior abdominal wall to the edge of the small bowel, varies from 12 to 20 centimetres. The small bowel therefore is the most mobile part of the gut and can reach almost any part of the abdominal cavity, which is why it is the small gut which strangulates in a hernial sac or by volvulus.

Small bowel obstruction

The most important lesion which affects the small bowel is intestinal obstruction and it arises in three ways. It may be due to objects which block the lumen, such as large lumps of food or a gall-stone. Abnormalities may arise in the wall of the gut itself, such as tumours, or diverticula which may in addition become inflamed or twisted. Most frequently, obstruction can be due to the bowel becoming strangulated in a hernial sac or twisted on itself. The latter may be due to adhesions or rotation of the mesentery to produce a volvulus.

Symptoms and signs. The symptoms and signs of obstruction of the small bowel are colicky pain, vomiting and distension. The higher the obstruction, i.e. the nearer it is to the pylorus, the earlier will be the onset of the vomiting. If the abdominal wall is thin, as in a baby, visible peristalsis may be seen through it, passing across it in waves as the bowel tries to force its contents through the obstruction. Auscultation with a stethoscope over the abdomen reveals greatly increased bowel sounds with gurgling and rumbling. Such sounds are called borborygmi.

Treatment. The treatment of small bowel obstruction is always one of the greatest urgency. The patient is received into hospital as soon as possible and an immediate start is made to aspirate the contents of the bowel above the obstruction and to replace the body fluids by intravenous therapy. A nasogastric tube is passed into the stomach and the nurse can then apply intermittent or continuous suction. A specially long nasogastric tube may be used in order to try and deflate the bowel. The contents of the bowel are often yellowish-brown, but if the obstruction has existed for some time the fluid may be dark and offensive and is traditionally called 'faecal'. It is not, of course, in any way composed of faeces.

The replacement of body fluids by intravenous therapy has already been discussed and it is precisely in such a patient as this that it is of most importance. Adequate water, sodium chloride and potassium are necessary and if they are given in correct amounts the patient remains fit and well for a number of days. Blood is sent to the laboratory for determination of the concentration of sodium, potassium and chloride. A specimen of urine is obtained and its specific gravity and chloride content determined. If the patient is unable to micturate the surgeon is informed, as it may be necessary to pass a catheter.

The patient's abdomen is likely to be so tender that it is inadvisable to prepare the skin by shaving or washing until the patient has been anaesthetized. The theatre staff is warned to be ready and the patient is then operated upon in order to relieve the obstruction as a matter of urgency. Postoperative treatment is no less exacting as there is always the possibility of peritonitis, which can lead to paralytic ileus. A late complication of peritonitis is the formation of adhesions and the necessity of a further operation.

Nursing care. Only ice or sips of water are allowed by mouth during the first day. When bowel sounds can be heard by placing a stethoscope on the abdominal wall, fluids can be given by mouth more freely. As soon as flatus has been passed, solids are introduced into the diet. In the absence of complications, thinly cut bread and butter and a lightly boiled egg may then be eaten as early as the fourth day and the diet is subsequently increased, as with patients following operations on the stomach.

Meckel's diverticulum

This is a blind pouch of bowel which arises from the terminal metre of the ileum in about 2½ per cent of the population (Fig. 15.5). Occasionally in its wall there is a little area of mucous membrane such as is found in the stomach and a peptic ulcer may develop here and bleed or perforate, just as in the stomach itself. Occasionally also the pouch may be the cause of a volvulus or start an intussusception (see chapter on paediatric surgery).

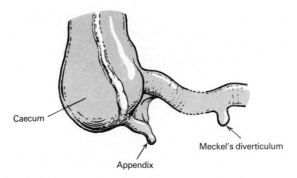

Fig. 15.5 Meckel's diverticulum.

Crohn's disease

This condition is a chronic inflammatory one typically affecting the last part of the ileum but also occurring in other parts of the small and large bowel and at times involving more than one segment. The bowel wall becomes grossly thickened and inflamed so that it resembles a rigid narrow tube; the mucosa ulcerates and bleeds. It produces chronic intestinal obstruction with the gradual onset of colicky pains and perhaps some distension. The bowel action is often fluid and frequent and it is common to see perianal abscesses. There is great loss of weight and anaemia. The condition occurs typically in young adults but the cause is not known. The treatment is conservative in the first place with prolonged bed-rest and a high protein, high carbohydrate diet with vitamins and iron. Cortisone may lead to a remission which is characterized by a gain in weight, feeling of well-being and fall in ESR. If the symptoms persist or the condition worsens the affected part of the bowel may be resected or by-passed. Careful follow-up studies show that a relapse is likely in almost three-quarters of the patients affected, but the disease may go into a long remission although it typically flares up at intervals over many years. Operation is best reserved for obstruction. In recent years there has been an increasing incidence of involvement of the large bowel by Crohn's disease but the reason for this is not known.

16
Appendix and
Large Intestine

The large bowel consists of the caecum, ascending, transverse, descending and sigmoid colon, together with the rectum. It starts at the ileocaecal valve and ends at the anus. The appendix arises from the caecum near to the ileocaecal valve (Fig. 16.1) and will be considered in this chapter. The function of the large bowel is very different from that of the small bowel. The contents are not sterile and the presence of bacteria is essential for health. The large bowel is of greater calibre, but has a thinner wall than the small bowel. The contents, which are fluid in the first part of the large bowel, slowly become of firmer consistence as they pass along, due to the absorption of water which is one of the main functions of this part of the gut. Finally the formed motions are passed through the rectum and anus at defaecation.

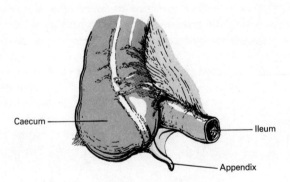

Caecum —— ———— Ileum

———— Appendix

Fig. 16.1 Terminal ileum, caecum and appendix.

Appendix

The appendix in man is a vestigial structure and serves no useful purpose. Its main importance to the surgeon is that it is frequently the site of inflammation and appendicitis, as it is called, is one of the most common and serious forms of inflammation of the bowel.

Appendicitis

Appendicitis can occur at any age, but it is rare before one year and after this age slowly becomes more common, its incidence reaching peaks around the ages of 10 and 20 years. With the passage of time the incidence is less, but it has to be remembered that appendicitis in the very young and the very old runs a much more acute or even fulminating course than in other age groups.

Symptoms and signs. The cardinal symptoms and signs of appendicitis are pain, vomiting and a moderate rise in temperature, which occur in that order. The pain is typically central abdominal in the first place and a child, if asked where the pain is, usually points to the umbilicus. The pain may be continuous or colicky, but soon localizes in the right iliac fossa. There is often acute tenderness over *McBurney's Point*, which is situated a third of the way along a line drawn from the anterior superior iliac spine to the umbilicus

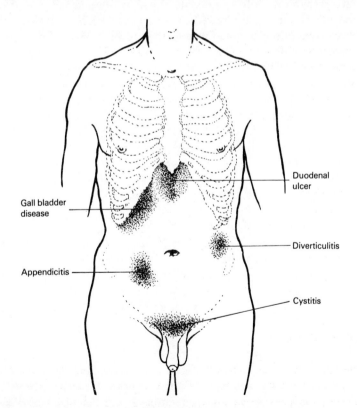

Fig. 16.2 Shaded areas show where pain is felt in abdominal disease.

(Fig. 16.2). If peritonitis develops, there will be muscle guarding and the patient will try to resist palpation of his abdomen. Rigidity of the muscles of the abdominal wall occurs later and as the inflammation spreads there may be tenderness in other parts of the abdomen. The breath is often foetid, the tongue furred and there is general malaise and frequently nausea. The temperature rises rather slowly, but there is often a more rapid rise in the pulse rate. The cause of appendicitis is unknown, but it has been observed that the disease is very much more common in Europe and North America than it is in those countries where the consumption of meat is minimal and the diet contains much fibre.

Surgical treatment. Once the diagnosis of appendicitis has been made, the patient is transferred to hospital as quickly as possible and preparations made for operation. Nothing is administered by mouth, no purge is given, nor is an enema administered, the patient being prepared for operation as described in an earlier chapter. The abdomen is not usually shaved or washed since it is so tender. The patient is encouraged to pass water and if unable to do so the surgeon is informed and may request catheterization or elect to do this on the operating table before opening the abdomen. Preparation of the skin is carried out on the operating table after anaesthesia has been induced. When the appendix is removed the peritoneal cavity may require drainage and it is important that the drainage tube be carefully watched and subsequently shortened as the discharge lessens. The nurse should dress the wound daily until it is clean and dry. If the disease is advanced and a large abscess present, it may only be possible to drain this, a further operation being performed some months later in order to remove the appendix.

Postoperative nursing care. After regaining consciousness the patient is supported in the sitting position. Nothing is given by mouth for the first 6 hours. If there is no vomiting after this time sips of water are permitted. Fluids and later food are gradually increased in amount so that by the fourth day a light diet is being taken. If the disease is uncomplicated the patient will be allowed out of bed after the first day and will be walking about quite comfortably by the eighth day, when the stitches are removed.

If there is peritonitis, a nasogastric tube will be passed through the nose into the stomach and the contents aspirated hour by hour. The fluid intake will be maintained by intravenous therapy. Antibiotics may be ordered when the infection is not localized and are administered intramuscularly once or twice in each 24 hours. A specimen of urine is obtained daily for routine tests until intravenous therapy is discontinued. A fluid balance chart must be used.

Caecum

The caecum derives its name from the Latin word for blind as it forms a blind pouch at the beginning of the colon. It varies very much in size in different people and is not often the site of disease. The two conditions affecting it are a simple ulcer, which is rare, and carcinoma.

Carcinoma

Carcinoma of the caecum is usually a bulky polypoid type of growth rather than the ulcerative and constricting variety which is so commonly seen in other parts of the large bowel. Because the contents of the caecum are fluid, a tumour in this part of the bowel does not cause obstruction until late The symptoms and signs of carcinoma of the caecum are very similar to those of subacute appendicitis, for which it is often mistaken in the older patient.

Treatment. The treatment of such a tumour is by an operation called right hemicolectomy in which the terminal 15 cm of the ileum, the appendix, caecum, ascending colon and hepatic flexure are all removed in one piece together with their mesentery and any involved lymph nodes. The continuity of the bowel is restored by anastomosing the terminal ileum to the transverse colon.

Nursing care. Before operation a four-day course of one of the insoluble sulphonamides such as phthalylsulphathiazole may be prescribed in 1 to 2 g doses four times a day and since anaerobic organisms are often the cause of postoperative infection, metronidazole (Flagyl) may be ordered. A simple enema is administered the night before operation to empty the lower bowel. Before operation a nasogastric tube is passed and the stomach contents aspirated.

Postoperatively the suction and intravenous infusion are continued until bowel sounds are heard, after which fluids are allowed by mouth. As soon as flatus is passed, a light diet is started. It is imperative that no enema is given in the postoperative period.

Colon

The various parts of the colon are described as ascending, transverse, descending and sigmoid and extend from the caecum to the rectum. The diseases to which the colon is subject may be grouped under the various ages at which they appear. In the newborn and in infants, Hirschsprung's disease occurs; in young adults, ulcerative colitis and Crohn's disease; after middle age carcinoma may develop as also may diverticulosis. Polyps occur at any age.

Ulcerative colitis

This condition, of which the cause is not known, is seen most often in young adults and only rarely in children. The individual develops diarrhoea and there is passage of mucus and blood in the motions. The bowel shows multiple small ulcers when inspected with the colonoscope, which are very loath to heal and the constant loss of blood and mucus with frequent stools leads to loss of weight, anaemia and general debility. Under a strict medical régime, salazopyrine by mouth and the local instillation of cortisone by enema, there is usually some improvement, but the condition, if severe, often relapses. Strict bed rest, a high calorie, low residue diet and correction of anaemia by blood transfusion and iron may produce a remission.

It is considered that ulcerative colitis in many patients is a psychosomatic condition and therefore the approach to the patient is most important. The nurse should try to win the individual's confidence by listening sympathetically to the account of all the worries and problems with which they are beset. In addition to an understanding manner, the nurse can also help by arranging for practical assistance with problems involving the family, the home and work from the medical social worker.

Surgical treatment. The surgical treatment of ulcerative colitis, though it leaves the patient with a permanent ileostomy, can be very successful in restoring health and is indicated when the disease frequently relapses and prevents normal life, or when a flare-up despite treatment threatens life.

A *colectomy* is often performed in two stages, the rectum being removed at the second operation. Total colectomy may however have to be done in one stage because of the life threatening loss of fluid, protein and blood from the ulcerated mucosa. In the desperately ill patient, a blood transfusion is given during and after the operation. The ileum is brought to the surface in the right iliac fossa.

The contents of the ileum, if allowed to come into contact with the skin of the abdominal wall, would excoriate it. Therefore the *ileostomy* is surrounded by a protective ring of 'Stomahesive' or similar material and is then fitted with a light polythene bag. By this means the skin is protected. The contents of the bowel collect in this bag, which can be renewed as necessary. It is easily disposed of down the lavatory. The apparatus used today is very neat and the patient can lead an almost normal life. The nurse can help by teaching the patient how to manage this apparatus. There are ileostomy clubs which patients can join, obtaining the latest information on appliances and gaining much moral support from fellow sufferers. In a few patients it is possible to join the terminal ileum to the stump of the rectum and so conserve the anus.

Carcinoma

Malignant disease of the colon is a common condition and occurs more often on the left side than the right (Fig. 16.3). Carcinoma of the sigmoid colon is the most frequent variety and the symptoms are usually those of obstruction. The disease takes the form of an ulcer with heaped up edges and the fibrosis which this produces in the bowel wall leads to narrowing of the lumen and eventually

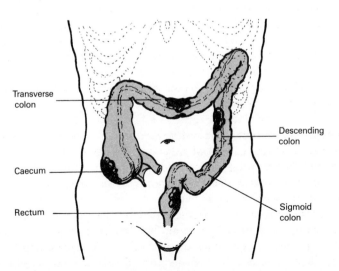

Fig. 16.3 Common sites of carcinoma in the colon.

complete obstruction. The diagnosis is confirmed by a barium enema which demonstrates the narrowing in the bowel, or with a sigmoidoscope or colonoscope, which may be passed to show the lesion, when a biopsy will be taken and sent to the pathology laboratory.

Pre-operative preparation. Because patients with carcinoma of the colon are usually in an older age group and because the disease has been present for a long time before it makes itself known, careful preparation before operation is necessary. Anaemia is corrected by giving iron or a blood transfusion. The operation is explained to the patient so as to overcome the natural repugnance which is usually aroused. For those patients who will have to wear a colostomy belt on leaving hospital, this is ordered as soon as the surgeon has decided to operate. The contents of the bowel are rendered sterile by oral administration of a non-absorbable sulphonamide, such as phthalyl-sulphathiazole, for this reduces the risk from soiling at operation. The drug is given every 6 hours in 2 g doses for 4 days. In order that the bowel be as well prepared as possible the nurse should see that the patient is given a low residue diet, which is one consisting mainly of milk, eggs, minced lean meat, chicken and fish. Fruit, except for fruit juices, vegetables and fatty foods are avoided as far as possible.

The skin of the abdomen is shaved and cleaned. A bowel washout is performed on at least two occasions; metronidazole (Flagyl) and neomycin may be ordered by the surgeon to be given by mouth during the 24 hours before operation. Antibiotics may also be given intravenously during the anaesthetic and postoperatively. This lessens the incidence of wound infection with anaerobic organisms and aids healing of the anastomosis.

Operation. At operation the affected segment of bowel is excised, together with the lymph nodes in the mesentery which drain it. The continuity of the bowel is restored by direct anastomosis wherever possible. If, however, too large an area of the bowel is involved, the proximal end is brought out and sutured to the abdominal wall to form a colostomy.

When carcinoma of the large bowel causes obstruction, excision is not always carried out, but an operation to relieve the obstruction is performed as an emergency. A loop of bowel proximal to the obstruction is brought to the surface and when opened forms a *colostomy* (Fig. 16.4). Underneath the loop a glass rod is placed to prevent the bowel slipping back into the abdominal cavity and a piece of rubber tubing is attached to each end of the glass rod so that

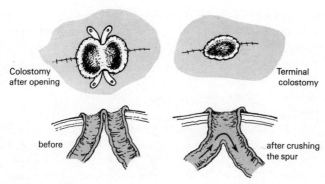

Colostomy after opening

Terminal colostomy

before

after crushing the spur

Fig. 16.4 Colostomy.

it remains anchored in place. On the operating table the colostomy is usually partly opened immediately to let out some of the gas or contents, but the full opening is not made until a few days later, so that the bowel becomes sealed to the peritoneum around the edges of the wound. The surgeon may tie a piece of glass tubing into the opening in the bowel and connect this up with some soft rubber tubing (Paul's tubing) to a container at the bedside. Most importantly the skin is protected with 'Stomahesive.'

Postoperative nursing care and the management of a colostomy. Frequent dressings may be required for the first few days after the colostomy starts to work and the nurse must hide any feelings of disgust when performing this task; indeed it is easy to do this when it is realized how much the patient dislikes the dependence. It is a satisfying duty to make such patients comfortable, and the nurse has a great chance at such times of reassuring and teaching the patient about the future management of the dressings.

The postoperative care of patients after a colostomy has been performed is aimed to produce a habit of regular bowel evacuation. Some patients are able to train the colostomy to work every morning after breakfast and the regular use of a methyl cellulose preparation (e.g. Celevac) helps in keeping motions to the right consistence. Others find it more suitable to wash out the colostomy before starting the day. The irrigation may be performed with a special irrigating apparatus or by a catheter size 10 to 12 (Jacques) attached by a glass connection and rubber tubing to an irrigating can. The orifice is dilated with a gloved finger and the catheter is gently inserted about 15 cm into the opening and water or normal saline is allowed to flow slowly into the bowel. It may be necessary to use up to 1 litre of the fluid to ensure an efficient evacuation. The patient learns how to carry out this procedure under supervision 10 to 14 days after operation.

After the colostomy has worked, the patient is encouraged to move about to hasten drainage. When all discharge has ceased the skin area is cleaned and a pad or bag applied with a light belt to hold it in place.

When carrying out treatment the nurse should endeavour to help the patient to adjust to the new circumstances. With a sound knowledge of what a colostomy means, it is possible to help the patient greatly by means of simple and tactful information, together with a sympathetic approach to the patient's problems. The dressings should be done whenever necessary to spare any embarrassment, and instructions given on the care of the skin. The patient should also be told to take only moderate amounts of food containing roughage in order to ensure regular action of the colostomy. Fruit and pips may irritate the bowel and should be avoided if they cause too frequent action of the colostomy. The motion can be made more solid by methyl cellulose granules, which are taken by mouth, as these swell in the intestine and give light but firm bulk to the stool. The patient should be shown how to apply a small dressing held in place with the colostomy belt and advised to take a bath daily. Alternatively a bag is used. The patient is encouraged to join a colostomy association.

Diverticular disease

Diverticula are small pouches in the wall of the bowel and they arise typically in the distal part of the colon (Fig. 16.5). They rarely occur

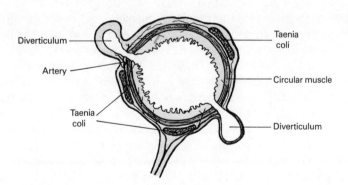

Fig. 16.5 Cross-section of the colon and two diverticula. Note the diverticula pierce the muscle coat where the arteries enter.

before the age of forty, but after that age are frequently seen in barium examinations of the bowel (Fig. 16.6). They cause no symptoms unless they become inflamed, but this they are quite likely to do and, if their contents stagnate, the organisms within may give rise to irritation. This condition is known as *diverticulitis* and causes crampy abdominal pain, diarrhoea and the passage of mucus and occasionally blood. Those who eat plenty of roughage in their diet seldom develop diverticulosis and the addition of one or two tablespoonfuls of bran daily to a western type of diet is good prevention and may relieve bowel symptoms. Certainly it usually prevents constipation and gives a regular well-formed stool. Those who have always eaten a low residue diet (white bread, little or no fruit or vegetables and salad) may take time to adapt to the change. Once an attack of diverticulitis occurs, the patient should be kept in bed and restricted to a fluid diet until the acute symptoms have resolved. Antibiotics such as tetracycline and metronidazole may be ordered.

The complications of diverticulitis are the formation of abscesses round the bowel and fistulas between the bowel and any of the surrounding organs, especially the bladder. When an abscess occurs, surgery is indicated in order to drain it.

When blood and mucus are repeatedly passed, colonoscopy is performed to exclude a polyp or carcinoma and if the symptoms are disabling the most severely affected segment of colon is excised, with immediate anastomosis of the ends using the same régime as described for colectomy in carcinoma of the colon.

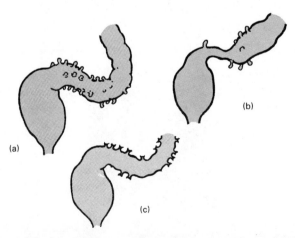

Fig. 16.6 Appearance after barium enema of: (a) diverticulosis of the sigmoid colon, (b) stricture of the colon, (c) diverticulitis, note saw-tooth appearance.

Polyposis

Polyps, which are benign growths looking sometimes rather like cherries on stalks, may occur in any part of the large bowel. In children they occur in the rectum and usually disappear spontaneously.

In adults any part of the large bowel may be affected and bleeding occurs. Later they may undergo a malignant change and for this reason it is necessary to excise them, including the stalk, using the colonoscope.

There is a rare variety of the condition which occurs in families, in whom multiple polyps arise in the large bowel in childhood, undergoing malignant change at an early stage. As a result the victims develop carcinoma of the colon at a younger age than is usually seen, for example between 15 and 25 years. The treatment of multiple polyposis is colectomy, since this is the only means of preventing the development of carcinoma. The patients require regular endoscopy postoperatively.

Rectum

The rectum, which is 20 to 23 cm long in an adult, is the terminal part of the large bowel and lies in the pelvis, ending below in the funnel-shaped anal canal. It is supported on each side by a strong muscular diaphragm made up by the two levator ani muscles (Fig. 16.7). The rectum is a common site for carcinoma to develop, especially in the male (3900 deaths per annum in England and

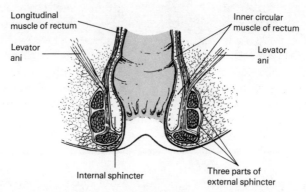

Longitudinal muscle of rectum
Inner circular muscle of rectum
Levator ani
Levator ani
Internal sphincter
Three parts of external sphincter

Fig. 16.7 Rectum and anus showing sphincters.

Wales). It is also the site of haemorrhoids, so that a careful investigation of the rectum is a most important procedure.

For examination of the rectum the patient is usually asked to lie on the left side, covered with a blanket, with the knees drawn up to the chin. First the anus is inspected to see if external haemorrhoids are present. These are varicosities of the veins underneath the anal skin and may be the site of a haematoma, which produces a painful subcutaneous swelling of a bluish tinge. Next, the surgeon usually takes a rubber finger cot, finger stall, or rubber glove, and having lubricated it with liquid paraffin, Vaseline or jelly inserts it very gently into the anus and rectal canal. This allows palpation of any lesion affecting the wall, and a carcinoma, if present, can be felt. A proctoscope, which has been previously warmed and lubricated, is then passed. The obturator is removed, the light switched on and the walls of the rectum carefully inspected as it is gently withdrawn.

Anal fissure or fissure in ano

This is a crack or linear sore in the anal canal usually caused by constipation and producing intense pain at defaecation with the occasional passage of small amounts of blood. At examination the anus is held in spasm and digital examination causes great pain, but with gentleness it is usually possible to reveal the fissure. Treatment is the relief of constipation and the application of an analgesic ointment such as nupercainal. If the condition becomes very chronic, the fissure has to be excised under general anaesthesia and allowed to heal by granulation after stretching the anus widely.

Anal fistula or fistula in ano

In this condition a fistula or track communicates from the skin beside the anus to the rectum. It is usually brought about by infection and is a particularly chronic condition which needs to be laid widely open by incision. The wound is dressed with tulle-gras and the bowels kept costive for 3 days. Subsequently the patient sits in an antiseptic bath after each defaecation until healing occurs. Fistula in ano is occasionally produced by a tuberculous infection, the result of swallowing infected sputum.

Haemorrhoids

Haemorrhoids, or piles, may be internal or external. *External* ones have been described above and are really varicosities of the anal veins. *Internal* haemorrhoids are also varicose venous enlargements and occur in the branches of the superior haemorrhoidal veins in the lowest part of the rectum and the anal canal. The veins are situated deep to the mucosa, and the piles can be seen with a proctoscope. Internal haemorrhoids cannot usually be palpated by a finger in the rectum because they are too soft. A proctoscope is a hollow speculum with an indwelling obturator which is lubricated and gently inserted into the rectum. An electric light is passed up the instrument and it is then possible to see the interior of the rectum. Haemorrhoids may be of three degrees. In the first degree they are only seen with a proctoscope inside the rectum; second-degree haemorrhoids prolapse out through the anus at defaecation, but always return of their own accord; third-degree haemorrhoids not only prolapse, but remain outside the anus unless they are replaced. Haemorrhoids are a source of great discomfort, pain and bleeding and their treatment is important as they cause so much minor ill health.

Treatment by injection. First-degree haemorrhoids are treated by the injection of 5 per cent phenol in oil, using a special syringe and a proctoscope. Second- and third-degree haemorrhoids require a surgical operation, haemorrhoidectomy or forcible dilatation of the anus under anaesthesia.

Pre-operative nursing care. The pre-operative treatment aims to clear the lower bowel. The patient is given a low residue diet for a few days and an enema the night before operation. The perineal and perianal area of the skin is shaved, the patient has a bath or shower and on the morning of the operation the rectum is washed out.

Operation. At operation the piles are dissected, ligatured and the greater part of them excised. This leaves a raw area at the site of each pile and this is likely to be painful for some days. Alternatively the anus is dilated by 4 fingers of each hand and the patient can usually go home the next day being warned that there may be some leakage from the anus for a few days.

Postoperative nursing care. The patient is nursed after haemorrhoidectomy, usually with two or three pillows. An air-ring or latex cushion may make for comfort. The diet is so arranged that the bowels will not be opened for 4 days and this is also assisted by giving medicine, such as chalk and opium, by mouth. Pain is relieved by an injection of morphia, which also has a constipating

effect. A small oil enema, which is retained for 4 hours and followed
by a simple enema, is given on the third or fourth day to help the
patient have a soft bowel motion and thereafter he sits in a bath each
day after the bowels act so that cleansing of the raw area is facilitated
and healing by granulation stimulated. After a week or ten days the
patient is usually fit enough to return home, but before doing so a
digital examination of the rectum is carried out to make sure that
there is no stricture formation. Some surgeons prefer the patient to
have a bowel action the day after operation and therefore prescribe
no constipating medicine. If there is any narrowing of the anus the
patient is given a dilator which he can lubricate with Vaseline and
gently insert each day.

Carcinoma

The rectum is a common site for malignant disease in the male and
the diagnosis of carcinoma is usually made when the patient reports
a change in bowel habit and pain. There may be alternating
constipation and diarrhoea, the passage of mucus and a little blood
and a feeling of fullness in the rectum which gives the patient the
sensation that the bowel is not properly emptied even after a motion
has been passed.

Diagnosis. The carcinoma is often diagnosed by the doctor
inserting a finger into the rectum, when the indurated edges of the
ulcer can be palpated and also its attachment to structures surrounding the rectum. It may be seen by passing a proctoscope,
sigmoidoscope or colonoscope depending on the level of the
tumour. The sigmoidoscope is a cylindrical speculum, 10 inches in
length, with a small glass telescope on the proximal end and an
electric light which can be passed down the instrument. It is
introduced into the anus with an obturator and then the obturator is
removed and the telescope put in its place. It is then advanced under
direct vision, the walls of the rectum being pushed aside by the
insufflation of air carried out by means of a small bellows attached to
the side of the instrument. An anaesthetic is not given for this
investigation, and if carried out in the left lateral or knee–elbow
position, it allows inspection of the whole rectum and part of the
lower sigmoid colon. A colonoscope is used somewhat similarly but
since it is introduced much further, being flexible, the bowel needs
irrigation to clear it of faeces.

Treatment. If a tumour arises high up in the rectum, it is possible to excise it and restore the continuity of the bowel, an operation known as conservative or *anterior resection*. The scope of anterior resection has been extended by the introduction of the stapling gun, which permits the anastomosis of bowel deep in the pelvis. When the tumour arises in the lower part of the rectum or anal canal it is necessary to remove the whole of the rectum and the tissues surrounding the anus and to bring out the proximal part of the large bowel in the left iliac fossa as a colostomy, an operation described as *abdominoperineal*. This operation must be carefully explained to the patient beforehand, as usually he is distressed when it is first mentioned. However, if the patient can talk to another who has already had a colostomy, he soon discovers that it can easily be managed and that it is not such a source of inconvenience or embarrassment when properly looked after. As the operation is accompanied by a considerable blood loss and shock, the patient's blood will be grouped and a supply of matched blood put aside for transfusion.

Pre-operative nursing care. Before the operation of excising the rectum, the patient should be given a low residue diet and have the lower bowel washed out for 1 or 2 days. The skin of the abdomen and the perineum is shaved and cleaned. Phthalylsulphathiazole (1 to 2 g three times daily) is given to sterilize the large bowel and often neomycin and metronidazole.

On the morning of operation a nasogastric tube is passed and the stomach contents aspirated. The surgeon may require a self-retaining catheter to be inserted in the bladder before the patient is taken to the operating theatre.

The operation. This is usually an abdominoperineal one and consists of removing not only the rectum but a large ellipse of skin in the perineum and all the surrounding soft tissues. Usually two surgeons work simultaneously, one dealing with the abdomen, the other the perineum. After the operation the dead space may be obliterated by loosely bringing together the flaps with sutures and applying suction, or a light pack may be inserted. The colostomy is dressed with 'Stomahesive' and a bag.

Post-operative nursing care. The patient is nursed supported with pillows in the sitting position. An air-ring or latex cushion is an advantage.

The catheter in the urethra is left in place for a few days, the bladder being emptied at regular intervals or continuous drainage maintained. A bag is placed over the colostomy in the early days after operation to collect the bowel contents before such time as it settles down to a regular action. Fluid and electrolyte balance is maintained by intravenous infusion and nasogastric suction is used for the first postoperative days while the anastomosis is healing.

The abdominal wound is left untouched, unless there is reason to think it is infected, and the sutures are removed after 10 days.

Care must be taken to keep the perineal wound clean, and a daily bath is given after the tenth day following operation. As soon as the colostomy action is established, the diet is increased from fluids to solid foods which will stimulate one bowel action daily. After 3 days the patient is sat up out of bed and for a longer time each day thereafter. Two to three weeks after operation the patient should be ready for convalescence.

17
Liver, Gall Bladder, Pancreas and Spleen

Liver

The liver is the largest organ within the abdominal cavity and lies more on the right than on the left side, the right lobe being much the larger. Its upper and convex surface is applied to the under surface of the diaphragm, to which it is attached by ligaments. The liver may be likened to a large chemical factory, all the blood from the bowel passing back into it and the breakdown products of the food being dealt with there. In addition the liver stores glycogen, which is a substance from which glucose can be readily released, and also manufactures bile, which passes into the duodenum to help in digestion and especially the absorption of fats. Since the liver also makes the serum proteins, albumin and globulin, it is important in immunology and the protection of the body from infection and invasion by foreign protein as in grafting operations. This organ when diseased is more often the subject of investigation and treatment in the medical wards, but there are a few conditions affecting the liver which call for treatment by a surgeon and these are described below.

Rupture

The liver, being a large and rather friable organ, is liable to rupture in crush injuries of the abdomen or lower chest. The signs and symptoms are those of severe pain and shock, the latter being due in part to the loss of blood from an organ which is so vascular. The treatment is to combat the shock and replace blood loss by transfusion. It may be possible to repair the injury under a general anaesthetic, but if damage is extensive the non-viable part of the liver is excised and the raw area is oversewn. A drainage tube or tubes will be necessary and the postoperative treatment will aim to prevent peritonitis and also lung collapse and infection due to impaired movement of the diaphragm. Since there will almost certainly be other injuries the patient is likely to be nursed in an intensive care unit.

Abscesses

There are two varieties of abscess occurring in the liver which may, on occasion, require operation.

(i) The amoebic abscess is seen in patients living in hot countries. The amoeba is a protozoon which is a contaminant of food. It passes through the bowel wall and lodges in the liver where it gives rise to an abscess, usually in the right lobe. The abscess is often large and contains pus which is brownish and thick, resembling anchovy sauce. The patient is ill and toxic, and as the abscess spreads the diaphragm is involved and often the right pleural cavity, producing signs of an effusion and possibly consolidation in the right lower lobe of the lung. The treatment of this condition is by metroni-dazole (Flagyl) 400 mg t.d.s. for 5 days or intramuscular injection of emetine 65 mg daily for a week, but it is also occasionally necessary to drain the abscess. This is done by making an incision between two of the ribs in the mid-axillary line and passing a wide-bore tube into the cavity.

(ii) The other condition producing multiple abscesses in the liver is due to inflammation in the bowel, such as appendicitis. This infection spreads to the liver by veins or lymphatics and leads to multiple green abscesses throughout the liver substance. The patient has a severe toxaemia with a high swinging fever. The condition is of surgical importance because the source of infection in the abdomen requires drainage. In all liver abscesses secondary infection is common and is treated by penicillin and streptomycin, or whatever is the appropriate antibiotic (see chapter 2).

Neoplasm

New growths of the liver (hepatoma) are rare, but in certain countries, for example among some of the coloured people of South Africa, they are seen more frequently. The patient usually has anorexia followed by loss of weight, becomes jaundiced and usually dies within a space of months after the initial symptoms have presented. It is unfortunately not always possible to excise part of the liver containing a tumour because such tumours are usually already large before they are diagnosed, the liver is very vascular and wide excision is difficult and leakage of bile and blood after operation is a real problem. The CAT scanner is valuable for diagnosis.

Portal hypertension

One form of cirrhosis (of which there are many kinds) produces an increase in fibrous tissue around the portal veins as they pass through the lobules of the liver. This strangulation of the blood returning to the liver from the bowel causes it to be dammed back and the pressure within the portal vein to rise. Because the portal blood is unable to pass from the bowel, anastomoses develop between the portal and systemic veins in other parts of the body. The most important are the connections which occur in the lower end of the oesophagus and these dilated veins are called *oesophageal varices*. Very rarely anastomosis occurs between the two kinds of vein at the umbilicus and a mass of varicose veins, called a caput medusae, is then seen in the abdominal wall around the navel. Portal hypertension is made more severe by thrombosis in the splenic vein and may be accompanied by increase in the size of the spleen, a condition called *splenomegaly*.

The patient will present for treatment in one of a number of ways. If an oesophageal varix ruptures there will be severe bleeding with haematemesis and melaena. There may be *ascites* with the abdomen distended by fluid. There may be general anorexia with loss of weight.

Portal hypertension can be brought about in a number of ways including severe attacks of infective hepatitis and the accidental ingestion of substances toxic to the liver, such as carbon tetrachloride, which is used sometimes for cleaning clothes.

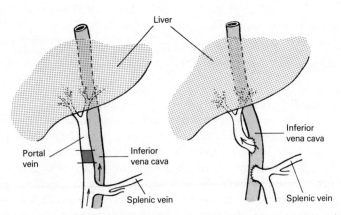

Fig. 17.1 Treatment of portal hypertension by anastomosing the portal vein to the inferior vena cava.

Treatment. The aim is to reduce the pressure in the portal venous system by anastomosing the portal vein to the inferior vena cava: a porta-caval shunt (Fig. 17.1). Before this can be safely carried out the serum proteins albumin and globulin must be estimated to determine whether the liver function is good enough to handle the portal blood. Subsequently the patient's protein intake is restricted because a rise in the nitrogen compounds in the blood may cause encephalopathy with fits and coma—so called meat intoxication.

Gall bladder and bile ducts

Bile, which is a greenish-yellow fluid, contains bile salts and bile pigments. The pigments are derived from the breakdown of red blood cells. Bile passes down the right and left hepatic ducts to the common bile duct, which opens into the duodenum at the ampulla of Vater. Also communicating with the common bile duct is a more narrow channel, the cystic duct, which drains the gall bladder, a small pear-shaped sac lying under the right lobe of the liver. Within the gall bladder, water is absorbed and possibly other substances are added to the bile increasing its concentration some eight-fold. The gall bladder serves as a reservoir for bile and its emptying is brought about reflexly by the hormone cholecystokinin when food enters the duodenum. Thus concentrated bile is passed into the duodenum exactly when it is required. Bile helps in the absorption and digestion of fats, and it is the presence of oil or fat in the duodenum, which most vigorously stimulates the gall bladder to empty. The anatomy of the bile ducts is extremely variable and because of this, operations on the gall bladder and bile passages are always fraught with some danger.

Cholecystitis

Inflammation of the gall bladder is called cholecystitis, but the word is also used to include many conditions where the wall of the gall bladder is abnormal. Probably many of these conditions are due to metabolic derangements rather than inflammation. In a typical attack of cholecystitis the patient has severe vomiting and loss of appetite with a particular dread of fatty food. The temperature is raised, often quite high, and there may be shivering attacks or rigors. When the attack is very severe there may be a mild icteric or jaundiced tinge to the skin due to the presence of an abnormal amount of bile pigment in the circulating blood.

The treatment of acute cholecystitis is rest in bed with clear fluids (especially glucose drinks) as the only form of nourishment permitted by mouth, until the acute symptoms have worn off. Subsequently cholecystectomy can be performed, the gall bladder being excised and the cystic duct doubly ligated and divided. Some surgeons prefer to remove the gall bladder during the acute attack, and this certainly saves time. Operation is however never done during the period of recovery from an acute attack. The cause of cholecystitis is rarely discovered but it would appear that certain people are much more prone to develop it. Usually they are obese. 'Fat, female, fertile and forty' epitomizes the typical patient.

Cholelithiasis (gall-stones)

Gall-stones are of three kinds named according to the major constituent, although most gall-stones contain a combination of all three.

The commonest type of gall-stone is formed in the gall bladder and is referred to as a *mixed* infective stone, being made of bile pigments and their calcium salts together with cholesterol.

Occasionally a solitary stone, or solitaire, is discovered which is oval, rough and pale in colour and made of almost pure *cholesterol*.

The third variety consists of pure bile *pigment* and therefore appears soft and black. Pigment stones may be accompanied by putty-like masses and debris called biliary mud. They are seen most commonly in patients with acholuric jaundice, in whom the red blood cells are abnormally fragile and are therefore being broken down at a greater rate than in normal people. The excess haemoglobin produces much bile pigment, which then appears in this form.

The signs and symptoms of gall-stones depend on the site at which they are found (Fig. 17.2). If a stone tries to leave the gall bladder it may become impacted in the outlet and produce intense colicky pain. The stone may pass further into the common bile duct, where it may cause not only pain but jaundice by obstructing the flow of bile into the duodenum and causing the excess to be absorbed into the bloodstream. Large stones may lie quietly in the gall bladder, incapable of leaving it and causing minimal symptoms. Gall-stones are seen much more often in women than in men and can be associated with obesity, chronic constipation, overeating and lack of exercise. Many gall-stones cause no symptoms at all and if their presence is discovered accidentally during ultrasound or X-

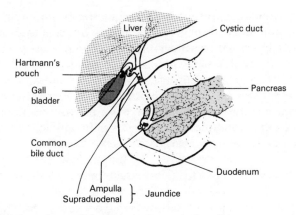

Fig. 17.2 Sites where gall-stones are commonly found.

ray examination of the abdomen it is often better that the patient should not be told about it.

Gall-stones are typically associated with flatulent dyspepsia, heartburn, palpitations and eructations. There are attacks of pain which may be of two kinds. If a stone engages in one of the bile ducts there will be severe colicky pains causing shock and the patient will recall the exact time of the onset of the condition. Alternatively, there may be chronic pain under the right costal margin which though not severe is made worse by eating, especially fatty foods. Occasional attacks of fever with rigor are also seen.

Special tests. In a patient suspected of having gall-stones but in whom the diagnosis remains in doubt, examination using ultra-sound is the best way of demonstrating them, requires no special preparation and is non-invasive. In many clinics, however, a cholecystogram will be ordered. The patient has a fat-free meal at night and two hours later takes capsules of a drug containing a high concentration of iodine. This drug, or dye, is excreted in the bile and X-ray pictures taken the following morning outline the gall bladder if it is still functioning satisfactorily and concentrating bile. Stones may be demonstrated and when the patient is given a fatty meal the gall-bladder will contract or empty if it is still capable of so doing. In patients in whom the gall bladder does not concentrate any dye, or in those in whom the gall bladder has already been removed and who are suspected of having stones in the bile-ducts, another variety of dye called 'biligrafin' is administered intravenously. This is concentrated in such amounts by the liver that it outlines the ducts.

If a patient is jaundiced, the problem will arise as to whether the jaundice is due to obstruction by a stone or by a tumour of the bile ducts or pancreas. It may also be due to some form of liver disease, such as hepatitis, which does not allow the bile to reach the biliary tract. It is unwise in the jaundiced patient to perform cholecystography, as the liver is damaged, and ultrasound is then most helpful. Diagnosis is aided by tests of liver function performed on specimens of urine and blood and also by determination of the serum alkaline phosphatase, because this substance is greatly increased in the bloodstream in obstructive jaundice.

Pre-operative treatment. It is unusual for the surgeon to operate on a patient who is jaundiced if this can be avoided, but when it becomes necessary, precautions are taken to prevent undue haemorrhage at operation. A jaundiced patient bleeds much more freely, because the damaged liver is unable to form prothrombin, which is necessary for blood clotting. Therefore the patient is given vitamin K by injection (22 mg) before operation to make good this deficiency since it is only absorbed from the bowel when bile is present.

The skin of the abdomen is shaved and the patient prepared for a general anaesthetic.

Operation. The treatment of gall-stones is their removal; this means the removal of the gall bladder and in addition, if there has been jaundice, the exploration of the common bile duct to remove any stones from it. After the common bile duct has been opened, it is drained by means of a T-shaped tube (Fig. 17.3) which allows some of the bile to run down into the duodenum and the remainder to pass out into a bottle placed at the patient's bedside. The purpose of this is to allow the free drainage of bile for a week or 10 days after

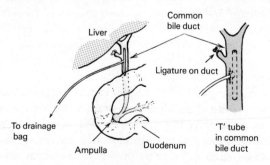

Fig. 17.3 T-tube for draining the common bile duct.

operation and then the tube may be removed with safety, allowing the common bile duct to heal over. Usually at operation, dye is injected into the bile ducts and X-rays taken to see if any stones have been left behind.

Postoperative nursing care. As soon as the patient is fully conscious she is sat up if this is found to be the most comfortable position. Pain and abdominal discomfort are particularly common after gall bladder operations and so analgesics will be ordered by the doctor and if there is much distension, the passage of a flatus tube into the rectum. The amount of bile drainage is noted. Before the T-tube is removed from the common bile duct the patient goes to the X-ray department and a small amount of opaque dye, such as diodone, is injected down it to show that the common bile duct is free from stones and that bile can drain normally into the duodenum. There is no risk of leakage of bile into the peritoneum after a week has passed, because adhesions will have formed around the indwelling tube. There may also be a tube to drain the gall-bladder bed, this tube is shortened daily and removed after 4 to 5 days.

Patients with obstructive jaundice cannot digest fats and they are best given large quantities of fruit drinks with the addition of glucose; they are also unable, because of liver damage, to deal with the usual doses of drugs such as morphia and phenobarbitone, therefore these must be used very sparingly and, since they have a cumulative effect, must be given at longer intervals than normal if they do not at once produce the desired effect. Such patients often feel mentally depressed and the nurse needs to be especially sympathetic and tactful with them.

It might be thought that after cholecystectomy the patient would be unable to digest fats normally, but it is found in practice that the diet does not need to be restricted. The patient is usually ready to leave hospital after 10 days.

Pancreas

The head of the pancreas lies in the curve formed by the duodenum and the tail of the organ extends to the left side, where it comes into contact with the hilum of the spleen (Fig. 17.4). The pancreas has two main functions: the production of internal secretions (into the bloodstream) and an external one (into the duodenum). The most important internal secretion is insulin, which controls the level of

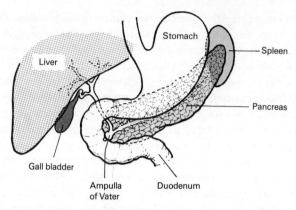

Fig. 17.4 Relation of the pancreas to the duodenum and spleen. Note the common bile duct and the pancreatic duct.

blood sugar. It is the absence of insulin which leads to diabetes mellitus. It also secretes a number of other hormones, the most important of which is gastrin. The external secretion is made up of the ferments trypsin, lipase and amylase. These break down the three main constituents of the diet: protein, fat and carbohydrate. These digestive ferments are secreted into the main duct of the gland, which opens into the duodenum at the ampulla of Vater, into which the common bile duct also drains.

Fibrocystic disease

This is a condition of the pancreas in which the gland does not develop properly and, therefore, the normal digestive ferments do not pass into the gut. As a result a newborn baby presents with intestinal obstruction due to plugging of the lumen of the bowel with meconium (the contents of the intestine which are present during foetal life and at birth). This condition necessitates immediate operation, when emptying of the bowel and an ileostomy or resection and anastomosis are performed, subsequently Pancreatin is given by mouth to make good the deficiency. The lungs are also usually affected because the secretions of their mucous glands are not fluid enough. The child, being unable to bring up the sputum, develops bronchitis and bronchiectasis.

Pancreatitis

Acute pancreatitis is a disease which usually affects obese patients after middle age who may previously have had symptoms due to gall-stones. The precise cause of the condition is not known, but the patient has sudden severe abdominal pain, vomits and suffers from shock. The appearance of a patient with slightly bluish lips, pale sweating face and grunting respiration is very striking and may be mistaken for that of coronary thrombosis. The release of pancreatic ferments into the peritoneal cavity causes widespread fat necrosis and there may be a blood-stained peritoneal effusion.

The laboratory estimation of serum amylase, which is greatly raised in this condition, is diagnostic.

When the diagnosis of acute pancreatitis is made no operation is performed. Shock is treated and intravenous therapy started. The stomach contents are aspirated and nothing allowed by mouth until the acute signs have passed off. When gall-stones are implicated, removal of the gall bladder and exploration of the common bile duct are done at a later date.

Chronic pancreatitis, an uncommon disease in Great Britain, causes recurrent attacks of central abdominal pain with vomiting. X-rays may show patches of calcification in the pancreas. This condition is often related to chronic alcoholism, but the connection between the two is not well understood. Treatment consists of various palliative measures aimed at improving pancreatic drainage into the bowel. Division of the sphincter at the ampulla of Vater, sphincterotomy, is one of these measures; anastomosis of the duct in the tail of the pancreas with the small bowel is another. Division of the sympathetic nerves into this area, i.e. splanchnicectomy, may relieve the pain.

The pancreas is occasionally affected in mumps, when it may swell up and cause central abdominal pain. Rarely the pancreas is injured, as for example by the tailboard of a vehicle which in backing strikes the central abdomen. The usual complications of haemorrhage, inflammation and accompanying shock occur, but most important is the development of a cyst of the pancreas due to digestion of the surrounding tissues by escaping pancreatic enzymes. The condition, which is called a pseudopancreatic cyst, requires surgical drainage into the gut, i.e. an internal fistula is created.

Carcinoma of the pancreas

Malignant disease of the pancreas is not uncommon and usually arises in the head of the organ. It obstructs the common bile duct and the patient develops painless jaundice. This is usually the first sign of the disease. The patient is prepared for operation and given vitamin K because of the biliary obstruction. The operation carried out will depend on the extent of the tumour. If the tumour is small and mobile then an operation called pancreaticoduodenectomy is performed (Figs. 17.5, 17.6). In this operation the stomach is divided at the pyloric entrance and the pylorus and the whole of the duodenum round to the jejunum is excised, together with the head and body of the pancreas and the lower part of the common bile duct. Continuity is restored by anastomosing the common bile duct, the stomach and the main pancreatic duct in the stump of the pancreas into a loop of upper jejunum.

The operation is not well tolerated by an ill and jaundiced patient and there are many complications which may arise.

If the disease has progressed further and it appears to the surgeon that the pancreas cannot be excised, a short-circuit operation is performed. The gall bladder is anastomosed to a loop of small bowel so that the obstruction to the flow of bile is relieved. As a result the

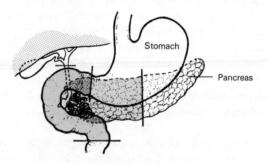

Fig. 17.5 Pancreatico-duodenectomy, shaded area is excised.

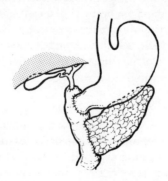

Fig. 17.6 Pancreatico-duodenectomy, completion of operation.

jaundice slowly disappears and the patient therefore feels much more comfortable although the tumour is left behind and death occurs in a few months.

Insulinoma

An adenoma of the pancreas may arise from the islet cells which manufacture insulin. When this occurs the patient has attacks during which the blood sugar level falls precipitously and this produces a syndrome resembling an epileptic fit. Some patients discover that eating sweet things relieves the symptoms or prevents an attack and they become very obese. The mental changes caused by the hypoglycaemia may lead to the patient's admission to a mental hospital. The treatment is the removal of the adenoma. A gastrinoma is a tumour of the G cells which causes hypersecretion by the stomach and a severe form of duodenal ulcer, the so-called Zollinger-Ellison syndrome, often treated by Cimetidine and if necessary, total gastrectomy.

Spleen

The spleen lies between the left leaf of the diaphragm, the stomach and the left lower ribs. Its artery is particularly large and it is a very vascular organ. Its functions, which are probably multiple, are not entirely known, but it has two which are of importance. It has a sponge-like structure in the meshes of which much blood is held and when a patient suffers from shock, the spleen contracts and empties this blood into the circulation. The spleen also has numbers of cells of the reticulo-endothelial system, which are found distributed through many parts of the body. These cells destroy waste matter and also manufacture some of the immune bodies which are so important to the health of the patient. As a result splenectomy in a young patient reduces the resistance to infection and long-term prophylaxis with antibiotics is necessary.

Rupture

The spleen may be ruptured by violent injury such as may occur at rugby football. More often it is already diseased when it is ruptured, and the commonest condition causing it to enlarge and become more friable is malaria. Occasionally when the spleen is injured the haemorrhage does not take place for some days afterwards because the capsule retains the clot.

Treatment of a ruptured spleen is immediate transfusion followed by an emergency operation to remove the damaged organ: splenectomy. The complications which follow splenectomy are mainly due to irritation of the left side of the diaphragm. This leads to difficulty in breathing and poor expansion of the left lower lobe of the lung.

Acholuric jaundice

In acholuric jaundice or spherocytosis, the patient has abnormally fragile red cells and therefore the spleen, which destroys red cells, becomes much enlarged. The patient is anaemic, suffers mild attacks of jaundice and may develop gall-stones due to the destruction of the red cells in the liver and the increased excretion of bile pigment. The treatment of acholuric jaundice is splenectomy since this cures all the symptoms. Often a whole family is affected and each member required to undergo splenectomy.

Thrombocytopenic purpura

This is a condition in which the spleen destroys platelets (thrombocytes), which are one of the essentials for the clotting of blood. As a result the patient has spontaneous haemorrhages, or bleeds following trivial injury. The condition may be improved by splenectomy. The operation has often to be performed while the patient is taking prednisone to control the thrombocytopenia; the anaesthetist has to be forewarned of this. In the postoperative period the patient may (very rarely) develop thromboses, which can be guarded against by early mobilization or giving heparin.

Splenectomy is an operation often followed by chest complications and in addition wound-healing may be affected. Sometimes the tail of the pancreas is injured and the liberated trypsin digests the sutures and leads to bursting of the abdominal wound. Irritation of the left dome of the diaphragm may cause intractable hiccough.

18
Genito-urinary System

In the foetus, the development of the urinary system, which consists of the kidneys, ureters, bladder and urethra, is so intimately connected with the development of the genital organs that disease processes affecting the one system often affect the other (Fig. 18.1). In the male this is especially the case, but in the female the study of diseases of the generative organs has become a specialty under the name of gynaecology and will therefore be found described in an accompanying book to this (entitled *Obstetrics and Gynaecology*).

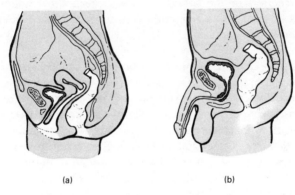

(a)   (b)

Fig. 18.1 Diagrammatic section through the female (a) and the male (b) pelvis. In the female, note the vagina and uterus lie posterior to the urethra and bladder. In the male, the rectum lies posterior to the bladder and prostate.

It is convenient to describe the particular symptoms, signs and special tests which apply to the genito-urinary system before going on to discuss each organ separately.

Pain. Pain may be felt by the patient in the region of the kidney, ureter, bladder or urethra. In the kidney it may be of two kinds, if there is some obstructing lesion, such as a stone or blood clot, the contractions of the renal pelvis to expel the obstructing agent produce intense *colic*. Such a pain is also produced when a stone or similar object tries to pass down the ureter. The pain is so severe that the patient often suffers from shock and becomes pale, sweats, has a raised pulse rate and is greatly distressed.

Another kind of pain, which is due to a non–obstructive lesion, can occur in the kidney. This is a dull ache constantly present on one side, and felt most severely over the loin.

Frequency. When a patient has to pass urine more often than usual, it is referred to as 'frequency'. A simple method of recording how often this takes place is to write down the number of times by day over the number of times by night with the initials D over N beside them, thus D/N = 5/0. A usual figure would be five over zero, but there are wide variations in the normal depending on the amount of fluid consumed and also the amount lost by other routes; for example in the tropics, with excessive sweating, there will be much less urine excreted. Frequency is caused by the presence of some irritant in the urine such as infection or blood. It may also be caused by obstruction to the passage of urine from the bladder, as in prostatic disease, or to reduction in the size of the bladder, as in tuberculous disease.

Haematuria. This is the presence of blood in the urine and is a sign of disease or injury to the genito–urinary tract. When urine is passed which is believed to contain blood, it is most important that it be saved and each specimen should be kept in a separate glass so that the progress of the haematuria can be seen. Injury to the upper part of the genito–urinary tract will lead to much more intimate mixing of blood and urine, which will be the same throughout the entire specimen. If the blood clots, its passage will cause colicky pain and, in the bladder, may obstruct the outflow at the urethra and so cause retention of urine. Small amounts of blood in the urine impart to it a smoky appearance, but it is necessary that the presence of blood be confirmed by chemical or other tests. This is especially so as urates, which are a normal constituent of urine, occasionally take on a pinkish or reddish colour and are mistaken by the patient for blood. Eating beetroot is also a cause of reddish urine in some patients.

Retention. When a patient cannot pass urine it is referred to as 'retention' and its treatment is a matter of urgency. Obstruction in men is most commonly found in the urethra or bladder neck and can be due to stricture, enlargement of the prostrate, a new growth, stone or blood clot. When the patient cannot pass water there is pain above the pubis as the condition progresses. If allowed to remain unrelieved, the back pressure on the kidneys causes secondary changes. In addition, the inability of the kidneys to get rid of those substances which they normally excrete, especially urea, leads to an increase in the blood level of these compounds which is eventually fatal. When there has been gradual obstruction to the outflow of urine over a long period of time, the changes in the kidneys may pass unnoticed until suddenly acute retention occurs. The patient is then much less fit to stand this additional trouble. This is particularly so in a patient who suffers from prostatic hypertrophy.

The *clinical examination* of a patient with genito-urinary disease is not complete until rectal examination has been carried out. By this means the finger palpates the area at the base of the bladder and part of the urethra; it is especially valuable in the male, where the prostate can be readily felt. Rectal examination can be carried out in the left lateral position with the knees brought up to the chin, or the patient may be asked to kneel on the couch with the shoulders well down, a position usually referred to as genupectoral or knee—elbow.

Special tests

The urine. Examination of the urine is of the greatest importance in diseases which involve the genito-urinary tract and not only are routine tests carried out in the ward and outpatient department, but further specimens should be sent to the laboratory.

The colour of the urine gives some indication of its concentration. The presence of gross infection imparts to the urine a hazy appearance and often a fishy smell due to the breakdown of urea to ammonia. The specific gravity also indicates the concentration and thus the capacity of the kidneys to concentrate urine. For this reason the specific gravity is measured with a hydrometer. The reaction is determined either by using litmus paper, which goes pink in acid and blue in alkaline urine, or by using indicators which give a much more precise indication of the pH. Normal urine is usually slightly acid, but the presence of infection may render it strongly alkaline or less often, strongly acid according to which variety of organism is present. If a specimen is required for culture to show what micro-organisms it contains, it must be obtained under sterile conditions or it will be contaminated with those bacteria normally found about the skin and urethral meatus. For this reason the specimen is obtained in midstream or rarely with a catheter and collected in a sterile bottle.

The blood. As a result of genito-urinary disease many substances in the bloodstream will be found to be altered in amount. The most important is the level of urea, which normally lies below 6.5 mmol/l in health. The body's method of getting rid of nitrogen consists of converting ammonia into urea, which is readily soluble and passes out in the urine. With most diseases of the kidneys, or obstruction to the outflow of urine, the level of blood urea rises.

Cystoscopy. A cystoscope consists of a hollow metal tube fitted with an internal telescope and an electric light which enables the bladder interior to be seen. It can be passed after local analgesia has rendered the urethra insensitive, although most urologists prefer the patient to have a general anaesthetic for this investigation. To facilitate examination of the bladder with a cystoscope, distension of the bladder with clear fluid is necessary. A quantity of fluid, usually 0.9 per cent sodium chloride is introduced through an irrigating system which is specially designed for attachment to the cystoscope. The sodium chloride used is available in either 1 or 3 litre bags and commercially produced for irrigation purposes only. It is not to be confused with intravenous preparations of sodium chloride. About 240 ml (8 oz) of solution are left in the bladder and then its interior is inspected with the cystoscope. This allows an examination of the mucosa, the openings of the two ureters and any abnormalities such as diverticula or stones which may be present. Very fine catheters (ureteric catheters) may be passed up the cystoscope and introduced into the ureter on each side. By means of these catheters, specimens of urine can be obtained from each individual kidney and this is of importance if infection is only present on the one side. If it appears that one kidney is not secreting urine, an injection of indigo-carmine is made into a vein. This substance is very quickly secreted in the urine and the bluish spurts which appear from the ureteric orifice show if secretion is taking place normally.

Urography. There are substances which can be injected intra-venously and when excreted by the kidneys can be demonstrated by X-rays. This method, called excretory urography or IVU for short, is useful in showing the function of the urinary tract and in mapping out its pattern. The patient has a laxative two nights before the investigation and as far as possible is encouraged to walk about, especially on the day of the examination, so that too much gas does not accumulate in the bowel. In order that the dye shall be well concentrated, he is told not to take any fluids by mouth for 6 hours before being X-rayed. The patient empties his bladder and is then given an intravenous injection of diodone. An intramuscular form is available for babies, which is excreted more slowly. Radiographs are then taken after 3, 5 and 15 minutes have elapsed and, if excretion is slow, after half an hour. The patient is instructed to empty his bladder and a further X-ray picture is taken to demonstrate that organ. The resulting pictures should show the outline of the calyces and pelvises of the kidneys, the ureters and bladder.

Radio-opaque fluid is injected under certain conditions into the ureter and renal pelvis before X-raying the patient, a method described as *retrograde urography*. In order to demonstrate ureter and pelvis a ureteric catheter has first to be passed by means of a cystoscope. Much clearer X-ray pictures are obtained by this technique than by the intravenous method, but they give no indication of the capacity of the kidney to concentrate.

Ultrasonography. Ultrasound offers an excellent way for diagnosing calculi in the kidney or lower renal tract because the patient does not have to take radio-opaque material by mouth or injection. It is ideal for outlining cysts in the kidneys.

The kidneys

Trauma

The kidneys are sometimes injured by direct trauma, especially in road and air accidents. A tear in a kidney leads to bleeding into the renal pelvis and haematuria. When this occurs each specimen of urine that is passed must be saved so that a careful watch can be kept as to whether the bleeding is increasing or diminishing. There may be severe pain from the passage of clots down the ureter and this requires relief by an injection of pethidine or morphine, which may be given with atropine. The latter relieves spasm.

Treatment. When the bleeding continues, blood is cross-matched in readiness for a transfusion and an IVU performed to show the injured kidney and also the function of the kidney on the opposite side. The usual treatment for a ruptured kidney if the bleeding continues is nephrectomy so long as a healthy organ exists on the other side.

Postoperative nursing care. On regaining consciousness the patient is supported with pillows in the most comfortable position, usually leaning towards the affected side. This position allows any fluid to escape through the drainage tube and the dressings are renewed as required. The tube is turned and shortened according to the surgeon's instructions and removed when the discharge ceases, usually on about the third or fourth day, but in some cases it may be required for longer. The nurse should note the amount of urine passed and report any abnormality without delay so that the surgeon may gauge the function of the remaining kidney.

Care of the mouth is particularly important and frequent mouthwashes should be given. The drinking of fluids should be encouraged and nourishment gradually increased until the patient is taking a full diet.

Infection

We are concerned here not with nephritis, about which information should be sought in a textbook of medicine, but with pyogenic infections occurring within, or just outside, the kidney proper.

Pyelitis. This is the term used to describe inflammation of the renal pelvis. It occurs commonly with infections which ascend the urinary tract and is associated with organisms and pus in the urine. The patient has pain in the loin, a high swinging temperature, is toxic and ill. The commonest organism causing this condition is *Escherichia coli* and this often leads to cystitis, i.e. infection in the bladder with its attendant frequency of micturition and scalding pain. If the infection is very acute, rigors will accompany the rise in temperature. Treatment consists of rest in bed, copious fluids by mouth and the administration of a suitable sulphonamide, which should be a soluble one. Septrin or Bactrim (Cotrimoxazole) 400 mg twice daily for adults is suitable.

When the acute infection has subsided, a search is made to find if any abnormality is present which might have predisposed to the infection. The commonest causes are hydronephrosis, calculus or some congenital abnormality such as a double kidney, or double ureter. When such an abnormality is found it is corrected; otherwise recurrence of the pyelitis is likely and the outcome of recurrent infection in the kidney is the final destruction of that organ.

Pyonephrosis. When the outflow of urine from a kidney is partially obstructed, the renal pelvis dilates and forms a hydronephrosis. If a hydronephrosis becomes infected, the condition is called a pyonephrosis. It is accompanied by severe damage to the kidney and nephrectomy is almost always necessary.

Tuberculosis. *Mycobacterium tuberculosis* is carried to the kidney by the bloodstream and therefore such an infection is secondary to a primary focus in some other part of the body, frequently the lungs. The presence of tuberculous infection in the renal tract is accompanied by frequency of micturition, the urine being acid in reaction and containing what appears to be sterile pus, since it grows no organisms by the usual cultural methods.

A specimen of urine examined under the microscope does not often reveal the presence of *Mycobacterium tuberculosis*; there is, however, a more reliable test by guinea pig inoculation. For this, urine from a 24-hourly collection or from three early morning specimens is centrifuged in the laboratory and the sediment injected into a guinea pig. The animal is examined in 6 weeks' time for infection.

Tuberculous infection in the kidneys destroys the renal substance and this can be detected in its early stages by an intravenous urogram (IVU) which shows deformation of one of the calyces of the pelvis. As times passes, if the infection is left untreated, more and more of the kidney will be destroyed. Fibrosis will take place and may be accompanied by calcification of the caseous material which fills the destroyed shell of kidney. Tuberculosis of the kidney and renal tract is a serious disease if it is not recognized promptly and treated thoroughly. When both kidneys are affected the prognosis is not so good.

Treatment. Treatment of tuberculosis of the renal tract has been revolutionized by the introduction of streptomycin, isoniazid (INAH) and para-amino-salicylic acid (PAS). A combination of these drugs given for a period such as 6 months preferably, combined with rest in bed under suitable supervision for the ill patient, encourages most of these lesions to heal. After 6 months, when the urine is free of tubercle bacilli the streptomycin is discontinued but PAS and INAH are usually continued for a further 18 months. Rifampicin by mouth may replace the injections of streptomycin but is expensive.

When much of one kidney is already destroyed while the opposite one is apparently healthy, it is usual to combine the course of chemotherapy with removal of the diseased kidney. It must be remembered, however, that the ultimate prognosis of a patient with only one kidney is considerably less good than that of a normal individual.

Hydronephrosis

Distension of the renal pelvis is due to slow obstruction, either continuously or intermittently applied, to the outflow of urine from the kidney. If the outflow from one kidney is suddenly blocked, hydronephrosis does not result, but the kidney swells, there is aching pain in the loin and within a few weeks the kidney is destroyed. Partial obstruction to the outflow of urine leads to dilatation of the renal pelvis and the calyces. If obstruction to the outflow of urine is in the bladder or urethra, the hydronephrosis will occur on both sides and will be accompanied by the dilatation of the ureters, called hydro-ureters.

Hydronephrosis can cause a dull aching pain in the loin which may be not at all severe. As the kidney gradually enlarges it will produce a palpable swelling in the loin and may cause a dragging sensation. Accompanying this enlargement will be a slow diminution in kidney function as the tissue of the organ is destroyed.

Intravenous urography may show the distended renal pelvis in the early stages of this condition, but where much of the kidney is destroyed not enough of the dye will be concentrated to demonstrate the abnormality. Under these circumstances cystoscopy and retrograde urography may be successful in forcing dye up through the obstruction into the renal pelvis and outlining the distended organ. Ultrasound will also demonstrate the lesion. The causes of hydronephrosis are many. Congenital lesions, such as narrowing at the junction between renal pelvis and ureter or at the lower end of the ureters, are common. A stone may, by partial obstruction, lead to this condition. Occasionally an abnormal renal artery passes across from the aorta and kinks the ureter so that it cannot empty properly. In many cases no cause is found. Where some obvious abnormality can be detected, the treatment is to correct this surgically, as for example a plastic operation to enlarge the opening between the renal pelvis and the ureter. If this operation is performed in a child it can be very satisfactory. Where no obvious cause is found and the kidney is largely destroyed, the treatment is nephrectomy, so long as the other kidney is healthy.

Calculus or stone

Renal calculi are produced by the deposition of crystals within the kidney tubules; these crystals migrate into the pelvis where they may grow in size and some pass down the ureter into the bladder. They are of three kinds: *phosphates*, *oxalates* and *urates*. Phosphatic stones, which are produced primarily as a result of infection in the urine are soft, friable, greyish-white stones which can grow to a very large size and fill the renal pelvis and calyces, giving the appearance of a stag's antlers; hence the term stag-horn calculus. Oxalate stones are sharp and cause bleeding so that they are dark in colour from the blood pigment which is deposited on their surface and it is with difficulty that they pass down the urinary tract. Stones formed of urates are smooth and dark in colour and can pass into the bladder, where the deposition of further salts increases their size.

Renal colic is the extremely acute pain accompanying the passage of a stone or blood clot down the ureter. The onset of pain is often sudden and it radiates down to the groin and sometimes the scrotum or thigh. The patient rolls about in agony, suffers from shock and may vomit, the pulse is rapid and of poor volume and the patient sweats. If the stone causes trauma to the urinary tract, blood is passed in the urine and the painful passage of blood-stained urine is referred to as *strangury*. The treatment of renal colic is the hypodermic injection of pethidine or morphine with atropine. Heat in the form of a hot-water bottle or a fomentation applied to the loin is of help, or the patient may lie in a hot bath. He should also be warned to look for the passage of a stone which, if small, may be voided in the urine.

Renal calculus is diagnosed by a plain X-ray picture of the abdomen or IVU. When there are no signs of onward movement of the stone for weeks or months and when there are signs of damage to the urinary tract by the obstruction, a decision is made to operate. The stone is removed by incising the kidney, ureter or bladder as the case may be. Sometimes part of the kidney is removed, *partial nephrectomy*, or it may be necessary to remove the whole kidney, especially in the case of a stag-horn calculus. Alternatively the kidney is cooled, the blood supply temporarily occluded by clamping the renal artery and the stone or stones entirely removed.

The treatment before and after operation is similar to that of a patient who has had nephrectomy. Some surgeons prefer patients who have had part of the kidney removed to rest in bed until the tenth or fourteenth day, in order to permit sound healing of the tissues and so prevent herniation.

Stones occur more often in people living in tropical countries where so much more fluid is lost by the body through perspiration. In certain parts of the world, stone formation is common, as in Thailand. It appears that the diet is also of importance; in Elizabethan times the incidence of urinary stones was high in England, whereas today it is relatively low. Patients who have had renal stones should always be advised to drink large quantities of fluid in order that their urine does not become concentrated.

Neoplasms

New growths of the kidney occur typically before the age of four and after the age of forty. In infants the commonest is a *Wilms' Tumour* or sarcoma of the kidney. It produces very little pain, but a large mass in the loin, which the mother may discover when bathing the child, and occasionally haematuria. The tumour is often fast growing but early diagnosis, removal combined with radiotherapy and actinomycin D can result in cure.

In adults over the age of forty the type of tumour which is most likely to occur is a *hypernephroma*, which produces a large golden coloured mass, usually in the lower pole of the kidney. The early signs and symptoms are haematuria, pain and a swelling in the loin.

The patient also may feel unwell and suffer from anorexia, a fairly common symptom in malignant disease. The diagnosis is made by intravenous or retrograde urography, and the treatment is nephrectomy. Tumours which are too large to be removed through the loin may be approached through the abdominal cavity via an anterior incision, or through a combined thoraco-abdominal incision.

In infants, renal tumours are usually approached via the peritoneal cavity at laparotomy; in adults the lumbar or thoraco-abdominal route is most commonly employed. Radiotherapy is ordered to follow the operation in order to destroy any malignant cells which have been left behind. A hypernephroma metastasizes by the bloodstream and the first sign that the patient is suffering from the condition may be the occurrence of a secondary deposit in a distant organ, usually in a bone or the lungs. The metastasis may be a solitary one and if so is removed when feasible by excising bone or a segment of lung, in addition to excision of the kidney and primary tumour.

Ureter

The ureter carries the urine from the renal pelvis to the bladder by active peristaltic movements. Its normal length is between 30 and 40 cm in the adult and the diameter is approximately 0.5 cm or a little less than a quarter of an inch. Very few diseases affect the ureter primarily, but it is often involved secondarily by conditions affecting the kidney and bladder.

Infection

Infection in the renal pelvis in the form of pyelitis usually passes down to involve the ureter by direct extension. Likewise, infection from cystitis may pass up the ureter to involve the kidney.

In tuberculous infection of the kidney it is common for the organism to appear also in the bladder and the epididymis. It is not certain if this infection spreads by the urine or whether it passes along the lymphatics which form a rich network in the wall of the ureter.

Hydro-ureter

Dilatation of the ureter may be unilateral or bilateral. In order for this condition to arise, there must be an incomplete obstruction to the outflow of urine from the lower end of the ureter or from the bladder. As the ureter becomes enlarged, not only does its lumen increase, but it also becomes tortuous. In male babies born with a congenital valve in the posterior urethra, the ureters may be enormously distended and even when adequately drained do not return to their proper size.

Calculus

A stone formed in the kidney or renal pelvis may pass down the ureter and produce attacks of renal colic. The likely sites for the stone to be arrested are at the junction between the pelvis and ureter, about two-thirds way down its length, and at its lower end where it passes obliquely through the bladder wall. The latter part of its course is referred to as the intramural part of the ureter. Most calculi eventually pass through the ureter and enter the bladder. If they are held up in their passage down the ureter, cystoscopy is carried out and a ureteric catheter is passed to try and dislodge the stone and thus help it pass on into the bladder, or a ureteric basket is coaxed past it and an attempt made to withdraw the stone in it. On those rare occasions when the calculus does not pass, the ureter is approached via an abdominal incision, which allows the peritoneum to be pushed unopened to one side. A further incision is made into the ureter a little above the stone, which is then milked out through the opening. In all such operations a drainage tube is passed down near the opening in the ureter. This may leak urine for a few days before the wound finally closes.

Congenital lesions

The commonest congenital lesion is a narrowing of the lower or intramural (i.e. in the bladder wall) part of the ureter. This leads to hydronephrosis and hydro-ureter and is treated by the transplantation of the ureter into a new and larger opening which is made in the bladder wall. The ureter may also be narrowed at its uppermost point and then hydronephrosis results. This requires a plastic operation to reunite the ureter through an adequate aperture with the renal pelvis.

Transplantation of the ureters

When the bladder is so involved by malignant disease that it must be removed, or when it is so fibrosed due to old infection that its volume is minute, it is necessary to divert the urinary stream. This is also necessary when a baby is born with an improperly developed bladder, the base of the organ opening on to the abdominal wall (extroversion of the bladder called ectopia vesicae).

In such conditions the ureters used to be transplanted by detaching them from the bladder and reinserting them obliquely through the muscle coats of the sigmoid colon. By this technique the urine was diverted into the large bowel and the patient learned to retain it and pass it at intervals. The main danger of the operation was that infection could spread back from the bowel up the ureter and eventually destroy the kidney.

The present day variation of this operation is to implant the two ureters into an isolated segment of ileum which is anastomosed to the abdominal wall and the patient then wears a small rubber ileostomy bag to collect the urine. By this means the risk of ascending infection from the bowel is eliminated and many of the problems of fluid and electrolyte imbalance, which resulted from absorption in the large bowel, are prevented.

Postoperative nursing care. When consciousness is regained the patient is nursed in the sitting position in order to encourage drainage of urine. Copious fluids should be drunk and everything passing in and out of the patient must be carefully documented on the fluid balance chart.

Bladder

The bladder has strong muscular coats, is covered over most of its outer surface by peritoneum and is lined internally with mucous membrane. The two ureters enter near its base and the internal urethral opening lies anterior to this. The three openings form a triangle with the apex pointing forward; this area, known as the *trigone*, is always studied carefully at cystoscopy. In an infant the bladder is situated above the symphysis pubis, but in an adult it is a pelvic organ.

Trauma

A sudden blow over the lower abdomen, especially when the bladder is full, may lead to a ruptured bladder. If the tear occurs through the peritoneal surface, the urine will enter the peritoneal cavity and lead to great pain, shock and a rigid abdominal wall. If the tear involves the surface not covered by peritoneum, the urine will be extravasated into the lower abdominal wall and down towards the thighs, where it will cause a red, brawny, tender mass. Treatment in either case is immediate surgical operation to close the tear and drain the bladder, the drainage being continued until the tear has soundly healed. If urine has entered the fascial planes of the abdominal wall it is let out by multiple incisions.

Inflammation

Infection in the bladder is called *cystitis* and it may arise by organisms entering the urethra and spreading upwards, or by their descent from infection in the kidneys. Alternatively there may be direct extension of infection from a nearby pelvic organ such as the colon, the organisms gaining entry via lymphatics or by a fistula which may follow diverticulitis. The signs and symptoms of cystitis are pain, which is often of a scalding variety at the end of micturition, frequency and a rise of pulse rate and temperature which is accompanied in severe infection by rigors. In many urinary infections the urine has a distinctive fishy odour.

The treatment of cystitis, like that for pyelitis, is rest in bed with the administration of copious fluids by mouth. The infection is treated by one of the soluble sulphonamides, e.g. cotrimoxazole (Septrin) 400 mg bd. and should the infection return after such treatment, a very thorough investigation of the urinary tract is carried out, since this is an indication that some abnormality is present. Tuberculous cystitis has already been mentioned; it leads typically to frequency and the passage of 'sterile pus in an acid urine'. In the late stages of the disease the bladder wall is replaced by fibrosis and its volume greatly decreased so that the patient has to pass urine every few minutes. The condition is also painful and a surgical operation may be called for to increase the volume of the bladder, for example by using an isolated loop of the ileum.

Occasionally infections do not respond to the sulphonamides and then other antibiotics are used: ampicillin, nitrofurantoin, nalidixic acid and oxytetracycline, or whichever antibiotic to which the organisms are sensitive.

Retention

When the patient is unable to empty the bladder the condition is called retention of urine and the signs of this were described earlier in the chapter. It now remains to discuss the causes and treatment of this condition.

The commonest cause of retention is obstruction to the flow of urine at the bladder neck, such as is produced by an enlarged prostate, a stone, or a retroverted gravid uterus. The internal urethral sphincter, which guards the passage of urine from the bladder, may be paralysed, as in injuries to the spinal cord. Such patients usually have a very distended bladder which empties itself by the urine dribbling away after the internal pressure has risen high enough. The condition is referred to as *overflow incontinence*. Many patients find themselves unable to micturate after an operation and this may be due to the unfamiliar position in which they have to perform the act, or to fear or postoperative pain. It should be remembered that some men are unable to void urine when others are present, owing to nervousness.

Treatment. The treatment of acute retention is always first to persuade the patient to try and pass water naturally. This may be encouraged in many ways; the most likely to succeed is sitting in a hot bath, or if the patient is being nursed in bed, allowing the legs to dangle over the side. It may help if the patient is permitted to stand up. In addition plenty of fluids should be drunk and a tap turned on so that the patient hears the sound of running water can help. Giving a simple enema sometimes relieves the condition. Certain drugs have the power of stimulating the bladder to contract, the most useful being carbachol, which is given by subcutaneous injection (1.0 ml ampoule containing 0.25 mg of the drug); however, it must only be used under close supervision since it may damage the bladder.

When all these methods fail, catheterization is carried out, but only on the instructions of the surgeon, because of the risk of introducing infection however carefully done. In some males it can be a most difficult manoeuvre. The type of catheter which is passed depends on the kind of obstruction. Catheters are made of plastic, latex, gum-elastic or, rarely, silver. Plastic and latex catheters are those in most constant use because their softness prevents them from causing injury to the delicate mucosa of the urethra and they are not as irritant as rubber. Gum-elastic catheters are stiff and may therefore pass difficult obstructions. Finally, silver catheters are only passed by a surgeon when other methods have failed. The most useful catheter for relieving retention in the male is Tieman's. Where an enlarged prostate has to be negotiated, the tip of a catheter may be given a bend (coudé) or two bends (bicoudé). In women, and especially when a self-retaining catheter is required, Foley's is used. This has a small rubber balloon near the tip which on inflation with water (or a dye, e.g. methylene blue, which colours the urine if the balloon should leak and become deflated) prevents the catheter from slipping out. A glance at Fig. 18.2 will most quickly describe the various types of catheter which may be used.

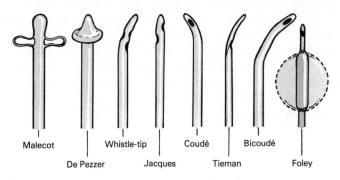

Malecot	Whistle-tip	Coudé	Bicoudé
De Pezzer	Jacques	Tieman	Foley

Fig. 18.2 Types of catheter.

Catheterization. This treatment should be done with great care to prevent the introduction of infection. Catheter, lubricant and gauze must be sterile, and the procedure is carried out as for a surgical operation, using the 'no-touch' technique.

The bed is screened and the patient made comfortable with a blanket covering the chest and the abdomen; the bedclothes are turned back to the level of the mid-thigh. A female patient is asked to flex the knees and abduct the thighs. A bell-lamp or torch is arranged so that the light falls on the external genitalia.

The nurse washes her hands, dries them and returns to the patient's bedside. After arranging sterile dressing towels over the lower part of the abdomen and thighs, the patient's genitalia are thoroughly cleansed with a weak antiseptic solution, e.g. Cetrimide 1 per cent or chlorhexidine (Hibitane) solution, 1 in 5000, using cotton wool swabs held in forceps which are then discarded; a fresh pair of forceps is used to pick up the catheter and introduce it gently into the urethra. A sterile lubricant, e.g. K-Y jelly may be used to lessen trauma to the mucous membrane and make the introduction of the catheter easier.

The female urethra is 4 cm (1½ in) long and if the catheter (size 8 English gauge, 30 International Standard) is held about 5 cm (2 in) from the eye, there should be no danger of introducing infection.

The male urethra is 20 cm long (7 to 8 in), and therefore the catheter (size 10 English gauge, 37 International Standard) used for catheterizing men is usually stiffened so that the part entering the urethra may remain uncontaminated. For male catheterization (which is usually performed by the surgeon or a male nurse) it may be necessary to use a local analgesic, e.g. 0.1 per cent amethocaine. For this a urethral syringe with a rubber 'acorn' for introduction and penile clamp is also required.

The distal end of the catheter is placed in a sterile receiver and should not be allowed to come into contact with anything which has not been sterilized. This is also important when a self-retaining catheter is introduced. All spigots, connections, drainage tubes and drainage bottles should be sterilized and will require changing at frequent intervals, using the aseptic technique.

When the catheter is withdrawn, the genitalia should be cleaned with cotton wool swabs or the dressing towel may be used to wipe the patient dry.

When catheterization is not possible and it is essential to empty the bladder, this is done by *suprapubic cystotomy*. Under an anaesthetic the surgeon opens the lower abdomen with a short vertical incision about two fingerbreadths above the symphysis pubis and plunges a knife and tube into the bladder. Alternatively, the bladder may be drained with a fine trocar and cannula passed straight through the anterior abdominal wall using local analgesia. In either case there is no danger of entering the peritoneal cavity because distension of the bladder carries its peritoneal reflection high up the anterior abdominal wall. The surgeon may ask that the bladder be decompressed slowly and this is most conveniently arranged by incorporating a drip connector from a transfusion giving-set in the tube leading from the bladder. All urine must be saved and its volume carefully noted.

Some surgeons prefer to treat retention due to prostatic enlargement by immediate prostatectomy, not draining the bladder first. It is claimed that by this method infection is prevented from entering the urethra and the convalescence is smoother.

Calculus

A stone in the bladder causes pain which is often referred to the tip of the penis at the end of micturition. There may be slight haematuria, which is more likely towards the end of micturition, and frequency which is made worse by exercise. The diagnosis is confirmed by cystoscopy and an X-ray picture will show an opaque stone. Ultrasound is a simpler way of demonstrating a calculus.

The treatment of vesical calculus is by the closed or open method. The closed operation is called litholapaxy and is not so often employed today. The interior of the bladder is first inspected with a cystoscope and distended with sterile fluid. A lithotrite is introduced and the stone manipulated blindly between its jaws. It is then screwed up, crushing the stone, the fragments of which are then removed with a Bigelow's evacuator.

Open operation for bladder stone consists of opening the bladder suprapubically, lifting out the stone, or stones, and closing it again around a drainage tube which is left in place for a few days. A urethral catheter is left in place so that the bladder may be washed out according to the written instructions.

Diverticula

Blind out-pouchings of the bladder wall are called diverticula and occur most commonly in older men who suffer from back pressure in the bladder due to prostatic enlargement. Infection or calculus formation may take place within a diverticulum and cause symptoms which necessitate operation. The diverticulum is removed by a suprapubic approach, usually being pulled inside out into the bladder and the neck cut across and closed.

Neoplasms

There are two growths which occur in the bladder: innocent, called a *papilloma*, and malignant, a *carcinoma*.

A simple papilloma looks like a small sea anemone at cystoscopy. The first sign it produces is haematuria. If it is solitary, it can be coagulated by diathermy through a cystoscope and the patient is then examined at 6-monthly intervals in case of recurrence. If the papilloma produces seedlings which partially fill the bladder, a portion (partial cystectomy) or even the whole of the bladder will have to be excised, the latter operation being called *total cystectomy*. The first step before total cystectomy is to transplant the ureters into an isolated loop of ileum or directly into the colon.

Carcinoma of the bladder is a condition which may arise by a malignant change in a papilloma or as an ulcer which is malignant from the start. It requires wide excision or total cystectomy, alternatively it may be treated by the implantation of irradiated tantalum wire or gold seeds. Considerable success is now obtained by irradiating the bladder with a supervoltage machine as by this means a very high dosage of radiation can be directed at the tumour through various 'ports' of entry. In all such patients the first step in treatment is usually drainage of the bladder by a suprapubic cystotomy and if total cystectomy becomes necessary, transplantation of the ureters as described above. Carcinoma of the bladder is particularly common among workers in the dye industry.

Prostate

The prostate gland is situated at the neck of the bladder and encircles the urethra at this site. In men over the age of fifty, enlargement of the prostate may lead to a typical group of symptoms, which are: difficulty in passing water, frequency (since little urine is passed at any one time) haematuria and acute retention. When obstruction has been gradual and the symptoms it produces disregarded, the patient may present with the signs of uraemia: malaise, headache, drowsiness, a dry discoloured tongue and offensive breath.

Enlargement of the prostate is occasionally malignant and such a cancer can spread directly into the pelvic tissues, but is also liable to metastasize to the bones of the pelvis and spine. The latter may be recognized on an X-ray film as being denser than the normal bones.

Prostatectomy

This may be carried out in one or two stages according to the condition of the patient and the particular technique adopted by the surgeon.

Transurethral prostatectomy (TUR). This is employed for most patients and in particular for those in whom obstruction to the urethra is caused by a malignant prostate. It is the commonest way of relieving prostatic obstruction.

The perineal area is prepared with antiseptic solution and after inspecting the bladder with a cystoscope, a resectoscope is passed incorporating a wire loop which can be heated by a current from a diathermy machine and the prostate is scooped out using this instrument. When resection is complete, a self-retaining catheter is inserted and attached to a continuous irrigation system. Although a Foley catheter can be used some surgeons favour the Porges due to its more rigid structure.

Suprapubic prostatectomy. The skin of the abdomen is shaved and the patient prepared for operation. The bladder is opened from above and the prostate enucleated by blunt dissection, usually with the index finger. If the *retropubic operation* is employed the prostate is approached lower down and the bladder is not opened. However, in this operation the urethra is laid widely open and if there is any remaining obstruction at the bladder neck, this is cut away at the same time.

Postoperative treatment. The postoperative problem with pros-tatectomy is haemorrhage and, therefore, the bladder may be drained both suprapubically and by a catheter left in the urethra. In the latter case a Foley type of catheter may be used and the inflatable balloon fills up the cavity and exerts gentle pressure on the raw surface from which the prostate has been enucleated, so reducing haemorrhage.

Postoperative nursing care. These patients require meticulous attention to all drainage tubes and if blockage occurs it should be reported at once (Fig. 18.3). The urinary drainage should be inspected at frequent intervals so that the amount of bleeding may be assessed and instructions may be given for irrigation through the catheter at intervals. The use of the KCH (Kings College Hospital) urine drainage bottle is helpful as it enables the amount of bleeding to be observed at regular intervals. Should the haemorrhage increase, this should be reported to the surgeon immediately as it may be decided to return the patient to the operating theatre.

The mouth should be carefully and frequently attended to. Many of these patients are elderly and so it is necessary to give particular attention to the pressure areas. Having undergone a major operation these older patients are occasionally liable to become disorientated especially at night time and the nurse should be on the look-out for

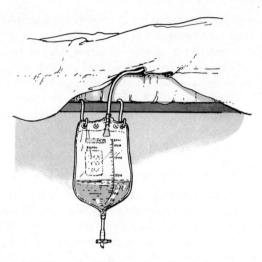

Fig. 18.3 Drainage bag hanging on bed rail.

this. Switching on the light and keeping it on throughout the night is often of the greatest help. Ideally a well-known relative or friend should be allowed to sit at the bedside. The patient is encouraged to drink copious fluids and the diet is gradually increased.

The fluid balance of these patients is most important and a record is kept of intake and output. Continuous intravenous glucose and saline are usually administered during the first 48 hours after operation. Since most of these patients are over seventy years of age and prone to postoperative complications such as pneumonia and thrombosis of the leg veins, they are encouraged to move about freely from the start and if possible are sat out in a chair on the first day after operation.

Malignant disease of the prostate

This causes the same signs and symptoms as benign prostatic enlargement, but the disease spreads to involve the base of the bladder and the adjoining pelvic tissues and also metastasizes to the bones. The metastases are dense and sclerotic and easily recognized by X-rays, the serum acid phosphatase is usually raised above the normal level of 170 nmol/l (3 King–Armstrong units). Treatment is palliative and consists of reducing the level of androgens in the blood by removing the testes and giving oestrogens by mouth.

Orchidectomy is first carried out. The skin of the scrotum and perineum having been prepared, the testicles are enucleated from within their capsules (*subcapsular orchidectomy*). In addition, the patient is given stilboestrol or ethinyloestradiol in tablet form by mouth. The patient is warned that the tablets will produce pigmentation of the nipples and development of breast tissue, i.e. gynaecomastia.

Urethra and penis

Trauma

The urethra in the female is short and therefore not usually injured, but in the male it may be damaged by direct injury from falling astride, or as a complication of a fractured pelvis. When the urethra is ruptured the patient is unable to pass water and blood appears at the urethral meatus. The treatment is immediate drainage of the bladder by suprapubic cystotomy and the urethra is explored so that the tear can be repaired surgically.

Inflammation

Acute urethritis is often due to gonorrhoea, but there are also other infections which may involve the urethra. The first symptom is intense pain, especially on micturition, and pus is discharged from the urethra. Treatment is by penicillin injections followed by careful supervision to ensure that if a relapse occurs treatment is carried out. A rare complication when antibiotic treatment has not been adequate is the development of a stricture requiring dilatation with bougies at regular intervals. Other forms of urethritis occur, the commonest being that produced by the irritation of an indwelling catheter.

Stricture

Strictures of the male urethra are much less common than formerly. This is because gonorrhoea is now readily treated by means of penicillin and therefore chronic forms of the disease which led to stricture are rarely encountered. Strictures of the urethra have to be dilated at regular intervals. They may be suitable for treatment by excision and reconstruction of the urethra.

Phimosis and paraphimosis

The normal prepuce or foreskin is adherent to the glans at birth and does not become free and therefore capable of being drawn back for many months. In some religious communities, e.g. the Jews, it is usual to remove the foreskin by circumcision. This practice is often used by races living in hot climates. The prepuce forms a protective cover for the sensitive mucous membrane of the glans and urethral meatus, so that when a baby develops a napkin rash the area is spared from inflammation. If, however, the prepuce has been pulled back or removed, the glans becomes affected in the inflammation and this can lead to ulceration of the urethral meatus, scarring and even stenosis.

Phimosis. This means narrowing of the preputial opening and is exceedingly rare in the newborn baby. It occurs however in children and adults as a result of repeated inflammation or balanitis, or as a complication of repeated stretching of the prepuce with accompanying tears and haemorrhage.

The treatment of phimosis is by circumcision, an operation in which a cuff of skin and mucous membrane is excised and the raw edges united with fine catgut sutures (Fig. 18.4). It is important that all haemorrhage is checked as if it should occur at this site it may exsanguinate a baby very rapidly. A dressing of gauze soaked in tinct. benz. co. is applied and this is soaked off in a bath after 5 days, no further dressing being necessary as the absorbable catgut stitches fall out spontaneously. In the newborn no anaesthetic is required but a brief general anaesthetic is desirable in older babies. Up to the age of one year admission to hospital for the operation is not usually necessary, but in children and adults it is very desirable that they be admitted for a few days and are given adequate sedation after operation to control the pain and discomfort.

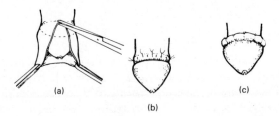

Fig. 18.4 The operation of circumcision. (c) shows the dressing tied in place using the sutures.

Paraphimosis. In this condition the tight prepuce is withdrawn behind the glans and cannot be returned to its normal position. It is accompanied by oedema of the glans and prepuce, the congestion leading to severe discomfort. It may be reduced by the application of ice compresses and gentle pressure. If this is not successful the constricting band must be divided on the dorsum by an operation referred to as a *dorsal slit*.

Hypospadias

This is a congenital abnormality due to lack of proper formation of the under surface of the penis. The penis is bowed downwards and the urethra opens at some point proximally on its undersurface. In addition the prepuce or foreskin is typically hooded. This lesion requires surgical correction which is carried out when the child is 4 years old. The operation is often performed in two stages, first to relieve the bowing and later to reconstruct the urethra.

Epispadias

A much rarer congenital deformity of the penis is one in which its upper surface is incompletely developed and the urethra opens part way along this aspect. In its most severe form epispadias is associated with incomplete development of the bladder, which opens directly on to the abdominal wall. The urine in this case leaks away continuously and there is maldevelopment of the bony pelvis anteriorly. Epispadias is a difficult condition to repair successfully, but some form of plastic operation is usually undertaken. When the bladder is extroverted it is usual to transplant the ureters into an isolated loop of ileum which opens on the abdominal wall and is fitted with an adhesive ring and a bag to collect the urine. The remnants of extroverted bladder are excised and the anterior abdominal wall reconstructed.

New growth

New growths of the urethra and penis are rare. In the female, a polypoid structure may develop from the urethra and present at the meatus. It is called a *urethral caruncle* and if it is discovered by a nurse when catheterizing a patient it should always be reported so that it may be treated by excision. In the male, *carcinoma of the penis* may occur and this requires surgical excision and radiotherapy to the affected lymph nodes in the groins.

Testis and epididymis

Undescended and ectopic testes

The testes develop during foetal life, high up on the posterior abdominal wall and descend via the inguinal canals to enter the scrotum before birth. The left one descends first and to a lower level than that on the right. Occasionally one or both testes fail to descend before birth and this condition of undescended testis is often accompanied by a hernia, which is commoner on the right side than on the left. When neither testis has descended, it sometimes happens that they both come down spontaneously at puberty, probably due to the increased secretion of male hormones. When one testis is undescended, operation is usually undertaken at about the age of eight and the testis brought down into the scrotum and secured there.

The testis may descend along a path other than the normal one and be arrested in an unusual or ectopic position, the commonest being just over the pubis. In this position the testis requires surgical correction because the organ has no chance of passing down into the scrotum by itself. This operation can be performed at any age. Undescended testes are more subject to malignant change than are normal ones.

Orchitis and epididymitis

These two names are given to inflammation of the testis and epididymis respectively.

Acute inflammation of the testis occurs as a result of infection by streptococci, staphylococci, *E. coli* or gonococci. It may also complicate an attack of mumps.

When inflammation goes on to suppuration, atrophy of the testis is the eventual outcome. The epididymis is involved in gonorrhoea, and after operations on the prostate it may become acutely inflamed due to spread of infection along the vas deferens.

Chronic infection of the testis and epididymis is usually due either to tuberculosis or syphilis.

Tuberculosis involves the epididymis first and is commonly associated with tuberculous infection in some other part of the urinary tract. The organ becomes swollen and the overlying skin oedematous, ulceration follows and results in a discharging sinus.

The treatment of inflammation of the testis and epididymis is rest in bed with support for the scrotum. Local application of a cooling lotion may relieve the pain. The infection is treated by antibiotics, i.e. penicillin for gonorrhoea, streptomycin, PAS, isoniazid and/or rifampicin for tuberculosis.

Hydrocele

This is the name given to a collection of fluid in the sac (tunica vaginalis) surrounding the testis and epididymis (Fig. 18.5). Little is known about the cause of this condition, which may arise at any age. The treatment is either by 'tapping' the sac with a trocar and cannula to drain off the fluid, which is often done in the outpatient department, or under an anaesthetic by surgical exploration and removal of the lining of the sac. If tapping is done, it usually has to be repeated at intervals. Hydrocele in the first years of life is due to peritoneal fluid draining into a patent processus vaginalis.

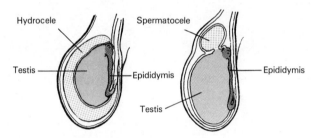

Fig. 18.5 Hydrocele (left) and spermatocele (right). The shaded area represents fluid; note its relationship to the testis and epididymis.

Varicocele

This name is given to a varicose dilatation of the veins in the spermatic cord which drain the testis. Treatment is rarely necessary, but when the patient complains of the condition a suspensory bandage often gives relief. Segments of veins may be excised.

Spermatocele

This is a cyst arising in the epididymis (Fig. 18.5) and may attain a large size. It can be treated by tapping, but is most satisfactorily dealt with by excision.

Tumours of the testis

Tumours of the testis are rare, but two varieties are seen. The commonest is a *seminoma*, which is a form of carcinoma and occurs in young and middle-aged men. It causes a painless heavy swelling of the testis and requires surgical excision (orchidectomy) followed by radiotherapy to the abdomen over the para-aortic lymph nodes, which are the first to be involved.

Teratoma of the testis is usually a cystic swelling and the prognosis is not so good as that of seminoma because the tumour may metastasize by the blood stream to the lungs and bones.

19
Peripheral Vascular Disease; Autonomic Nervous System

Peripheral vascular disease

Trauma

Direct injury to a blood vessel may wound its wall and by interrupting the normal flow of nervous impulses cause it to go into spasm. If the spasm persists, as it may in the brachial artery, ischaemia or defective blood supply to the muscles of the forearm and hand will eventually result in a condition referred to as *Volkmann's contracture*. Such spasm is relieved by exposing the artery at operation and applying papaverine to relax the arterial wall or, more often, repairing the damaged vessel.

More severe injury to an artery will cause a tear in the wall of the vessel which it is possible to suture or replace with a graft. Often the bleeding is stopped by pressure from without and a cavity in the tissues (false sac) arises in communication with the artery; this is called a *false aneurysm*. Alternatively, the vessel wall may not be ruptured but is so thinned by the injury that it dilates to form another variety of aneurysm.

An injury may occur to an artery and a vein running alongside each other with the result that the two communicate and form what is called an *arteriovenous aneurysm*.

Arteriosclerosis

Atheroma (patchy degeneration) and arteriosclerosis (hardening of the arteries) are responsible for more peripheral vascular disease than any other cause. The changes which they produce take place in the intima or lining of the vessel and produce a roughening upon which blood may clot, so that in time the lumen of the vessel is greatly diminished or even completely occluded. It is a change which takes place with age and is typically seen only in older patients. However, in the presence of diabetes it may occur in a younger age group. It affects men more severely than women and especially those who are heavy cigarette smokers.

When the blood vessels leading to the lower limbs become partially occluded, the pulses cannot be felt at the knee or the ankle and with exercise the patient complains of cramp-like pains in the calves. This pain is referred to as *claudication* and the distance which a patient can walk before the pain halts him is called his claudication distance. The extent of the disease is determined by arteriography, a fine catheter being threaded into the aorta from a femoral artery, dye injected and series of X-ray films of the legs taken called *femoral arteriography*. A non-invasive method which is replacing arteriography is the use of *Doppler* ultrasound. The instrument is moved over the surface of the limb and the diseased segments can be mapped out by ear.

Treatment. The surgical treatment of arteriosclerosis is by improving the flow of blood to the lower limb. If the narrowed part can be cored out and the vessel sutured or repaired with a vein patch the operation is called *endarterectomy* or sometimes disobliterative endarterectomy. If the narrowed area can be short-circuited by anastomosing a length of saphenous vein from iliac to popliteal artery it is called *femoropopliteal bypass*. Sometimes the bifurcation of the aorta to form the two iliac arteries is blocked (Fig. 19.1) and then it may be excised and a woven cloth tube made of an inert fibre such as Teflon sutured in place, an *aortic bifurcation graft* (Fig. 19.2). If these operations are not possible, a lumbar sympathectomy is performed, which allows the smaller vessels to dilate and gives symptomatic relief and a warmer foot and leg. It is usually considered preferable to nurse patients in the Intensive Care Unit immediately following major arterial surgery, so that continuous observation and monitoring of the patient can be carried out.

The obstruction to the arteries may progress and the most serious

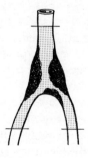

Fig. 19.1 Aneurysm of the abdominal aorta. The shading represents organised blood clot.

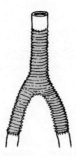

Fig. 19.2 Aortic bifurcation graft replacing the aneurysm.

complication is gangrene of the toes or foot. The treatment of this complication is described below.

Emboli

When a fragment of blood clot passes into the circulation it is referred to as an embolus and it may eventually block the lumen of a vessel, thus obstructing the circulation to some part of the body. Emboli occur most commonly at sites of narrowing or branching of arteries and one of the most usual of these is the bifurcation of the popliteal artery. A small embolus may block one of the main vessels going to the brain and produce paralysis. In some sites in the body the clot can be removed if the vessel is large enough, *embolectomy*, e.g. in the iliac vessels.

Raynaud's disease

This is a condition in which the smaller blood vessels, especially those of the fingers and hands, go into spasm when subjected to cold. It is a disease seen most commonly in young women and causes severe pain and eventually loss of the tips of the fingers through gangrene. It is usually treated by cervical sympathectomy.

Buerger's disease

This is a progressive condition seen in young men and affects the walls of the arteries leading to their blockage; it is often associated with cigarette smoking. Main vessels to the lower limb are usually the first to be affected and the condition is not greatly improved by any kind of treatment. Amputation of the gangrenous area is usually necessary and the patient may eventually lose both lower limbs.

The avascular limb

When the blood supply to the foot or leg is threatened by one of those diseases mentioned above which cause partial or complete blockage of the vessels, the foot becomes cold and painful. The pulses cannot be felt and the skin appears at first white and later a dusky colour due to stagnation of blood in the veins.

Under these circumstances it is necessary to reduce the oxygen requirements of the tissues of this leg to a minimum and this is done by cooling the limb by exposure to the air. At the same time the blood supply to the part is improved as much as possible and this is carried out by keeping the rest of the body warm. Warmed blankets and well-covered hot water bottles will help to do this. This causes reflex vasodilatation of the vessels in the affected limb. In addition, the patient may be given something by mouth to help dilate the blood vessels and one of the best substances is alcohol. Given in the form of whisky, gin or brandy it improves the patient's morale, deadens the pain and also improves the blood supply. If clotting occurs, heparin is administered intravenously every 6 hours.

When gangrene occurs, the dead tissue will have to be removed. If gangrene is seen in a patient suffering from diabetes, proper treatment of the latter disease may permit the gangrene to be fairly well localized and amputation of only that part of the tissue which is dead is sufficient. When, however, the block is due to atherosclerosis, it is known that the blood supply to the whole of the lower limb is impoverished and amputation carried out below the middle of the leg is unlikely to heal. For this reason the limb is usually removed at the site of election, which leaves some 10 cm of tibia. Often the atherosclerosis is so extensive that a mid-thigh amputation eventually becomes necessary.

Amputation

Pre-operative nursing care. The skin over the healthy part of the leg is shaved and thoroughly cleaned before operation. A patient about to lose a leg may be very distressed unless the pain is so severe that they welcome the relief it will afford. The nurse will require great tact and can give real encouragement if she has seen how successfully an artificial limb (prosthesis) can be fitted.

Postoperative nursing care. On return to the ward the patient's wound should be constantly observed for signs of bleeding. Such patients need especial care to prevent pressure sores. It is usual to support the remaining limb with two slings attached by springs to a Balkan Beam or similar type of bed frame. This limb should be exercised and observed carefully for any signs of impairment of the circulation. It is important that the stump should not be allowed to become flexed on the trunk and the nurse should keep the bandage applied firmly in order to maintain a shape which will eventually fit into a prosthesis. The patient is propped up comfortably on pillows and analgesics are given to relieve any pain. This pain may seem to the patient to be coming from the removed limb, the so-called 'phantom limb'. The amputee is sat out of bed after 48 hours if the general condition allows, the stump being supported on a pillow. As soon as the wound is healed a temporary support or pylon leg is used to encourage the patient to start learning to walk again. Finally, limb-fitting is usually carried out at special centres such as the one at Roehampton, and the patient has to be taught to walk with it.

Varicose veins

Varicose veins are a tortuous enlargement of the veins, usually of the legs. They are commoner in women than in men and especially so in those who do a lot of standing. They may occur or become more severe in pregnancy or when any structure within the pelvis presses on the great veins, e.g. fibroids. They are often familial and may occasionally be seen in quite young people.

Symptoms and signs. Varicose veins lead to aching after long standing, a feeling of tiredness in the legs and swelling of the ankles. Patients may also complain of the unsightliness of the veins and often come for treatment for this reason. More fortunate patients have no symptoms at all, only unsightly legs.

Complications. The common complications are varicose eczema, weeping and ulceration. A *varicose ulcer* is much more likely to complicate those varicose veins which occur after thrombosis of the deep veins in the leg. Varicose ulceration is a condition which is indolent and difficult to treat, and even after the varicose veins have been adequately treated by surgery the ulcer may persist.

Treatment. The treatment of varicose veins is either by the injection of sclerosing agents or by excision, but patients have to be warned that the complaint is likely to recur in 7 or 8 years no matter what treatment is used. *Injection* therapy consists of isolating a length of the varicose vein by pressure applied with the fingers above and below and then injecting a sclerosant such as sodium tetradecyl sulphate into the empty vein followed by firm bandaging with elastic or crêpe bandages over a sorbo rubber pad, which needs keeping in place for at least two weeks, the patient walking on the leg as usual. The removal of varicose veins is usually done under general anaesthesia by *stripping* them out via two small incisions, one at the groin and one at the ankle. This operation is combined with division of the internal saphenous vein and all its branches where it enters the femoral vein at the groin. When this is not possible, multiple ligatures with division of the vein between them are carried out at different levels in the leg, or short lengths of vein are removed.

Postoperative nursing care. After operation early ambulation is essential to encourage the collateral circulation and avoid thrombosis. The patient is allowed out of bed the day after operation and is encouraged to walk. The patient is fit enough to go home within 24 hours and can return later to have the stitches removed. They often require a few injections to complete the treatment.

Many patients with varicose veins are greatly helped by wearing *elastic stockings* or bandages which are put on before getting out of bed in the morning and removed before going to bed at night. These support the legs and prevent the veins filling so that there is very little swelling and the patient feels less tired.

Varicose ulcers. When a varicose ulcer complicates this condition, the application of a bandage impregnated with gelatine and other medicaments, such as Unna's paste, is very useful as this combines support with substances helpful in the healing of the ulcer. The bandage needs renewing every one or two weeks until the ulcer is healed when the patient should wear an elastic stocking.

Autonomic nervous system

Surgery of the autonomic (often called sympathetic) nervous system requires a working knowledge of its physiology and anatomy. It is convenient to think of the autonomic nervous system as being the earliest nervous tissue to evolve as it controls bodily functions like digestion, defaecation, sex, blood pressure and heat regulation. The central nervous system made up of the brain and spinal cord controls muscles, sensation and the intellect. Both are closely linked and with the endocrine system complement each other.

Anatomy

The autonomic or involuntary nervous system is made up of two parts, the parasympathetic and the sympathetic, which can be considered as being mainly antagonistic to each other.

The *sympathetic* nervous system is made up of a series of ganglia joined together by chains of nervous tissue which run down on either side of the vertebrae from the cervical to the lumbar region. The chains are made up of white and grey rami communicantes (i.e. joining branches). The white rami, containing medullated fibres, convey impulses from the spinal cord (via spinal nerves) to the sympathetic ganglia. The grey rami, or non-medullated fibres, connect the sympathetic ganglia to the spinal nerves. It is by way of these fibres, which link with cranial nerves, III, VII, IX and X and the spinal nerves, grouped especially in the cervical and sacral outflows, that impulses pass from the CNS to the blood vessels of the limbs and trunk via the peripheral nerves and to many other organs.

The nerve fibres of the *parasympathetic* nervous system pass with certain cranial and sacral nerves to ganglia which are situated in or near the organs that they supply.

Physiology

Impulses passing along the sympathetic nerves can cause constriction of the peripheral blood vessels and speed up the action of the heart. They also diminish bowel movement and at the same time bring about contraction of most sphincters in the body. In other words, activity of the sympathetic nervous system prepares the individual for attack.

Activity of the parasympathetic nerves, on the other hand, causes dilation of blood vessels, slowing of the heart beat, and increased peristaltic activity of the bowel. In brief, the parasympathetic nervous system is more important during sleep and is particularly responsible for what are often called the vegetative functions of the body, digestion, reproduction and sleep.

The autonomic system, in addition to supplying the smooth muscle of the blood vessels, intestines and heart, is responsible for the innervation of the sweat glands. It also carries painful impulses, including those from the heart.

Sympathectomy

This operation consists of removal of parts of the sympathetic chain, and the two most important portions removed are the cervical and lumbar sympathetic ganglia.

Cervical sympathectomy is carried out (1) through a small incision made over the clavicle, (2) by a posterior incision beside the scapula or (3) through the axilla by separating two ribs and pushing the lung out of the way. It is principally used for patients who have poor circulation to the hands or suffer from excessive sweating in the upper limbs.

Lumbar sympathectomy is used primarily to increase the flow of blood to the legs and feet. The operation is carried out either through a lumbar incision, as for operations on the kidney, or through a transverse abdominal incision. The peritoneum is pushed out of the way and two or three lumbar ganglia, together with the nerves between them, are excised. When it is necessary to operate on both sides at once, this can be done most conveniently by a paramedian incision opening the peritoneal cavity.

The limb should feel much warmer immediately after operation and the veins should be prominent due to increased flow of blood.

Some patients suffer severe pain when the coronary vessels supplying the heart muscle are narrowed and the myocardium does not receive adequate blood supply; the pain is called angina pectoris. It can be relieved by dividing the sympathetic fibres carrying the painful impulses from the heart, but is more satisfactorily treated by a coronary venous bypass graft which improves the blood supply to the heart muscle or myocardium.

20
The Endocrine System

The endocrine system consists of the glands of internal secretion, the largest of which are the pituitary, thyroid, adrenals and parathyroids, all of which manufacture hormones which pass into the bloodstream and thus reach all the tissues of the body unlike the nervous system which only supplies part of it. During the evolution of animals the endocrine glands were among the earliest specialized tissues to evolve, thus their secretions regulate the more primitive functions in man. The endocrine glands are closely related to each other, the secretion of many of them exerting some action on the others. They are all largely dominated by the secretions of the pituitary, which is itself under the control of the higher centres and especially the hypothalamus.

Pituitary

The pituitary or hypophysis is a cherry-like structure with a stalk which is suspended from the base of the brain and lies in a small bony cavity, the sella turcica, in the floor of the skull. The pituitary has two lobes, the anterior and posterior, which subserve different functions. The hypothalamus sends releasing hormones to the pituitary via veins surrounding its stalk.

The *anterior lobe* manufactures a great number of hormones. They are known as trophic hormones (Greek *'trophe'* = nourishment) since they regulate the growth and activity either of the body as a whole or of other endocrine glands. Thus the thyrotrophic hormone (TSH) stimulates the thyroid gland, adrenocorticotrophic hormone (ACTH) stimulates the adrenals and follicle stimulating hormone (FSH) stimulates the ovaries. In addition, a number of other hormones have been isolated which control basic metabolic processes such as growth hormone (GH).

The internal secretions of the *posterior lobe* of the pituitary control the level of the blood pressure and the secretion of the urine (ADH, antidiuretic hormone); oxytocin plays an important part in the contractions of the uterus during childbirth.

A tumour of the anterior pituitary is capable of producing increased growth so that a child becomes a giant and an adult undergoes those changes referred to as *acromegaly* with increase in the size of the skull and hands and a characteristic coarsening of the features. Such a tumour may also press on the optic nerves at the base of the skull and lead to blindness. The treatment of pituitary tumours is described in the chapter on the surgery of the central nervous system; in brief, such tumours may be excised via the skull or the nose, or they may be irradiated with X-rays or by the implantation of radon or other radioactive substances.

The pituitary gland in a woman is sometimes destroyed by thrombosis of its vessels because of severe haemorrhage following childbirth. The resultant disease is called *Simmonds' disease* and is characterised by loss of body hair, low blood pressure, loss of weight and amenorrhoea.

At the present time patients with widespread malignant disease, especially that due to cancer of the breast or prostate, are sometimes subjected to hypophysectomy (destruction of the pituitary) in order to try and arrest the progress of the disease and this can be done by inserting pellets of radioactive yttrium through a cannula passed up each nostril into the sella turcica. The aftercare of such patients includes the giving of cortisone and thyroxin daily as the secretion of ACTH and TSH has been destroyed.

Thyroid

The thyroid gland is shaped like the letter 'H' with two lateral lobes and a connecting isthmus. The isthmus crosses the first two or three rings of the trachea and the lobes lie on each side of it and to the sides of the larynx. The thyroid secretes a hormone, thyroxin, which stimulates the metabolism of all the cells of the body causing increase in the uptake of oxygen and a greatly increased output of heat and energy. In order to make this hormone, the thyroid gland needs a supply of iodine.

Endemic goitre

In those parts of the world where iodine is lacking in the diet, the gland becomes hypertrophied to compensate for this lack and the enlarged thyroid is referred to as a *simple goitre*. In certain mountainous places, such as the Swiss Alps, Himalayas and Andes, goitre is widespread and is then said to be endemic. In such areas most of the population are affected and the swellings in the neck increase with age giving rise to pressure on the trachea, oesophagus and great vessels and causing much ill health. In addition, goitrous mothers in such areas may give birth to *cretins*, who are of low mentality and have stunted bodies. Simple goitre can easily be prevented by the addition of iodine to table salt. Many countries such as Switzerland, New Zealand and the United States have introduced the use of iodized salt with a striking diminution in the incidence of goitre. In Great Britain there are areas where goitre occurs and the Medical Research Council has recommended that salt be iodized, but this unfortunately has not yet been done.

Toxic goitre

The thyroid gland may become overactive and produce too much of its hormone. This condition is referred to as hyperthyroidism, thyrotoxicosis or Graves' disease and it produces a characteristic clinical picture. The patient, usually a young woman, is nervous and has palpitations. The hands are warm and moist with sweat and the eyes are prominent. The appetite is increased though there is loss of weight and bowel motions are frequent, due to the increased metabolic rate.

Pre-operative treatment. Such a patient is treated by being given a drug which prevents the thyroid gland from making too much of its hormone, so that the metabolic rate returns to normal with a loss of the excitability and apprehensiveness. Antithyroid drugs like carbimazole (5 to 10 mg every 8 hours) or methyl thiouracil (100 to 200 mg every 8 hours) may be used in this way, and when the patient's condition has returned to normal she is usually admitted to hospital for subtotal *thyroidectomy*. Many surgeons give a course of Lugol's iodine in the immediate pre-operative period to reduce the vascularity of the gland. Propanolol, a parasympathetic nerve blocker, 40 mg, 8 hourly may also be used to control the heart rate, sweating and nervousness.

Operation. In this operation a transverse incision is made in the neck and after tying the superior and inferior thyroid arteries which supply the gland, some seven-eighths of each lobe is excised, together with the isthmus. Care is taken not to damage the recurrent laryngeal nerves which supply the vocal cords as injury to a recurrent laryngeal nerve causes hoarseness. It is also necessary to preserve the parathyroid glands, tiny structures lying on the posterior surface of the thyroid, since they control calcium metabolism and their loss leads to tetany. The neck wound is closed with fine sutures or Michel clips and often little drainage tubes are left at each end of the wound.

Postoperative nursing care. As the patient regains consciousness she is gradually sat up in bed supported by pillows and a careful watch is kept on the pulse rate. The drainage tubes are removed after 24 hours and the clips or stitches removed by the third day so that scarring is minimal. Wounds of the neck and face heal more quickly than those in other parts of the body. Patients are nursed in the sitting position, with the head carefully supported. They are sat up in bed the day following the operation and encouraged to walk about as soon as they are able. If bleeding occurs postoperatively causing pressure on the trachea, the wound is quickly opened in the ward and the patient returned to the theatre. For this reason, sterile clip removers should be kept by the patient's bedside during the postoperative period, for use in an emergency.

The ready availability of radioactive isotopes has made possible the treatment of hyperthyroidism using *radioactive iodine*. This is prepared in the pile at Harwell and can be given to the patient as a drink. The iodine is concentrated by the thyroid and its radiations destroy much of the gland and so controls the disease. This kind of therapy is usually reserved for older patients, those who are unfit for operation and those with a recurrence of the disease following a previous operation for hyperthyroidism. The main complication is hypothyroidism, which occurs commonly after isotope therapy. Its onset is insidious and may be delayed many months or years. Hence these patients should be seen at intervals for the rest of their lives. Radio-iodine therapy is not given to children, young women and those who are pregnant for fear of inducing a thyroid carcinoma.

Malignant goitre

Thyroid cancer is commoner in those parts of the world where goitre is endemic.

It occasionally occurs in young people, when it is usually slow growing and spreads by the lymphatic nodes (papillary carcinoma). The treatment for these patients is surgical excision of the affected thyroid and the lymph nodes of the neck. Such patients must, however, be examined at regular intervals in case of a recurrence; this is usually discovered by palpating a firm enlarged lymph node. These nodes are then excised. It is also important that these patients should take thyroxine by mouth for the rest of their lives since there is evidence that this discourages recurrence of their carcinoma while at the same time providing the hormone they need.

In some patients the thyroid may be involved by a malignant process which reproduces the pattern of the gland in its metastases and therefore these secondaries, which are often in bone or lung, may be capable of concentrating iodine (follicular carcinoma). Such patients, after removal of the whole thyroid gland together with the malignant tumour (total thyroidectomy), can be treated with radioactive iodine which is then concentrated in the metastases. They also must take thyroxin by mouth for the rest of their lives.

Finally, in patients over sixty, a much more malignant form of thyroid cancer is encountered which grows rapidly and obstructs the trachea causing dyspnoea and eventually asphyxia (anaplastic carcinoma). These patients may need a tracheostomy to allow them to breathe. The treatment of this variety of thyroid cancer is by radiotherapy which, however, may only cause a temporary remission.

Adrenals

The adrenals, or suprarenal glands, are situated above the upper poles of the kidneys (Fig. 20.1) and are highly vascular small glands made up of two distinct parts, an outer cortex and an inner medulla.

The *adrenal cortex* elaborates a great number of hormones, some of which control carbohydrate metabolism, secondary sexual characteristics, protein metabolism and electrolyte balance. The adrenal cortex is essential for life.

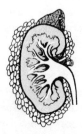

Fig. 20.1 Section through the right kidney showing the adrenal gland sitting on its upper pole like a cocked hat.

The *adrenal medulla*, on the other hand, is not essential for life, but it elaborates two hormones, adrenaline and nor-adrenaline, which help in maintaining the blood pressure and regulate the rate and contraction of the heart.

Adrenal cortex

Overaction of the adrenal cortices leads to three different clinical pictures, according to the type of cell which is affected. In the first, called *Cushing's disease*, the patient presents with increased fatness of the face and trunk, raised blood pressure, weakness and headache, together with amenorrhoea and the passage of sugar in the urine. The condition is due to overactive adrenals, but is often associated with a tumour in the anterior lobe of the pituitary which produces ACTH and thus stimulates the adrenals. The treatment of Cushing's disease is the removal of the pituitary tumour, if one is present, by an operation usually done by a microsurgical technique via the nose or by excision of the adrenals (bilateral adrenalectomy), the patient being maintained on cortisone by mouth. Irradiation of the pituitary may be used.

Another type of disease seen with hyperplasia of the adrenal cortex is called the *adrenogenital syndrome*. In this condition the patient, often a child and usually a girl, undergoes masculine changes with growth of hair on the face, deepening of the voice and redistribution of body fat. There is an excess of 17-ketosteroids in the urine. The cause of the adrenogenital syndrome is the inability of the adrenal cortex to make one of the essential hormones. As a result the adrenal is stimulated by the pituitary more and more and pours out other hormones which it can make in excess. This results in the masculinization of the child and the high level of 17-ketosteroids in the urine. The treatment of the adrenogenital syndrome is giving cortisone by mouth as this replaces the hormone which the patient's own adrenals cannot manufacture.

Occasionally an adult develops a tumour in one adrenal and this leads to a similar clinical picture. Removal of the tumour results in a cure.

The third type of syndrome seen with adrenal cortical disease is one in which there is a great loss of electrolytes, especially potassium, from the body with resulting weakness and eventually kidney damage. The hormone producing this change is called aldosterone and the condition *primary aldosteronism*. Treatment is removal of the adrenal which contains the tumour; this is golden in colour and quite small.

The principal hormones manufactured by the adrenal cortex have been isolated and are prepared commercially. The name of the most important of these is cortisone. This substance is essential when a patient has to have a bilateral adrenalectomy, for cortisone or its related substances (prednisone, prednisolone) are necessary for life. Reference to the companion book in this series, *Principles of Medicine and Medical Nursing*, gives information about cortisone and how it is given for a great many other conditions, such as rheumatoid arthritis, ulcerative colitis and other chronic inflammatory conditions.

Adrenal medulla

Tumours of the adrenal medulla are referred to as *phaeochromocytomas*. They manufacture nor-adrenaline and this produces enormous increases in the blood pressure which may be spasmodic or continuous. If untreated the patient eventually dies due to a ruptured blood vessel or damaged kidneys. Therefore the treatment is removal of the tumour. This may be followed by a sudden fall in the blood pressure and so it is necessary to prepare the patient with substances which block the effects of nor-adrenaline in the tissues (e.g. phenoxybenzamine, an α-blocker). It is also essential to be able to give rapid transfusion during and immediately after operation.

Adrenalectomy

When an adrenal is to be removed because of the presence of a tumour, the incision can be the same as for nephrectomy or the patient may lie face down so that both can be visualised. In children a laparotomy is more suitable.

Postoperative nursing care. Following operation the patient is nursed sitting or on one side if there is a drainage tube in the wound. A careful watch is kept on the blood pressure and the nurse records this at regular intervals as instructed. Care is taken that the intravenous infusion continues, since if the blood pressure falls it is by the intravenous route that drugs (e.g. nor-adrenaline) are given to restore it.

When both adrenals are to be removed, this may be performed in two stages, the second gland being removed about 10 days after the first. Some surgeons prefer to remove both at one time using an anterior approach through the abdomen or a posterior approach through the bed of the eleventh rib on each side. It is necessary in these patients to provide replacement therapy with cortisone before and after operation and a typical programme for doing this is as follows:

2 days before operation,	50 mg, 6 hourly, IMI.
1 day before operation,	50 mg, 6 hourly, IMI.
Day of operation,	100 mg by mouth 3 hours before operation.
1st post-operative day,	25 mg, 6 hourly, IMI.
2nd—4th post-op. day,	25 mg, 6 hourly by mouth or IMI.
5th — 10th post-op. day,	12.5 mg, 6 hourly, by mouth.
Subsequently,	12.5 mg, by mouth, or more.

On leaving the hospital, patients are generally issued with a card as shown in Fig. 20.2.

Parathyroids

The parathyroids are four small pea-like glands which are situated behind the four poles of the thyroid gland. They regulate calcium metabolism and may be the site of a tumour.

Hyperparathyroidism

When a patient has a parathyroid tumour there is great loss of calcium from the skeleton which leads to cyst formation and fractures. The excretion of calcium may lead to stones forming in the urinary tract and can cause calcification in the kidneys and lungs, which is eventually fatal. Treatment is removal of the tumour through an incision exactly the same as for thyroidectomy. In the convalescent period the patient is given calcium by mouth to replenish the stores in the skeleton and if necessary Vitamin D to help to absorb it.

Thymus

Although it is debatable whether the thymus gland produces an important internal secretion, it is convenient to consider the organ here. Great interest has developed in the thymus in recent years because it has been discovered to produce a special type of

STEROID TREATMENT

Hospital: _____

Name: _____

Address: _____

_____

Phone No. _____

Family Doctor

_____

Drug

Date				
Daily Dose				

1. **DO NOT STOP** *taking these tablets except on medical advice. Always have a supply in reserve.*

2. *In case of acute illness, accident or emergency operation the treatment* **MUST** *be continued. A* **LARGER** *dose may be necessary at such times.*

3. *If the tablets cause indigestion, consult your doctor* **AT ONCE.**

4. **ALWAYS CARRY THIS CARD.**

Fig. 20.2

lymphocyte (the T-lymphocyte), especially in the early part of life, which is essential for the immunological defences of the body.

The thymus is situated in the upper and anterior part of the thorax in the mediastinum, is greyish pink in colour and is quite large at birth, remaining prominent until puberty. After this age it appears to shrink so that only a small and inconspicuous structure is normally seen in the adult. Its exact functions are not known, but it is occasionally the site of a tumour or of hyperplasia, either of which may be associated with a condition called *myasthenia gravis*. In this the patient has progressive weakness of the muscles. The removal of the thymus (thymectomy), by an operation at which the sternum is split vertically, may produce a great improvement in muscle power. This combats the weakness of the muscles of respiration, without which the patient would be unable to breathe or expectorate and might thus die of asphyxia. Patients with a thymic tumour are treated with radiation in the first place and only subjected to thymectomy at a later date.

21
The Skull, Brain, Vertebral Column and Spinal Cord

Today most patients who require surgical treatment of the central nervous system are sent to special neurosurgical centres. There are always, however, patients who sustain head injuries who are treated in general surgical wards, and there are a number of conditions affecting the central nervous system which may be encountered as complications of infection or of malignant disease.

The skull consists of a bony box which has three membranous layers within it surrounding the brain. The outermost layer is called the dura mater, the middle layer the arachnoid mater and the inner, the pia mater. The dura is lightly adherent to the inner surface of the bony skull and the pia dips down into the sulci, or furrows, of the cerebral cortex. Between the arachnoid and pia there is a space containing the cerebrospinal fluid, which circulates from the ventricles where it is manufactured by the choroid plexuses, passing out over the surface of the brain and down over the spinal cord. It may be tapped in the lumbar region by inserting a needle between two of the lower lumbar vertebrae, as described below under lumbar puncture.

The cerebrospinal fluid acts partly as a vehicle for carrying the necessary nutriment to the nervous tissue and also as a buffer to reduce shocks which might otherwise damage the extremely delicate nerve cells. The ventricles are cavities within the brain substance and they contain cerebrospinal fluid (CSF).

Head injuries

Injuries to the scalp bleed profusely because of its great vascularity. The bleeding can be easily arrested by firm pressure along the edges of the severed scalp and finally by sutures which hold these edges together.

Injuries of the head are usually described as open or closed. A closed head injury is one in which the skull remains intact although it may be fractured. In an open head injury the brain or its covering membranes are exposed in the wound. The difference is an important one because if the head injury is an open one, there is unlikely to be a rise in the intracranial pressure which brings with it a definite pattern of symptoms.

Fractures of the skull may be linear, depressed or comminuted, and the treatment will vary according to the type. The vault is more elastic than the base of the skull and therefore the base is more often fractured.

Depressed fractures often occur in children and the fragment of bone may require elevating. Such a fracture can occur during birth because the bone is very soft at this time. Because of its shape it is referred to as a pond fracture. Treatment is by elevating the fracture, a burr hole being made near by and the bony fragment being levered into position.

Symptoms and signs

Concussion. This is the result of a blow on the head which causes injury to the nerve cells and loss of consciousness. The depth of the unconsciousness varies and if light the patient can be roused by a loud command, but if deep even painful stimuli will not produce any response.

Compression. If there is raised pressure within the skull it causes loss of consciousness and as the pressure rises, so the unconsciousness deepens, the patient eventually passing into coma.

Pressure on the medulla results in a slowing of the pulse and a rise in the blood pressure. In addition the breathing becomes slower and eventually of Cheyne–Stokes type. In this condition the patient takes a number of deep breaths which succeed in removing the carbon dioxide from the bloodstream and then, without this stimulus to the respiratory centre, breathing stops and a pause ensues before a number of very deep breaths is taken again. If the rising intracranial pressure is left unchecked, death occurs following deep coma.

Occasionally a tracheostomy may be performed before an operation on the brain is undertaken so that good ventilation of the lungs is obtained and pulmonary congestion prevented in the postoperative period.

Amnesia. This word means loss of memory and after a head injury it is usually of a retrograde type, that is the loss of memory is for events immediately preceding the injury. Usually the more severe this loss of memory, the more severe the injury.

Cerebral irritation. When patients start to recover from concussion they usually pass through a phase of cerebral irritation in which they lie curled up in bed avoiding light and resenting any kind of intrusion. The reactions to stimuli are exaggerated and all the tendon reflexes are very brisk. Such patients are not in a position to co-operate properly, though they respond to simple requests such as 'put out your tongue'. The condition is due to increased irritability of the cerebral cortex, and during this period it is advisable to nurse the patient in a quiet room, with the windows shaded and with as little interference as possible.

Management of head injuries

All patients with a history of loss of consciousness, extensive scalp laceration or fractured skull should be admitted to hospital for a period of observation of at least 24 hours for fear of development of intracranial haemorrhage. This also applies to the intoxicated or confused person who smells of drink, as the confusion may be due to injury. The most important thing to determine on admission is the level of consciousness.

The general nursing management of a patient with head injury calls for skill and patience. While the patient is still unconscious he will be nursed and supported in the lateral position and turned from side to side at regular intervals with careful attention to pressure areas. It is important to ensure that the limbs are supported and put through a full range of normal movement to encourage circulation and prevent joint stiffness and deformity. A close watch is made for vomiting or the voiding of urine, which may take place into the bed without any warning. The surgeon may introduce a self-retaining catheter into the bladder for continuous or intermittent drainage. The nurse's duty will then include those precautions designed to prevent urinary infection, i.e. tubing sterilized and changed twice daily, sterile spigot and sterilized syringe for intermittent aspiration. It is an advantage to have a closed system of drainage such as that described in Chapter 17. Particular attention to the eyes of these patients is important. During unconsciousness the eyes are insensitive and are at risk to foreign bodies. If they are kept closed this risk is minimized.

The pulse rate is recorded regularly and any change, either slowing or speeding up, is reported at once to the medical officer, since it indicates a change in the cerebral state. Observations of temperature and respiratory rate should also be made. In the event of hyperpyrexia, special nursing treatments will be ordered to reduce the temperature. Fans may be effective, tepid and cold sponging, the application of ice bags or even more drastic measures such as the use of ice packs.

The blood pressure is recorded at regular intervals; a rise in blood pressure is a sign of increasing pressure within the skull. The size of the pupils is also noted by making little sketches of their relative diameters on a sheet of paper at regular intervals. The level of consciousness of the patient should be observed and recorded at regular intervals to provide a guide of the patient's progress. This is best achieved by the use of an accepted guide to measuring consciousness levels, in order to provide continuity of assessment by different nursing staff.

When the pressure increases in one side of the cranium, due for example to a bleeding meningeal vessel, the irritation stimulates the pupil on that side to contract. If the mounting pressure is left unrelieved, it eventually paralyses the nerve supply to the pupil, which then dilates (Fig. 21.1). This may be the only guide as to which side of the skull should be opened in order to find and control the bleeding.

SIDE OF COMPRESSION (R)		OPPOSITE SIDE (L)	
Slightly contracted	●	Normal	●
Moderately dilated. Reacts to light	●	Normal	●
More dilated. Does not react to light	●	Moderately dilated. Reacts to light	●
Widely dilated and insensitive	●	Widely dilated does not react to light	●

Fig. 21.1 Record of the size of pupils during increasing cranial pressure on the right side.

When unconsciousness continues for days, the maintenance of the patient's fluid balance and nutrition must be carried out by tube feeding and for this a nasogastric tube is passed, via the nose, into the stomach and a liquid diet introduced by means of a funnel or syringe. Alternatively, the insertion of a feeding line into the subclavian vein or vena cava may be preferred for long-term alimentation.

Special tests. Special investigations will be called for in complicated head injuries. All patients require X-ray pictures of the skull in two planes to show if a fracture is present. Rarely, it may be necessary to carry out a *lumbar puncture* and this will be done using careful aseptic technique. The patient lies in a lateral position and after injecting a local analgesic such as lignocaine, a lumbar puncture needle is passed between the third and fourth lumbar vertebrae. After removing the stilette, a spinal manometer is connected to the needle so that the pressure of the cerebrospinal fluid can be measured. In health this is usually between 100 mm and 120 mm of water, but it may be greatly raised after head injuries. In addition the CSF may be stained with blood and the amount of blood present may be of help in assessing the extent of the injury. The spinal fluid is collected in a sterile bottle and at normal pressure appears at the rate of one drop per second. Very little fluid is removed for fear of 'coning' the medulla into the foramen magnum with a fatal result.

Lumbar puncture is often performed as a diagnostic test in patients suspected of disease in the CNS. If headache follows the procedure it is due to a leak of the CSF from the spinal theca and is treated by elevating the foot of the bed on high blocks for at least 24 hours. In the early stages the patient will be nursed in a bed with the foot raised, and later the head of the bed may be raised if it is considered desirable to lower the intracranial pressure.

Convalescence. As recovery takes place the patient will regain consciousness and may need much tactful handling to help him to adjust to his surroundings while the memory of previous events is slowly returning. Relatives should always be warned that they may not be recognized at first, but there is often progressive improvement over a long period. Frequently the patient talks in a rambling way and relatives should also be warned not to attach too much importance to what is said.

Eventually the patient is allowed out of bed and progressively encouraged to get up and walk about, slowly rehabilitating himself, a process which may take weeks or months according to the severity of the injury and the type of individual. Some patients suffer from headaches and attacks of dizziness for months or years after head injury, but it is notable that those patients who were prone to have headaches, or were not well adjusted to life before the injury, are those who suffer most in this way. These disabilities are often referred to as the *postconcussional syndrome* and are often the subject of medicolegal action.

Complications

Intracranial haemorrhage. Bleeding within the skull may take place either outside the dura, inside the dura, or within the substance of the brain itself (Fig. 21.2).

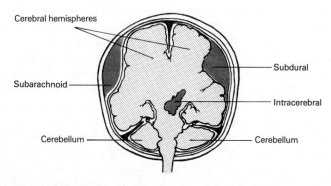

Cerebral hemispheres

Subdural

Subarachnoid

Intracerebral

Cerebellum

Cerebellum

Fig. 21.2 Intracranial haemorrhage.

Extradural haemorrhage. Haemorrhage between dura and skull is referred to as extradural and the commonest cause of this is a torn middle meningeal artery. This leads to slowly increasing intracranial tension; the pupil on the injured side at first contracts and later dilates; there is slowing of the pulse rate, a rising blood pressure, deepening coma and finally Cheyne–Stokes breathing.

Treatment is an immediate craniotomy, the skull being opened over the site where the bleeding is taking place. The artery is secured by tying or diathermy coagulation, or the bony foramen through which it passes is plugged with a small piece of wax.

Subdural haematoma. A collection of blood deep to the dura usually occurs as a gradual process and may not cause signs and symptoms for many months. The collection of blood clot produces its effects due to the space it occupies and this may change size from time to time due to alterations in its osmotic pressure. The result is that the patient presents signs which may vary from day to day but which usually increase in severity progressively. There may be weakness of some particular movement, an impediment in the speech, or alteration in the personality.

The diagnosis is confirmed by a CAT scan and by electroencephalography (EEG). In this investigation small electrodes are placed on the scalp and the potentials which occur in the underlying brain substance are amplified and recorded as a tracing on graph paper. The presence of a subdural haematoma, any severe injury, or a tumour, usually presents an unusual pattern of electric potentials. The blood clot is carefully removed and good recovery of function can be expected after this operation.

Intracerebral haemorrhage. A blow on the skull may impart momentum to the underlying brain, which may tear blood vessels within the substance of the brain itself and cause a collection of blood. Sudden changes in pressure, as may occur due to a nearby explosion, or indriven fragments of bone or metal may all produce a similar effect. Damage within brain substance, or any intracerebral collection of blood, is not amenable to surgical treatment except in so far as it may be drained. If foreign bodies have been introduced, they can be removed, but once the tissues of the central nervous system have been destroyed, they never regenerate. Any improvement which is subsequently noted is due to the recovery of nearby tissues affected by oedema which only temporarily interferes with their normal activity.

Late effects of head injuries. As mentioned below, the greatest problem in the rehabilitation of patients who have had cerebral injury is in those who before injury showed some signs of mental instability or poor adjustment to their surroundings. Such patients are prone to have headaches, dizzy attacks and great intolerance of alcohol. Their treatment is usually more in the province of the psychiatrist than the surgeon since they have to be trained to adapt themselves once more to the problems of life. Very little can be done medically or surgically to improve their condition.

Occasionally a scarred area acts as a focus of cerebral irritation and may produce epileptic attacks. In such patients it is sometimes justifiable to excise the scarred area in the hope that the scar will not recur as healing takes place and that the fits will be abolished.

Infections

Scalp. When infection occurs in the scalp it usually spreads in the loose areolar tissue deep to the pericranial aponeurosis and thus the whole scalp is lifted by a layer of pus. This condition is often referred to as Pott's puffy tumour, after Percival Pott, the surgeon who first described it. The treatment of infection in this area is wide incision to drain the pus and the giving of a suitable antibiotic, such as penicillin.

The scalp being vascular, heals rapidly and it is most unusual for any area of it to slough.

Skull. Infection of the bony skull is a form of osteomyelitis which is rarely seen. It typically follows a blow on the head in a patient who has a staphylococcal lesion in some other part of the body, e.g. a boil. There is severe pain, a high temperature and fast pulse rate with swelling of the scalp over the affected area. Treatment is by giving large doses of penicillin or other antibiotic at once and by draining the pus which collects under the periosteum of the outer table of the skull. Subsequently any dead bone (sequestrum) will have to be removed at operation.

Meninges. Infection which involves the meninges is called *meningitis* and the space in which the infection usually spreads is the subarachnoid, in which the cerebrospinal fluid circulates. Such infection may be acute or chronic and is introduced either by the bloodstream or by some nearby focus of inflammation, as may occur in the middle ear. This rarely demands surgical treatment except in that form which arises from infection in the middle ear. In these patients it is necessary to drain the abscess, which entails a mastoid operation and usually exposure of the temporal lobe of the brain, since this is the route by which the infection enters the skull. Carcinomatous metastases may invade the meninges and produce symptoms of meningitis.

Brain. Cerebral or brain abscesses may arise by extension from neighbouring infection, the commonest being the middle ear, as a result of open injuries or wounds, or by infection spreading via the bloodstream, as in the pyaemia which complicates empyema, bronchiectasis, osteomyelitis and certain fevers, e.g. typhoid.

The symptoms and signs of a cerebral abscess are headache, vomiting and papilloedema. Papilloedema is swelling of the optic nerve where it enters the retina, an area which can be seen with an ophthalmoscope. There may be attacks of giddiness and speech may be affected; it is often slurred.

Treatment is to open the skull over the suspected area. If pus is found it may be possible to drain it and leave a tube in situ for the instillation of penicillin. Occasionally the abscess is opened to the surface as after bullet or shrapnel wounds.

Venous sinuses. The large venous sinuses which drain blood from the brain may be involved in infection of neighbouring structures, e.g. middle ear disease, sepsis of the face, or infection of one of the air sinuses of the skull. The symptoms are those of any acute infection; high temperature with rigors, sweating and prostration, severe headache and vomiting together with the signs of the primary infection.

Lateral sinus thrombosis. This produces localised pain over the mastoid process and when the thrombosis spreads to the internal jugular vein, the latter can be palpated as a tender firm cord in the neck. There is a high swinging temperature.

Cavernous sinus thrombosis. This leads to protrusion of the eye and great oedema of the eyelids. Infection usually comes from a boil or carbuncle of the face, especially if this is situated near the nose. Treatment is with antibiotics and drainage.

Cerebral tumours

Tumours arising within the skull may develop in the meninges or the brain itself and may be benign or malignant. In either case they lead to a pattern of symptoms which is diagnostic and which is produced by increasing pressure within the cranial cavity.

Symptoms and signs. The three main symptoms are those of headache, vomiting and failure of vision. In addition there may be mental changes and attacks of drowsiness and apathy. According to the site in which the tumour arises there may be localising signs. Tumours of the meninges, called meningiomas, may press on the motor area of the cerebral cortex and cause attacks of epilepsy and later localised paralysis.

Tumours of the brain substance arising in the speech area lead to strange jumbling of the spoken words and inability to speak clearly. Tumours in the occipital area of the brain, lead to change in the field of vision and eventually blindness, while tumours of the cerebellum lead to attacks of dizziness with the patient often falling to the side on which the lesion is situated.

Special tests. Diagnosis is usually obtained with the CAT scanner and may be aided by X-raying the skull, especially after the introduction of air into the subarachnoid space, which shows up the position of the ventricles, a procedure called *air encephalography*.

Electroencephalography (EEG) may help in localising the site of the tumour. Cerebral *arteriography*, which is carried out by injecting radio-opaque fluid into the carotid artery, may reveal an abnormal pattern of vessels in the tumour, but carries the risk of further damage. The use of Nuclear Magnetic Resonance is a new technique which can outline the tumour.

Treatment. The prognosis of a patient with a brain tumour is not good, but many meningeal tumours and some pituitary tumours are removable and may not be followed by recurrence. Tumours arising in the brain substance are called *gliomas* and one which offers a hopeful outlook is the astrocytoma, but many of the others are very malignant and operation is not often useful in prolonging life, although the use of chemotherapy is helping to improve the results.

On the other hand, *craniotomy* does give an opportunity to relieve the tension within the skull and thus to make the symptoms less severe. In this operation, referred to as a *decompression*, a wide opening is left in the skull and the scalp closed over it. The nursing care after these operations is modified according to the condition of the patient, but it is imperative that careful observations are made, as in the nursing of patients with head injuries. It is usual to nurse such patients lying with the head supported on the side opposite to that of the operation until the general condition improves.

Spinal cord

The most important congenital condition involving the spinal cord which is amenable to surgical treatment is spina bifida.

Spina bifida

This is a deficiency of the posterior wall of the bony spinal canal and is common in the lumbar region, but may occur throughout any part of the spine. If there is only a bony deficiency and all the soft tissues are normal, the condition is referred to as *spina bifida occulta*. When, in addition, there is a swelling in the region which is associated with a cyst of the meninges, the condition is referred to as a *meningocele*. If as well as the cystic dilatation of the meninges, there is also a defect of the spinal cord and the nerve roots are stretched out over the walls of the cyst, the condition is called a *meningomyelocele*. This is a serious condition because it is usually associated with paralysis of the lower limbs and of the sphincters controlling the urethra and rectum so that the baby is incontinent of urine and faeces. There are varying degrees of this paralysis, but if the condition appears to be compatible with life, operation is performed as soon as possible after birth to remove the cyst and replace the nervous tissue within the spinal canal. Little improvement results, except that the swelling is removed. The skin over the meningomyelocele is often thin and almost transparent.

Fractures and fracture-dislocations of the vertebral column

The three main divisions of the vertebral column, cervical, thoracic and lumbar, are affected by trauma in different ways and the greatest care should be exercised when moving a casualty with a suspected spinal injury for fear of increasing the damage.

Cervical spine

Fracture–dislocation is more common than simple fracture in the cervical spine and often follows a diving accident or similar type of injury. The atlas or axis may be fractured or dislocated and injuries in this part of the spine are often associated with damage to the spinal cord with paraplegia due to contusion or compression. If there is no nervous lesion the neck is supported by a padded collar which extends up under the chin and the back of the skull. If there is damage to the spinal cord treatment is by traction using metal callipers, rather like ice tongs, inserted into the skull, a weight of about 15 to 20 lb then being applied.

The nursing care should aim to prevent the formation of pressure sores and the limbs should be supported in a comfortable position.

After a few weeks the neck is supported in a plaster of Paris or light plastic collar and this may be retained for 2 to 3 months or until union has taken place.

Thoracic spine

Injury to this part of the spine is usually due to falling from a height, and compression of one or more vertebral bodies takes place. Vertebral injuries are treated by nursing in a bed fitted with fracture boards so that the patient lies quite flat. Fracture boards are simply strong pieces of wood laid beneath the mattress and extending over each side of the bed. If there is spinal cord injury and the fracture is unstable it must be treated by traction or internal fixation at operation.

Lumbar spine

Crush fractures in the lumbar region are also common (Fig. 21.3). A transverse process or spinous process may be fractured or avulsed by direct violence or muscle action. Such injuries are treated by rest. If pain becomes chronic, it may be necessary to remove an injured vertebral process. A prolonged course of exercises to improve the muscles and progressive rehabilitation completes the cure.

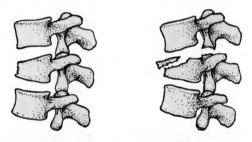

Fig. 21.3 Crush fracture of a lumbar vertebra with some dislocation.

Infections of the spinal column

Acute osteomyelitis. This infection, which is usually due to the staphylococcus, is rare in the vertebrae and difficult to diagnose and so it is often recognised late. Treatment is by giving penicillin and draining the pus. Adequate rest in bed or in a plaster jacket is necessary until consolidation has taken place. The treatment of pressure areas is important, and the nurse should report any signs of constriction or pressure caused by the plaster jacket.

Chronic osteomyelitis. The only chronic infection of the spine of any importance is tuberculosis and this is usually referred to as *Pott's disease*. It is seen in children, but may occur at any age, the infection reaching the vertebrae by the bloodstream from some other focus of tuberculosis in the body. The signs and symptoms of the disease are localised pain of an aching character with board-like rigidity of the muscles overlying the lesion. Thus a child will be quite unwilling to bend down, as for example to pick up toys from the floor. As bone destruction progresses, so the vertebral bodies collapse and become wedge-shaped causing an angular kyphosis of the spine. The prominent part of this angular process is usually referred to as a *gibbus*. It is treated by antituberculous medicines, surgical clearance of the abscess and bone grafting. A full description of this condition will be found in the chapter on bone.

Tumours

Tumours may occur in the meninges surrounding the spinal cord or within the substance of the cord itself. They are similar in pathology to those occurring within the brain and its coverings. The symptoms they cause are due to pressure on the nerve tracts or nerve roots, with resultant changes in sensation and motor power. Their removal is greatly assisted by the use of a laser instead of a scalpel.

22
Orthopaedics – Muscles, Tendons and Bursas

The word orthopaedics is derived from two Greek words meaning straight and children and was first used in the seventeenth century to describe work which was done primarily for the correction of congenital deformities in children. Orthopaedics today embraces the whole subject of treating injury, deformity and disease of the limbs together with that of the spine. Thus this branch of surgery is concerned with the treatment of those conditions affecting bone, muscle and tendon and all the structures associated with them.

Muscles

Injury

If a muscle is traumatized it results in tearing of some of the fibres with the extravasation of blood and the formation of a clot. There is severe pain at the time of the injury which often feels to the patient like a blow, followed by disability which is proportional to the amount of muscle that has been injured. For example, when playing tennis, part of the gastrocnemius or plantaris muscle may be torn and this leads to severe pain in the calf and limitation of movement at the ankle. The adductor longus muscle may be injured in riding and this leads to a similar disability in the thigh. Finally there may be calcification in the muscle where it is attached to the femur.

The treatment of a torn muscle is to rest the affected part for 2 to 3 weeks and then, when the haematoma has become organized and fibrosis has started, to institute movements, both active and passive. The resolution of the injury may be speeded up by the application of local heat in the form of infrared or short-wave diathermy. Subsequently, active physiotherapy will assist recovery.

Tumours of muscle

These are rare and since the muscles are derived from mesoderm, the malignant neoplasm is usually a sarcoma. Sarcomas may arise in both children and adults, they are usually very malignant and the prognosis is not good. Treatment consists of excision followed by radiotherapy.

Tendons

Injury

Tendons, like muscles are subject to injury, but less commonly, because they are stronger. Repair takes place by the formation of fibrous tissue, which usually leads to shortening, a condition referred to as a contracture.

A good example is the injury which may occur in the tendon and muscle of the sternomastoid at birth. The resulting fibrosis leads to shortening of the muscle so that the head is held to one side, a condition described as wry-neck or torticollis. The treatment of wry-neck is passive stretching of the sternomastoid, which the mother is easily taught to do, and provided this is carried out daily the muscle can usually be maintained at its proper length. If, however, the condition is not recognized and remains untreated, it will become necessary to incise the shortened tendon and stretch it, an operation called *tenotomy*. Occasionally the muscle may have to be excised if it is severely shortened.

When the tendons have been badly damaged, or the muscles have lost their power due to a disease such as poliomyelitis, other normally moving tendons may be transplanted to take their place. Such an operation is often performed on the tendons at the wrist joint where, due to paralysis of the radial nerve, wrist drop has occurred.

Nursing care. For operation on muscles and tendons in the limbs, a wide area of skin has to be shaved and cleaned pre-operatively. The wound is almost always clean stitched and the limb often immobilized on a splint or in plaster of Paris for several days or weeks. Sutures are removed on the eighth to tenth day. Active movements are superintended by the physiotherapist. Passive movements must never be attempted unless ordered by the surgeon.

Diseases of the tendons themselves are rare, but their sheaths are commonly involved in a variety of conditions, including injury, as described below.

Tendon sheaths

Inflammation of a tendon sheath is described as *tenosynovitis*. It may be the result of injury or inflammation.

Traumatic tenosynovitis. This follows excessive use of the tendons or may be due to the patient carrying out movements to which he is unaccustomed, such as the clerical worker who spends the weekend digging in the garden. The result is pain on movement and a grating sensation may be felt over the tendon, which is often described as *snowball crepitus*. Treatment is to rest and support the affected part for a few days, following this with active movements and physiotherapy. Warmth is soothing and encourages exercise.

Suppurative tenosynovitis. When infection enters a tendon's sheath the result is suppurative tenosynovitis. This is a serious condition for two reasons: firstly, the patient is ill and toxic with a high swinging temperature because pus is confined within the tendon sheath, and secondly, the inflammation if untreated is likely to destroy the tendon and the sheath in which it lies. Infection usually enters from a focus near the tendon, a good example being the whitlow which spreads to involve the flexor tendons of the finger. Treatment consists of incisions to let out the pus, splinting the affected part in the position of rest, and the giving of large doses of antibiotics to control the infection. The application of dry heat is soothing and may also speed resolution while the full resources of a Hand Clinic and the Physiotherapy Department will assist in regaining normal movement.

Tuberculous tenosynovitis. This may occur in the tendons of the wrist and palm causing a dumb-bell shaped swelling on the ventral aspect of the wrist. It usually contains loose fibrinous bodies described as melon seeds. The condition is insidious in its onset and may cause only slight disability. It is slow to heal, but recovery is often speeded by excision of as much of the infected material as can be removed. Such treatment is never undertaken until antituberculous drugs have been given for some weeks.

Stenosing tenosynovitis. This is a particular form of chronic fibrous involvement of a tendon sheath. It may occur around the extensors of the thumb at the wrist. In this position the constant friction caused by washing and wringing out clothes may cause chronic irritation and thickening of the sheath with the production of a painful nodule referred to as *de Quervain's* disease. Treatment is excision of the thickened area.

Ganglion. This is a swelling associated with a tendon sheath or a joint and contains a clear glairy fluid of the consistence of jelly. The cause of ganglia is unknown; they may arise at any age although they are especially common in children. Pain is unusual. Ganglia are often found arising on the back of the hand and the dorsum of the foot; when they enlarge they produce transilluminable swellings.

A ganglion may be dispersed by very firm pressure, aspirated through a wide bore needle or, best of all, excised. Excision is usually done in the day-surgery theatre and it is rarely necessary to admit these patients. Ganglia have a tendency to recur.

In children a particular form of ganglion occurs in the popliteal fossa and is referred to as a semimembranosus bursa because the swelling is associated with the tendon of the semimembranosus muscle. This bursa may be excised, but if left alone it will often resolve in time. The fluid contained within it is identical with that seen in a ganglion and may be expressed through a tiny incision.

Bursas

A bursa is a sac containing a viscid fluid which is interposed between two layers of tissue where friction is likely to occur. Bursas are found most commonly over bony protuberances which are subjected to much pressure, e.g. the elbow, olecranon bursa (miner's elbow); in front of the knee, prepatellar bursa (housemaid's knee); ischial tuberosity, ischial bursa (weaver's bottom). They also occur between muscle layers.

Bursas may become chronically inflamed, when they enlarge and are usually tender, although occasionally they are free from pain. Tuberculous inflammation of a bursa is occasionally seen and if untreated leads to a discharging sinus, the edges of which appear unhealthy, undermined and rather bluish in colour. In such a bursa there may be loose bodies made up of fibrin, the so-called melon seeds.

Acute inflammation may occur in a bursa and cause an exquisitely painful, red swelling. For example if a housemaid's knee becomes infected, the prepatellar bursa is distended with pus and the patient may have a high temperature and be toxic. Treatment is by incision to let out the pus. Giving an antibiotic may abort an attack. Later the bursa may be excised.

23
Orthopaedics – Bones and Joints

It is important to remember that bone is a living tissue, its cells and calcium salts constantly being mobilized and laid down afresh. It is enclosed in periosteum, which is mainly a fibrous sheath but is also capable of laying down new osseous tissue and moulding the shape of the whole bone. Bone is richly supplied with blood vessels, but being a rigid structure, the changes which it undergoes when it becomes inflamed or involved in other disease processes are different from those seen in the soft tissues of the body. Diseased bone usually takes a long time to undergo repair and the convalescence of patients suffering from such conditions is therefore protracted.

Since diseases of bone are likely to run a long course, the orthopaedic outpatients' department is one which sees great numbers of patients. In addition, because these patients require prolonged rehabilitation, it is usual for there to be close liaison between the orthopaedic and physiotherapy departments.

A typical long bone is made up of a shaft or *diaphysis* with, at each end, a growing area or *epiphysis* surmounted by a cap of bone and cartilage which articulates with the adjoining bone (Fig. 23.1). The region between diaphysis and epiphysis is a most important part of the bone; it is called the *metaphysis*. It has a richer blood supply than the remainder of the bone because it is an area where active growth

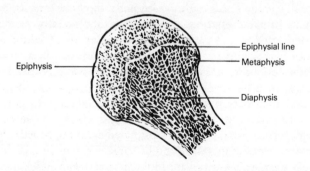

Epiphysis

Epiphysial line
Metaphysis

Diaphysis

Fig. 23.1 Diagram of a section through the end of a typical long bone.

takes place, for this reason it is one of the commonest sites of disease. The hard outer shell of the bone is called the *cortex*, and the soft interior the *medulla*.

Bone may be the site of inflammation which can be acute or chronic. If mainly the periosteum is involved it is called *periostitis*; when the medullary cavity is also involved, it is called *osteomyelitis*.

Acute osteomyelitis

This is typically a disease of children and infection is almost always due to the staphylococcus. The infection reaches the bone via the bloodstream and it is usual to find the causative lesion, such as a boil, in some other part of the body. The infection usually starts in the metaphysis and then spreads in one of three directions: (1) outwards through the cortex to the periosteum, where a subperiosteal abscess may arise producing a red, acutely painful brawny area in the tissues overlying the bone; (2) it may spread along the medullary cavity and subsequently reach the surface at other levels; (3) least commonly, the infection may break through the epiphysis into the joint cavity and cause a purulent arthritis.

The local signs and symptoms are those of acute inflammation with great pain, tenderness and redness over the affected part. The general signs are usually severe, the child having a high temperature and possibly rigors, toxaemia, sweating and even delirium. Staphylococci can usually be found in the bloodstream, i.e. *septicaemia*, which is confirmed by blood culture. If clumps of bacteria pass into the bloodstream, i.e. *pyaemia*, these may settle anywhere in the body to cause metastatic abscesses in other organs or other parts of the body.

Early diagnosis is important because if the correct treatment is started soon enough, severe bony changes can be prevented. The clinical signs are the most important guide to the diagnosis, but the presence of an abscess in some other part of the body, a raised white cell count and a positive blood culture provide confirmatory evidence. X-ray changes do not appear for about 2 weeks and are therefore no help in the diagnosis of acute osteomyelitis.

Treatment is the immediate administration of large doses of an antibiotic, such as penicillin, 200 000 units intramuscularly every 6 hours. When the organism is resistant to penicillin, one of the other antibiotics, such as tetracycline, must be used but this follows culture of the pus and determination of its sensitivities.

When pus forms it is evacuated under general anaesthesia, a wide incision being made over the area and all the pus mopped out from under the periosteum. If the bone appears unhealthy, it is drilled to allow the pus within the medullary cavity to escape. Subsequently the limb is immobilized in a light plaster cast, and if there is any risk of a nearby joint being involved this also is protected. In the case of the hip joint, which is particularly prone to pathological dislocation, light skin traction applied to the leg will prevent this happening and the nurse must take care that the traction apparatus works properly and does not chafe the skin.

Nursing care. The patient, who is usually a child, is nursed in bed with the affected part splinted and, if antibiotic treatment is started early enough, no other treatment may be necessary. The antibiotic is given for a minimum period of 3 weeks, but it may be required for longer if the symptoms persist. It is most important that it be given at the correct time so as to maintain a steady blood level.

A child with acute osteomyelitis must be encouraged to drink as much as possible and fruit drinks well sweetened with sugar or glucose provide a readily available source of calories. As the fever subsides the diet is increased and made as attractive and full as possible. Convalescence is of necessity protracted so the child's interest is stimulated with toys, books and, if possible, daily visits by the parents or relatives. It is often an advantage if the bed can be moved into the open air on fine days, so a country hospital is ideal. Schooling should be provided when possible; it not only occupies the child's mind, but makes it easier for him when he returns to his own school.

The incidence of acute osteomyelitis used to provide a good index to the general standard of public health in any district. Today it is a disease which is much less common and this is considered to be due to the improvement in the standard of living.

Chronic osteomyelitis

This is usually a sequel to acute osteomyelitis, but occasionally results from infection from less virulent organisms. Typically it is seen in a limb bone which has been inadequately treated for acute osteomyelitis.

A wound is present which breaks down from time to time to discharge pieces of dead bone or *sequestra*. Often there are sinuses from which pus will escape. As the growth of new bone in the limb usually prevents the easy escape of the sequestra, treatment consists of an operation to lay open the cavity in the bone and remove all the dead pieces. The operation is referred to as guttering or saucerizing.

The cavity is then left to heal up from the bottom so that no further discharge will occur. The bone, which is greatly weakened by this cutting away, has to be suitably splinted by a plaster of Paris cast for some months. Penicillin, or a suitable antibiotic, is usually given for a prolonged period to prevent a flare up of the original infection. There is an aphorism which says that surgery is the handmaiden of penicillin in the treatment of acute osteomyelitis, but that penicillin is the handmaiden of surgery in chronic osteomyelitis.

Brodie's abscess

When a low-grade infection enters a bone it may result in a localized lesion which is called a Brodie's abscess. This produces boring pain and from time to time a swelling over the underlying tissues. Diagnosis is made by radiography which shows a localized area of rarefaction surrounded by dense or sclerosed bone. Treatment is by laying open the cavity widely and then allowing it to heal from the bottom. The lower end of the femur is the usual site.

Tuberculosis of bones and joints

Tuberculosis of bones and joints is usually seen in children and young adults, and is always secondary to tuberculous disease in some other part of the body, such as the lungs or cervical lymph nodes. Tuberculosis is usually insidious in its onset and leads to the formation of tubercles in the bone which then break down to form cheesy or *caseous material*. The absorption of this diseased material and the decalcification which accompanies it is referred to as *caries*. Dead portions of bone or sequestra may lie in these areas and are readily recognised on an X-ray film because of their greater density. In the long bones tuberculosis first affects the epiphysis and thus more frequently breaks through into the adjoining joint by erosion of the articular cartilage than does acute osteomyelitis, which strikes at the metaphysis. In the phalanges and tarsal bones the infection often starts in the middle of the shaft or centre of the bone, probably because this is the point of entry of the main or nutrient blood vessel.

Tuberculosis of the joints arises either in the synovial membrane or in the articular surface of the bone. Certain joints are more prone to tuberculosis than others, especially the hip, knee, ankle and elbow, in that order. The onset is insidious and pain is rarely severe. Usually there is much wasting of the surrounding muscles, which are particularly prone to spasm.

The diagnosis of tuberculosis of bone and joint is greatly aided by

X-ray pictures, which show rarefaction and the typical moth-eaten appearance of the affected area.

Treatment. The treatment of this disease can be considered under two headings, general and local. The general management is best achieved in a sanatorium or special open-air hospital where the patient can rest in bed so that all of the body's energies can be deployed in combating the disease. Daily injections of streptomycin and the taking of isoniazid and PAS by mouth soon bring the infection under control and in various combinations may be given for up to 2 years. More expensive, but given by mouth, Rifampicin can replace streptomycin and PAS.

Local treatment consists in immobilization of the part by splints or plaster of Paris. Joints are splinted in the position of function which is best for them should fixation or ankylosis occur. Operation is only used to remove dead tissue where this is hindering treatment, or to introduce fresh bone where it is considered that it will stimulate healing. In elderly patients amputation may be called for since their powers of recovery are less good and they do not stand prolonged immobilization so well. Any bone or joint in the body may be affected by tuberculosis, but the two commonest sites are the hip joint and the spine and they are therefore dealt with in more detail below.

Nursing care. The day's programme should be organized with suitable rest periods. Mental relaxation is just as important as bodily rest and the nurse should endeavour to obtain the patient's confidence so that any problems that may be worrying him are discussed. The help of the medical social worker may be enlisted to overcome difficulties and it should be remembered that visiting by relatives, friends and the chaplain are of enormous importance to the long-stay patient.

The nursing of the patient will include general attention to the skin and pressure areas and frequent visits by the physiotherapist to ensure that the muscles keep their tone and do not waste. It is especially important that the position of the patient is regularly changed, otherwise stasis of the urine in the renal pelvis may lead to stone formation. Kidney stones were a common complication before the necessity of regularly moving the patient was appreciated.

Fresh air and sunshine are very important, also a liberal, well-balanced diet. The patient's appetite should be stimulated by variety in the food, which should include plenty of dairy produce, e.g.

butter, milk and cream, as these are valuable for their vitamin content as well as being highly nutritious.

The atmosphere should be one of cheerful optimism. Hobbies should be cultivated, while radio and television help to provide entertainment. Schooling for children should continue if it can be arranged.

Tuberculosis of the hip joint

This is most commonly seen in children during the first ten years of life. The disease starts just deep to the articular cartilage, either in the acetabulum or in the head of the femur, especially on the underside of the neck. There is breakdown of bone and radiographs show this as a rarefied area.

The disease then spreads to the synovial membrane, thus involving the joint proper. The muscles surrounding the joint go into spasm and the hip is held in the position of adduction and flexion.

If the disease is not arrested, there is destruction of the upper and outer part of the acetabulum so that the head of the femur dislocates and travels up on the ilium. Thus there is shortening of the limb, which is now held flexed and adducted and the patient is unable to bear weight on this leg.

The mother notices that her child limps and complains of pain in the hip or knee. The muscles are wasted and to compensate for the shortening and flexion the child develops compensatory curvature in the spine (Fig. 23.2). This takes the form of a lordosis or exaggeration of the normal lumbar convexity forwards and a scoliosis, which is the lateral curvature of the spine above this. Caseation leads to the formation of tuberculous abscesses which may track to the surface and burst. There is then a chronically discharging sinus which may become secondarily infected.

Treatment. This is of two kinds, general and local. The general treatment is that provided by a sanatorium with the daily administration of streptomycin, isoniazid and PAS; the local treatment is designed to overcome the spasm in the muscles and relieve the pressure on the joint surfaces. The leg is placed in extension, which is usually done by applying adhesive plaster to the limb and attaching a weight by means of a cord which runs over a pulley at the foot of the bed. The limb can be supported on flannel slings in a Thomas's splint. This corrects both adduction and flexion, and when the pain and spasm have been relieved, both lower limbs are

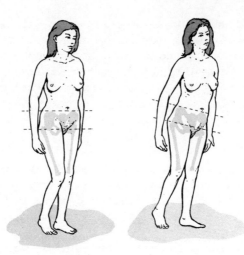

Fig. 23.2 Disease of the right hip joint. At first flexion, later apparent shortening of the limb, note the tilted pelvis.

immobilized in a plaster cast which takes the form of a double hip spica.

Nursing care. The nurse's main care is to keep the limb in exactly the position which the surgeon has put it. Dropped foot should be prevented by a suitable support to the sole and the limb must be kept warm and the skin healthy. The skin can be helped by gentle rubbing with oil and removal of dead skin.

If the disease can be arrested in its early stages a fair amount of movement and stability may be retained in the hip joint. If the joint is severely damaged by the infection it can be fused by an operation in which fresh bony surfaces are brought together. This operation is referred to as an arthrodesis.

Tuberculosis of the spine

Tuberculosis of the spine may occur at any age, but is commonest in children and young adults. The disease usually affects the body of one or more vertebrae in the thoracic region and this leads to softening of the bone. The body of the vertebra then collapses and gives posterior angulation of the spine with a very prominent deformity referred to as a *gibbus*.

The onset of the disease is insidious and the first complaint is usually one of an aching back pain which is made worse by jarring, as for example when riding a bus. The pain may radiate to the front of the body, due to pressure on the nerve roots where they emerge from their intervertebral foramina.

The muscles lying over the spine go into spasm in order to protect it from injury; this spasm can be readily felt and is best described as *boarding*. In addition, the child is most unwilling to bend the spine and this is seen typically when he picks up an article from the floor, for instead of stooping, he flexes his hips and knees and squats in order to reach down.

If a number of vertebrae are involved and collapse, each becomes wedge-shaped so that the angular kyphosis which is very noticeable behind is accompanied by crowding of the ribs anteriorly and the sternum bulges forward to produce a pigeon-chested deformity. Abscesses form and track along the fascial sheaths of the muscles. In the thoracolumbar and lumbar regions, the abscess tracks along the psoas muscle and may appear at the surface under the inguinal ligament, on the inner side of the thigh or even near the knee as a *psoas* abscess.

Tuberculous disease can affect the cervical spine and the patient may sit supporting his head in his hands; there may be torticollis or wry-neck. In the thoracic spine the most prominent deformity is a gibbus over the angular kyphosis. In the lumbar spine there is marked lordosis, which can result in the patient developing a waddling gait.

Treatment. When the diagnosis has been confirmed by X-rays the treatment is similar to that of tuberculosis in any other bone or joint. The patient is nursed in a sanatorium and antituberculous drugs are administered. The spine is immobilized in extension by placing the patient on a frame which is angulated opposite the site of the lesion. Subsequently a plaster cast is prepared in two parts: a posterior shell in which the patient normally lies and an anterior shell in which he can be turned so that the skin may be treated and kept in good condition. As soon as the lesion is well controlled an operation can be undertaken to remove dead carious bone and caseous material and insert bone grafts and bone chips in the resultant defect. Healing and bone union usually follows in a period of months.

Nursing care. Pressure sores are prevented by frequent turning, using the anterior shell, and gentle massage with talcum powder. Cheerfulness and good morale are particularly necessary with long-stay patients and visitors should be encouraged. Occupational therapy is most important. After recalcification occurs the patients is allowed to get up wearing a spinal brace for support.

The most serious complication of spinal tuberculosis, or Pott's disease, is paraplegia due to the involvement of the spinal cord. This may be caused by pressure on the cord due to the presence of an abscess, to granulation tissue, or to involvement of the blood supply to the spinal cord. *Pott's paraplegia*, as this complication is called, usually resolves spontaneously, but on occasion surgical decompression of the cord is carried out by an operation referred to as *costotransversectomy*, i.e. removal of part of the neck of a rib and the adjoining vertebral transverse process in order to drain the abscess, or by an anterior approach to the disease. The operation is completed by inserting a bone graft and bone chips.

Syphilis

Syphilis now being a rare disease, not many patients are seen with bony involvement. In the congenital form it causes periostitis, especially of the long bones in babies, but this usually is symptomless. In adults a gumma may arise in the clavicle or sternum, forming a painless spherical swelling which bursts through the skin to leave an ulcer with sharp edges and wash-leather base.

When tabes dorsalis occurs in the tertiary stage of syphilis, the lesion in the spinal cord leads to the development of neuropathic joints, often called *Charcot joints*. There is gross disorganization of the joint, which is unstable and flail and can be moved abnormally in any direction. The X-ray appearances may be bizarre. A Charcot joint is, however, painless and often produces surprisingly little disability considering the amount of destruction which has occurred. The VDRL test is always positive.

Osteo-arthritis

This disease is common after middle age and is typically a degenerative condition with slow loss of joint space, overgrowth of bone in the neighbourhood of the joint and progressive deformity. It may affect any joint, but is most crippling in the hips. The first symptom is pain and in the lower limbs this is followed by limp, muscle wasting and progressive loss of movement. Treatment in the early stages is by physiotherapy, which takes the form of heat and exercises designed to improve muscle tone. When changes have taken place which are so severe that the patient is unable to get about, operative measures may be employed.

Operative treatment. Various methods have been designed to refashion the hip joint, an operation described as *arthroplasty*. In the operation of *hip replacement* the joint is excised and the acetabulum and femoral shaft prepared for implantation of a new total hip prosthesis. This consists of two components, the femoral and acetabulum, the former usually made of vitallium, the latter of polypropylene. The operation is often performed in a theatre with special provisions to avoid the introduction of organisms into the wound.

Nursing care. A wide area of skin is prepared before operation, and the surgeon may ask for it to be painted with antiseptic such as 2 per cent iodine in 60 per cent spirit and then covered with a sterile towel. Great care is necessary in the postoperative period in order to retain as much movement as possible in the joint and maintain muscle tone. Mobilization is encouraged at the surgeon's discretion and can begin from two days postoperatively when the wound drains have been removed to one or two weeks. The patient is given a walking frame for support when first getting about. Intensive exercises to regain muscle strength are essential. Particular care of pressure areas is important, since patients undergoing this form of surgery are usually elderly and more prone to develop pessure sores. Another important point to remember in the postoperative nursing of these patients is the prevention of dislocation of the new hip joints, which can be caused by overadduction. The use of a pillow between the legs when rolling or turning the patient is useful.

The bony dystrophies

Osteochondritis (epiphysitis). There is a whole group of conditions affecting various bones in the body which is seen especially in adolescence and is characterised by a fragmentation and slow destruction of the epiphyses.

The first symptom is usually pain which, however, may only be slight. X-ray changes are often much greater than the symptoms suggest and the following are some of the better known forms of this group of diseases.

Perthes' disease. This is epiphysitis affecting the head of the femur, which becomes fragmented and mushroomed, the underlying neck being also affected so that it is shortened and the angle between it and the shaft lessened (coxa vara). Young boys are often affected and there is slight pain and limitation of movement at the hip joint. The condition is treated by immobilization with traction on the femur to prevent pressure on the femoral head. This usually produces great improvement clinically, although the X-ray changes may still be gross. There is a tendency in these patients to develop osteo-arthritis in later years.

Köhler's disease. This is avascular necrosis of the navicular bone of the tarsus, which becomes tender on pressure and enlarged, usually in the first 10 years of life. There is no treatment other than rest for pain and resolution is usually complete.

Kienbock's disease. This is a similar condition affecting the lunate bone in the wrist.

Osgood – Schlätter's Disease. This follows an avulsion of the tubercle of the tibia and is seen in children and young adults. X-rays show that the tubercle is lifted away from the shaft of the bone and there is tenderness and swelling.

Calvé's disease. This is an affection of the epiphyses of the vertebral bodies in children and produces a kyphosis.

Scheuermann's disease. This occurs in late adolescence as an epiphysitis of the secondary centres of a number of vertebrae; it produces a painful rounded kyphotic back.

Paget's disease (osteitis deformans)

This disease occurs after middle age and is more common in men than in women. There is a patchy porosis of the bones, especially of the pelvis, lower limbs and skull. Later there is deposition of much denser bone which is shown on an X-ray to have rather a woolly texture. The spine becomes curved, the tibias bowed forward and the skull enlarges so that the patient has to buy bigger hats. Deafness is common. The condition carries with it the risk of developing malignant disease in the form of osteosarcoma of bone. Injections of calcitonin relieve the pain and arrest progress of deformity.

Achondroplasia

This is a familial condition in which the bones developing in cartilage do not form properly so that the individual is a dwarf with a very typical large bossed head. Such people are often seen in circuses and may be very intelligent.

Rickets

Though this is not a true dystrophy since it is due to a vitamin deficiency, this disease can conveniently be included here. It is uncommon today because most babies and children get an adequate intake of vitamin D in the diet. This vitamin belongs to the fat-soluble group and is present in milk, eggs, butter and especially in halibut and cod liver oil. In addition, sunlight enables the body to manufacture its own supply of vitamin D. A rickety child appears unhealthy and lacks energy. The bones are tender to touch and their epiphyseal ends are swollen, especially those of the wrists and the junctions of ribs and costal cartilages (rickety rosary). When the child starts to walk the softened tibias bend outwards and produce bow legs. Treatment is provided by giving a well-balanced diet containing vitamin D, a healthy outdoor life and as much sunshine as possible.

Bone cysts

Solitary cyst. This may occur in any of the long bones and is seen typically in the upper end of the humerus and femur. It is often symptomless, but if a pathological fracture occurs through it, the resulting healing may lead to cure. Treatment is by curetting the cavity and filling it with bone chips, which act as a form of bone graft and consolidate the area.

Fibrocystic disease of bone. This condition is due to a tumour of a parathyroid gland, the secretion of which causes mobilization of calcium from the skeleton and its excretion in the urine. The body becomes generally decalcified and cysts appear in many bones, especially in the lower jaw and small bones of the hand. Treatment is removal of the affected parathyroid gland followed by the administration of calcium and vitamin D by mouth to assist the patient in recalcifying his skeleton.

Simple tumours of bone

Osteoma. An osteoma is an innocent or simple tumour of bone and consists mainly of dense or cortical bone, *ivory osteoma*, or of loose cancellous bone, *cancellous osteoma*. Treatment is its removal if it is causing symptoms.

Osteoclastoma. This is a giant-cell tumour of bone and although locally destructive it rarely metastasizes, being usually of a low grade malignancy. It occurs in the ends of long bones, just deep to the articular cartilage, and as a result of rarefaction and destruction produces cyst-like spaces which are full of blood clot. X-rays show a typical soap bubble appearance at the end of the bone. Treatment consists of scraping out the contents and filling in the cavity with bone chips. When, because of its size, it is impossible to deal with the tumour in this way, resection of the bone or even amputation of the limb has to be employed.

Chondroma. This tumour is conveniently included here although not arising from bone. It is a non-malignant or simple tumour due to a localized overgrowth of cartilage cells. Chondromas may appear on the surface of the long bones or within the medullary cavity. They show as clear areas on an X-ray film since cartilage is radiolucent. When they cause symptoms they are excised.

Malignant tumours of bone

Malignant tumours of bone are primary or secondary according to whether they arise in the bone itself or are brought by the bloodstream from a primary focus elsewhere.

Osteosarcoma. This is an extremely malignant tumour of bone which occurs characteristically in children or young adults before the age of twenty. It causes local destruction of one of the long bones of the limbs with some new bone formation around the lesion; very occasionally it is seen in a rib or other bone. Pain may be severe and the tumour grows relentlessly. The diagnosis is made only after a portion has been removed at biopsy and examined histologically. Treatment is irradiation, wide excision and when necessary, amputation. Frequently the cells have already spread to other parts of the body and secondaries develop. They are especially common in the lungs, where they form circular deposits which, when seen on an X-ray picture, resemble cannon balls. Radiotherapy is occasionally of value in reducing pain and regional perfusion may also be used.

Ewing's tumour. This is another malignant tumour of bone which arises typically in the middle of the shaft of a long bone and spreads by the bloodstream. It is a tumour arising in the endothelial osteoblasts. X-rays show an onion skin pattern of new bone. Treatment is by radiotherapy and occasionally excision but the prognosis is poor.

Multiple myeloma. This malignant disease involves the bone marrow and may produce severe pain in the bones, anaemia and loss of weight. The X-ray appearances are very typical and show multiple small punched-out areas in the cortex of the bones throughout the body, the skull, pelvis and ribs usually being the first to be involved. Diagnosis is confirmed by marrow puncture, when the malignant cells can be seen in a smear under the microscope. On heating a specimen of urine a precipitate resembling albumin may appear, only to redissolve as the temperature reaches boiling point. The substance precipitated is called Bence-Jones proteose and when present it is diagnostic of myeloma. Abnormal serum proteins are found in the blood of myeloma patients and can be demonstrated by the technique of electrophoresis in the laboratory. Treatment is given by cytotoxic drugs and steroids. Radiotherapy is helpful for localised areas of bone destruction. The anaemia which accompanies the condition often requires correcting by blood transfusion and renal failure is common.

Secondary deposits. Metastases in bone are common and the organs from which they usually arise are the kidneys, thyroid, prostate, lung and breast. Diagnosis may be difficult when the primary lesion has been overlooked. Attention may first be drawn to the existence of a primary tumour by the occurrence of a pathological fracture; for example, a woman with carcinoma of the breast may slip when boarding a bus and fracture her femur. When this is X-rayed a secondary deposit is seen to be present at the site of the fracture, having weakened the bone by local destruction. Such fractures will often unite if immobilized, but they may take a long time to do so.

24
Fractures

A fracture is a break in a bone due to violence; it may only be a crack or the ends may be widely separated. The blow may be a direct one and the bone then breaks at the point where it is struck. With indirect violence the break occurs some distance from the point of impact and the line of fracture is then likely to be spiral or oblique. Muscle action is another cause, for example the quadriceps femoris may, by sudden contraction, fracture the patella transversely.

Varieties of fracture

Closed fracture. This is often called a simple fracture. It is one in which the bone is broken without any involvement of the overlying skin or mucous membrane.

Open or compound fracture. This communicates with the exterior through a wound in the skin or mucous membrane and is therefore liable to become infected.

Greenstick fracture. This is a self-explanatory term which well describes the kind of fracture seen in a child. There is incomplete separation of the two fragments, which may be a little splintered and bent rather than broken. Greenstick fractures heal more rapidly than ordinary ones and do not require prolonged splinting.

Comminuted fracture. When a bone is broken into more than two parts it is said to be comminuted. Such a fracture is more difficult to reduce and less easy to maintain in a good position once reduction has been achieved.

Complicated fracture. This is one in which injury involves some other important neighbouring structure such as a nerve or blood vessel.

There are a number of other descriptive terms applied to fractures: an *impacted fracture* is one in which the bony fragments are jammed one into another so that force is required to free them before the position can be improved; a *crush fracture* is one in which a bone is compressed, as occurs in the vertebrae; a *fissure fracture* occurs when a crack is present in the bone without displacement, seen typically in the skull and the patella; *pathological fractures* occur where the bone has been previously weakened by disease or injury. If there is a secondary deposit in the bone, fracture is likely to occur at that site even when the stress is minimal. Similarly, if the bones are unduly fragile, as in the inherited condition *fragilitas ossium*, fractures follow trivial injuries.

Symptoms and signs

The three cardinal signs of a fracture are pain, swelling and loss of function. In addition bruising is often seen. Mobility may be abnormal, but it is unwise to test for this since a simple fracture may be converted into an open one by careless handling. There may be obvious deformity of the part due to angulation of the fragments. *Crepitus*, or the grating of the bony ends, may be felt, but this should not be sought for as it can only lead to further damage. Finally X-ray pictures will have to be taken, not only to confirm that the bone is broken and to see the position of the fragments, but also for medicolegal reasons since many injuries lead to claims for compensation.

Complications

It is convenient to consider these under two major headings of local and general.

Local complications. These will include infection when the fracture is an open one. Haemorrhage may occur due either to direct involvement of blood vessels or secondarily to destruction of the blood vessels by infection, i.e. secondary haemorrhage. Adjacent nerves may be traumatized and lead to paralysis or loss of sensation, but often much of this loss may be temporary, due to bruising and oedema.

A nearby artery may be put into spasm by contact with an irregular bony fragment, as is seen in a supracondylar fracture of the humerus in a child. If untreated this reduction in the blood supply can cause necrosis of the muscles of the forearm, a condition described as Volkmann's contracture. Gangrene may likewise occur due to injury to the main artery or pressure upon it by injudicious splinting.

In a similar manner, nerves may be injured by the pressure of a plaster cast, as may occur in the leg when the external popliteal nerve is damaged where it winds round the neck of the fibula. This injury leads to foot drop.

General complications. The general complications of fractures include *pneumonia*, which is seen most often in older people who have to stay in bed for a protracted period and so develop congestion at the bases of the lungs. *Delirium tremens* is seen in chronic alcoholics if they suffer a severe injury and is especially common after fractures; they require alcohol in moderation if this is to be prevented. *Pressure sores* may develop because the patient has to lie in one particular position. *Fat Embolism* may occur; the emboli are particles or droplets of fat which pass to the lungs or brain and produce complications which may be fatal in the severely shocked patient with extensive soft tissue injury.

The nurse should be on the look out for any of these complications, reporting them at once to the surgeon or preventing them, whenever possible, by the appropriate care.

The healing of a fracture

The first stage in the healing of a fracture is clotting of the blood which is extravasated around and between the bone ends. This haematoma becomes organised, and as a result a temporary firm calcified mass forms between the bone ends, called *callus*. This callus is invaded in subsequent weeks by bone cells or osteoblasts, which lay down new bone in thin bars or trabeculae. The callus is then absorbed and finally a moulding process takes place which shapes the bone much as it was before injury.

Many factors may delay union of a fracture. Movement of the broken bones, if it cannot be controlled, prevents deposition of calcium salts and delays healing. Lack of an adequate blood supply, which may be due to the original injury, leads to necrosis of the bones and delays union. Generalised debilitating diseases such as malnutrition, anaemia and intercurrent infections such as tuberculosis will all delay satisfactory healing of a fracture. The bones of children will heal more rapidly than those of adults, which in turn heal more quickly than those of elderly people. As a rough guide it should be remembered that the small bones of the fingers and toes unite in about 2 weeks, the forearm bones in a month, the humerus in 6 weeks, tibia and fibula in 8 weeks and femur in 12 weeks. These are all minimum times for an average healthy adult.

Treatment

First aid. Nurses are not often required to give first aid in hospital, but it is most important to know how to do so since they are often appealed to for help in public places. Good first aid should aim at treating shock and preventing any further damage due to unnecessary movement. Every care should be taken that a closed fracture is not converted into an open one and this means that some form of splintage must be used. Fractures of the upper limb can be immobilized by bandaging the arm to the trunk, and fracture of the lower limb immobilized by tying the two legs together, both above and below the knees.

The use of a *Thomas's splint* is by far the best method for fractures of the femur and such splints are usually kept at first-aid posts. The introduction of this splint in the 1914—1918 war enormously reduced the mortality from fractures of the thigh and its correct use should be understood by all. The ring of the splint is slid over the foot and up the thigh and is padded with any soft material so that it does not press unduly in the crutch or groin. Slings of flannel are put underneath the limb from one side of the splint to the other to support the leg, these are usually loosely attached to the splint before the ring is slipped over the leg. Traction is applied to the foot and maintained by fixing it to the end of the splint. A skewer may be passed through the shoe or boot just above the sole under the instep, or a bandage may be tied securely round the footwear. The bandage is then secured to the end of the splint and can be tightened by passing a stick or pencil between the two portions, twisting them up and finally securing the stick. This traction on the foot holds the femur firmly in position and helps to reduce the overriding fractured ends. This lessens pain and shock and also makes it much safer to move the patient.

First-aid kits often contain pneumatic splints. These are tied gently round the limb and inflated *by mouth* when they give excellent support. Too fierce inflation may restrict the blood supply.

If a fracture of the spine in the cervical (neck) region is suspected, the patient is kept quite flat with a small pillow in the hollow of the neck so that the head is extended.

Fracture of the spine below this level is best cared for by turning the patient gently on his face and putting a pillow under the upper chest. In this position it is safe to transport the patient.

Reduction and setting. The old term of 'setting' when applied to a fracture means aligning the broken fragments so that they are in good position. This used to be a great art among bone setters, but today the use of radiography and anaesthesia has turned the art into a science and it is generally possible to get perfect reduction. Usually a general anaesthetic is given and after reduction the fracture is immobilized by the application of a plaster of Paris cast (Fig. 24.1).

In the case of *Colles' fracture* of the wrist, for example, after reduction a piece of stockinette is applied over the forearm and a slab, made up of about six layers of plaster of Paris, is applied to the dorsum of the forearm and wrist. Light turns with another plaster bandage are then made around the forearm and into the palm and when this sets it effectively immobilizes the wrist. The patient is, however, able to move the fingers and so maintain good function during the 3 or 4 weeks that the fracture must be immobilized. In the case of many greenstick fractures no anaesthetic is required and a light plaster slab is all that is needed.

It is most important after a plaster cast has been applied that the patient be instructed to say if there is any pain or loss of sensation in the fingers or toes distal to the splint. Best of all, he should be given a printed card of instructions to take home with him such as that

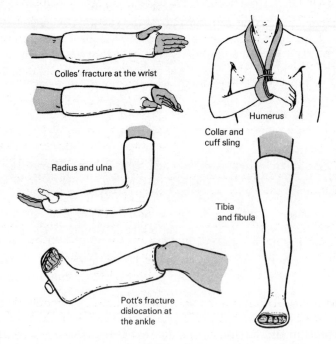

Colles' fracture at the wrist

Humerus

Collar and
cuff sling

Radius and ulna

Tibia
and fibula

Pott's fracture
dislocation at
the ankle

Fig. 24.1 Typical plaster splints for fractures.

```
┌─────────────────────────────────────────────────────┐
│  INSTRUCTION TO PATIENT WITH FRACTURE                 │
│    of...................on...................          │
│                                                       │
│  1. Do not go away from the Hospital until the Doctor │
│     says you may do so.                               │
│                                                       │
│  2. Your next visit to the Hospital must be within 24 │
│     hours, i.e., at................on................ │
│                                                       │
│  3. You should attend the Fracture Clinic             │
│     at................on................              │
│                                                       │
│  4. You should come to the Hospital at any time if the│
│     limb is painful, swelling has increased, or       │
│     fingers or toes gone numb, or changed colour.     │
│                                                       │
│  5. Do not undo bandages, move splints, or cut plaster,│
│     but come to the Hospital if something seems wrong.│
└─────────────────────────────────────────────────────┘
```

Fig. 24.2

shown in Fig. 24.2. The nurse should carefully watch the skin of toes and fingers for signs of congestion, which will show as red or blue discoloration. These should be reported to the surgeon immediately.

At the first sign of such interference with the circulation, the cast is split up with scissors or knife and the limb elevated so that swelling is reduced. If this is not done the injury to the circulation may be irreversible and gangrene or loss of function result.

It is often necessary to apply a new plaster splint after the initial swelling subsides, therefore any loosening of the cast should also be looked for and reported. No patient should be allowed to go home until the circulation is seen to be satisfactory and instructions are clearly understood that he must return if anything is amiss.

Maintenance of reduction. The maintenance of correct position of the bones by the simple methods of splinting described above may not be possible and it then becomes necessary to apply continuous skin or skeletal traction to the fracture.

Skin traction. For skin traction, the skin must be carefully shaved and then painted with tincture of benzoin to prevent the growing hairs sticking to the adhesive plaster. Long strips of adhesive plaster are then applied and bandaged firmly in place. A small wooden spreader is necessary to carry the extension cord, which is then attached to a weight over a pulley. An alternative method is to place perforated strips of foam rubber on each side of the limb and hold them in place with crêpe bandages.

Skeletal traction. Skeletal traction may be carried out by means of a Steinmann or Denham pin driven through one of the fragments of bone with the application of a stirrup and the addition of weights on an extension cord passing over a pulley (Fig. 24.3).

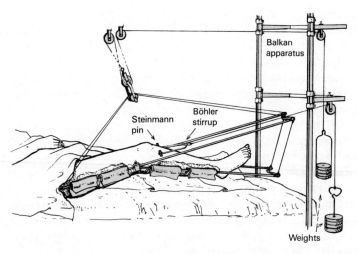

Fig. 24.3 Skeletal traction for a fractured femur. Kirschner wire with Steinmann pin in the tibia with a stirrup. (Footrest omitted for clarity.)

Nursing care. When a pin is used, a complete aseptic technique must be observed and the skin shaved, washed with soap and water and then painted with an antiseptic such as tincture of iodine. The patient is nursed in a bed prepared with fracture boards to keep the injured part level, and it is most important that the extension applied to the limb is kept up throughout the whole 24 hours of the day and night.

Pressure sores are a particular danger in such patients since they cannot move freely and great care has to be taken of the skin. Also, a foot must not be allowed to drop when the leg is in extension and a small stirrup with cotton wool and padding must be kept in place to keep it at right angles to the leg. Movement of the joints above and below the fracture should be encouraged as far as is possible without interfering with the immobilization of the affected bone.

Internal splinting. Internal fixation of a bone may be practised as opposed to the forms of external fixation described above. In internal fixation the patient is taken to the operating theatre and the fracture exposed. The bones are then properly aligned and a metal plate, or plates, screwed into position to secure the fractured parts. Bleeding during surgery is controlled by a tourniquet. The AO technique employs special plates and screws to hold the fractured ends together under tension.

An alternative method can be used in some long bones, e.g. radius and femur, an intramedullary or Küntschner nail being driven down the medullary cavity across the fracture site so immobilizing the fractured bone. After either kind of fixation a plaster cast may be applied and retained for some weeks to ensure complete fixation.

The nursing of patients with fractures, especially when the femur is involved, is made much easier by the use of a bed with a Balkan beam. This is a horizontal metal bar supported on uprights at the foot of the bed and the head; it gets its name from the Balkan war of 1903 when it was introduced by a Dutch Red Cross ambulance unit. From it the Thomas's splint or other apparatus can be supported by cords carrying small counterweights run over pulleys. By this means the patient has much more opportunity to move than if the splinted limb lies in the bed. Alternatively, metal frames may be used and are attached to the foot and head rails of the bed, they are easy to fix and less cumbersome than the wooden frame.

Rehabilitation

Restoration of function after a fracture has united is no less important than care in obtaining union of the bone in good position. As soon as possible after the fracture has been immobilized or has started to consolidate, the patient is encouraged to use his muscles and a skilful physiotherapist will see that wasting does not occur. Movements at first may have to be passive ones, i.e. the physiotherapist actually moves the joint for the patient. As soon as possible, however, active movements (i.e. ones made by the patient himself) are encouraged as these are the only ones which prevent wasting.

When the plaster cast or fixation apparatus can be removed, exercises are increased, but care has to be taken that too much strain is not put on the fracture site, since final consolidation is unlikely to take place for some months. For example, a patient who has had a fracture of the femur will not be allowed to put his whole weight on the leg when he is first out of bed, but will be given a walking frame, which allows the weight to be carried by the arms, or a walking caliper, which enables the weight from that foot to be carried by the bony points of the pelvis.

Fractures of the fingers, wrist and forearm are particularly prone to lead to stiffness of the hand, and great care is necessary in the re-education of hand movements.

When a good anatomical position cannot be obtained it is often possible to help the patient to return to the activities to which he was previously accustomed by the use of quite simple pieces of apparatus.

Occupational therapy

Many occupational therapy departments aim to produce the type of surroundings which the patient will find on returning home and to work. A model kitchen helps the patient to overcome difficulties in preparing a meal. Dressing and undressing may present problems which can be overcome by various gadgets quite easily made in the workshop. Typewriters and tools may be adapted to suit individual requirements.

It is important that the patient should regain full confidence in the use of his limb before being finally discharged from the care of the hospital.

25
Deformities and Amputations

Most of the abnormal conditions seen in the body can be classified into two large groups: congenital and acquired. The acquired conditions can be subdivided into those which are due to trauma, those due to infection and those due to neoplasm. This classification is most convenient when considering the many different kinds of deformity which are encountered in the human body.

Congenital deformities

Congenital deformities are those which are present at birth. They may be inherited from the parents, as for example web-toes, or they may be due to injury to the mother, as occurs if rubella is contracted during the first 3 months of pregnancy, when there is considerable risk of the infant being born with cataracts and heart disease. Some medicines taken in early pregnancy may be teratogenic; hence the tragedy of thalidomide, which caused phocomelia or failure of the limbs to develop properly, fortunately, very rarely.

Injury may occur during the birth of the baby, thus if the blood supply to the brain is seriously impaired, the child may be spastic.

Acquired deformities

These are seen in bone, as for example knock knees; in nerves, when as a result of poliomyelitis, there may be paralysis; in the skin, where gross scarring and contractures may result from burns; or in muscle when there may be spasm, as in the adductors of the thigh.

Most of these deformities are amenable to correction by surgical operation under anaesthesia. In addition to the general nursing care such patients need encouragement in regaining full use of the affected part.

Below are listed some of the more common deformities, but it must be remembered that no list can ever be complete and therefore only those which are likely to be seen are mentioned here.

Torticollis

This condition, which is also known as wry neck, is frequently due to injury to one of the sternomastoid muscles at birth. A swelling arises in the lower third of the muscle during the first week of life and as this resolves, fibrosis shortens the muscle and pulls the head down on that side. As a result the head is held constantly to one side and if left uncorrected, asymmetry of the face will develop. Treatment is daily manipulation which, under the supervision of a physiotherapist, the mother is very easily taught to do. If left untreated in the first years of life it requires an operation to lengthen or excise the muscle.

Upper thoracic outlet syndrome

This title covers a group of conditions a number of which are due to congenital deformity affecting the area bounded by the clavicle in front and the first rib posteriorly.

There may be an extra rib, usually called a *cervical rib*, which is really an abnormal growth of the seventh cervical vertebra. It passes forwards and can press upon the brachial plexus, the nerves of which supply the upper limb. As a result there is often weakness of the small muscles of the hand and numbness over the little finger due to compression of those fibres which go to make up the ulnar nerve.

The scalenus muscles may press on the brachial plexus and cause a *scalene syndrome*. Occasionally the subclavian artery is compressed in this site and leads to an insufficient blood flow to the hand. The condition may be bilateral and symptoms usually do not arise until later life when, due to faulty muscle tone, the shoulders tend to droop.

Another cause of this syndrome is pressure on the nerve roots in the neck by arthritic changes in the cervical vertebrae; this is known as *cervical spondylosis*. The painful, numb hand often seen in overweight women past middle age can be caused by nipping of the median nerve at the wrist by the transverse carpal ligament, the so-called *carpal-tunnel syndrome*. The pain is often worse in the early hours of the morning and the patient has to put the hands outside the bed clothes; dividing the ligament relieves the pressure.

Dermoid

This is a congenital cyst which usually arises at the junction between two parts of the body that have developed from different dermatomes or blocks of tissue. One such cyst is commonly seen at the outer end of the eyebrow and is called an *external angular dermoid*. It requires removal for cosmetic reasons and is often found to lead down to a pit in the skull.

Spine

Scoliosis. This is a lateral curvature of the spine accompanied by rotation of the vertebrae (Fig. 25.1). There are many causes; in children it may be due to faulty posture and is then associated with poor muscle development and round shoulders. Treatment is by exercises. Poliomyelitis can paralyse the muscles to one side of the spine and the unopposed pull of the muscles on the opposite side will lead to lateral curvature. A suitable support in the latter condition is a spinal brace.

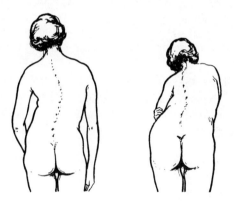

Fig. 25.1 Scoliosis. Flexing the spine also demonstrates that rotation is present.

Kyphosis. This is a curvature of the spine, the convexity of which is directed backwards. The curvature may be round or angular. It is commonly seen in the thoracic region and may be due to softening of the vertebrae by infection (e.g. tuberculosis) or malignant disease, degeneration of the intervertebral discs, osteochondritis of the vertebral epiphyses, rickets, Paget's disease or injury. Treatment is directed at the cause of the condition. When, however, the deformity is due to faulty posture, corrective exercises and the wearing of a supporting brace may be of help, or operation.

Lordosis. An exaggeration of the normal forward curvature of the lumbar spine is called lordosis. It is usually a compensatory deformity due to kyphosis in the thoracic region. It is commoner in women than men and is often seen in the obese. It frequently occurs in pregnancy. Physiotherapy to strengthen the back muscles and a supporting belt are all that are required.

Spondylolisthesis. It occurs when the fifth lumbar vertebra slips forward on the sacrum. It is usually due to congenital absence of part of the posterior portion of the fifth lumbar vertebra. The signs are lordosis with a hollow area above the sacrum, the patient complains of severe backache. Manipulation under general anaesthetic followed by immobilization in a plaster of Paris jacket may cure the symptoms in young patients.

Klippel–Feil syndrome. This is a congenital abnormality in which one or more cervical vertebrae are absent. There is thus a short neck with a low hair line and the neck movements are restricted. No treatment is possible.

Upper limb

Sprengel's shoulder. This congenital lesion is an elevation of one shoulder to a higher level than the other. It is due to the scapula on one side of the body being sited above the usual position. The condition does not require treatment.

Volkmann's ischaemic contracture. This crippling deformity follows injury to the brachial artery at the elbow and is usually due to a supracondylar fracture of the humerus. This fracture occurs in children falling from a height. In the early stages the hand is swollen, blue and painful, but with the passage of time the muscles on the front of the forearm become replaced by fibrous tissue and eventually the wrist is flexed, the fingers extended at the meta-carpophalangeal joints but flexed at the interphalangeal joints. The condition is one which can often be prevented if injuries to the brachial artery are recognized early and treated by an open operation. Great care should always be taken when treating injuries around the elbow joint to prevent the blood supply to the forearm being obstructed.

Madelung's deformity. This deformity is often familial and consists of a subluxation, or incomplete dislocation, of the ulna from the radius at the wrist joint. The lower end of the ulna thus projects backwards on the dorsum of the wrist in a rather unsightly way. Treatment is rarely called for.

Dupuytren's contracture. This affects the fascia of the palm, which becomes thickened and indurated. It causes a fixed flexion of the little and ring fingers and occasionally the middle finger. The patient is therefore unable to straighten his fingers. Treatment consists of excision of the greatly thickened palmar fascia.

Mallet finger. This common condition is due to an injury of the extensor tendon at its insertion into the terminal phalanx of the finger. As a result, the last joint of the finger is flexed and cannot be straightened. Treatment is by immobilizing the finger in extension.

Trigger finger. Also called snap finger, this is due to a thickening (stenosing synovitis) of the sheath of the flexor tendon where it crosses the metacarpophalangeal joint. It produces a snap when the finger is straightened and is treated by excision of the thickened part of the tendon sheath.

Lower limb

Congenital dislocation of the hip (CDH). This disabling congenital lesion often runs in families and is particularly common in Italy, Spain and parts of the Western Highlands of Scotland. The cause is a failure in development of the head of the femur and the acetabulum into which it normally fits. As a result when the child starts to walk he limps and the head of the femur is pushed up on to

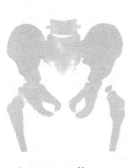
Appearance on X ray

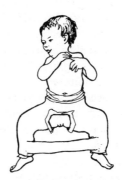
Frog plaster

Fig. 25.2 Congenital dislocation of the hip.

the side of the ilium. Treatment is manipulation of the hip joint into abduction, when the head of the femur can be made to re-engage the acetabular area. The position is maintained by a padded malleable splint or 'Frog' plaster spica (Fig. 25.2). The presence of the head of the femur in its proper place encourages further development of the joint and usually results in a satisfactory stable hip. The diagnosis should be made at birth when abduction of the hip is limited and a click can be felt by a finger placed just above the joint when full abduction is reached, *Ortolani's sign*. If, however, the condition is not treated until after the child has walked for some years, operation will be necessary to try to reconstruct the hip joint. If the condition is not seen until after puberty, the deformity is permanent.

Coxa vara. A reduction of the angle between the neck and shaft of the femur so that the thigh appears to be swung towards the midline is called coxa vara. It may be present at birth, develop later due to injury to the neck of the femur, or appear during adolescence due to slipping of the femoral epiphysis. Treatment in children consists of extension and abduction of the hip joint over a period of many months so that reduction and consolidation in the corrected position can take place.

Genu valgum or knock-knee. This consists of deviation of the legs outwards below the knees. There are many causes: rickets, poor muscle tone and trauma. Most cases respond to simple splinting at night time, wedging of the inner sides of the soles and heels or the wearing of a knock-knee brace by day. Severe knock-knee is seldom seen today, but its correction requires MacEwen's osteotomy of the lower end of the femur.

Genu varum or bow-leg. This also may be due to a number of different causes, such as horse riding and trauma. Treatment with splints is usually successful.

Genu recurvatum. Rarely the knee can be hyperextended. It is usually a congenital lesion but occasionally follows severe injuries. It is treated by means of a hinged knee cage which prevents overextension of the knee joint and thus gives stability.

Talipes. Talipes means club foot and there are a great many varieties of this condition, most of them congenital (Fig. 25.3). *Talipes equinus* means a club foot like the hoof of a horse with the toes extended downwards and the heel drawn up. *Talipes calcaneus* is

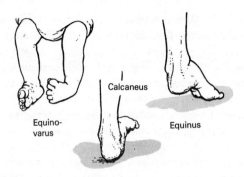

Fig. 25.3 Talipes.

the reverse of this, with the heel the most dependent part of the foot. Either of these two varieties may be further complicated by the foot being turned inward so that the sole points inwards and upwards in *varus* deformity, or the foot may be turned outwards in *valgus* deformity. The commonest congenital club foot is talipes equino-varus. Talipes in babies or young children can usually be corrected by the continuous application of splints such as those designed by Denis Browne. In adults, tenotomy is followed by the immobilization of the foot in an overcorrected position in a plaster of Paris splint, subsequently physiotherapy will be required.

Pes cavus or claw-foot. Accentuation of the longitudinal arch of the foot, often called high instep, is fairly common. In mild forms it is only a slight disability, except for the difficulty of obtaining comfortable footwear, but when severe it causes pain and difficulty in walking. It is occasionally seen complicating diseases of the central nervous system. Operative treatment consists of dividing all the tissues on the sole of the foot and forcibly flattening out the arch, which is kept in this corrected position for some weeks in a plaster of Paris cast.

Pes planus or flat-foot. This common condition may be congenital or acquired. *Congenital* flat-foot is usually painless and compatible with active exercises of every kind. *Acquired* flat-foot may be due either to lack of muscle tone (as for example when the patient has spent a long time in bed), or to injury or disease affecting the muscles or bones so that the foot becomes flat and rigid.

Treatment for the painless flat-foot is not called for. When the foot is flat, painful, but still mobile, exercises are given to strengthen the muscles and some kind of pad put in the shoe to hold up the arch.

The rigid form of painful flat-foot requires forcible manipulation under general anaesthetic, followed by physiotherapy.

Hammer toe. This occurs when two proximal phalanges, usually of the second toe, become acutely angulated on each other. The prominent joint pressing upwards on the shoe becomes the site of a callosity or *corn*. Treatment is by cutting away the adjoining portion of the two phalanges and fusing them together.

Hallux valgus. This common condition is one in which the great toe is turned outwards while its metatarsal is deflected inwards. Over the bony prominence of the metatarsophalangeal joint a *bunion* develops and when this becomes inflamed, due to the pressure of footwear, great pain may result. Treatment consists of wearing suitable shoes of adequate size, exercises to increase the tone of the small muscles of the foot and finally, when gross changes have taken place, osteotomy or wedge resection of the metatarsal to correct the deformity. It is caused by ill-fitting footwear.

Amputations

Amputations may be carried out either as an emergency or as elective operations. In the former case they are carried out immediately after the injury, and in the latter they are performed when it is convenient and the site of amputation can be chosen by the surgeon and not dictated by the injury.

Emergency amputations. An emergency amputation may be a life-saving measure, as for example where a miner has a limb crushed under a mass of fallen rock or timber. The operation performed will be the simplest that can be done under the circumstances and the soft tissues are cut across at exactly the same level as the bone is divided. This is called a guillotine amputation.

The conditions under which such an operation has to be done do not usually allow a careful aseptic or antiseptic technique and therefore the wound is left open, i.e. unsutured. In order that the soft tissue will not contact and leave a bare stump of bone in the centre of the amputation, adhesive plaster is attached to the skin and traction applied with a small weight and a pulley, so that in healing a conical stump is obtained. Delayed sutures may be inserted after a few days to bring the skin edges together if there is no obvious infection.

Elective amputation. Elective or late amputations are carried out so that the stump shall fit an artificial limb or *prosthesis*. The surgeon therefore plans to make the stump of a suitable size and length. The principles observed are that healing should be sound and by first intention, with no infection and no haematoma.

Postoperative care. Some surgeons advocate that for 24 hours following operation the patient is nursed with the stump slightly elevated on a firm pillow protected by a mackintosh cover. This position aids the venous return and so prevents excessive oedema. The use of an extension cloth supported with sandbags stops the twitching of the remaining part of the limb as this can be very uncomfortable for the patient. A bed cradle should be used to take the weight of the bedclothes, and if necessary the bed is made so that the dressings can be examined frequently in case bleeding occurs. It is important that the limb is not left too long in a position of flexion as this may cause permanent contraction of the flexor muscles. The patient may complain of severe pain which appears to come from the limb which has been removed and this pain in a phantom limb is a very real complication after the operation; morphia or other analgesic drugs will usually be ordered.

Nursing care. It is most important when dressing the stump to report at once: (1) if there is any indication that blood is collecting, (2) if there are signs of inflammation, (3) if there appears to be too much tension on the sutures. Stumps are constructed so that they shall not be end-bearing and limbs are made to fit around the surface of the stump so that the weight is distributed over a wide area. The stump is usually made as short as is compatible with the fitting of an artificial limb, for then the blood supply and nutrition is likely to be better. An amputation above the knee is usually made with about 25 cm or 10 in of femur in a woman and 30 cm or less in a man. Below the elbow 17 cm or 7 in measured from the tip of the olecranon is considered the most valuable, for if there is less than 10 cm no use can be made of the forearm stump. Above the elbow 20 cm or 8 in of humerus measured from the tip of the acromion is ideal.

The bandaging of the stump is a most important factor in its preparation for the subsequent fitting of a limb. The idea is to apply crêpe bandages so that pressure is distributed evenly over the whole stump. This encourages the absorption of the oedema and the stump is shaped to form a cone with a smooth surface.

In order to help the patient to use his new limb it is necessary that he develop his muscles, which is difficult to do when part of the limb

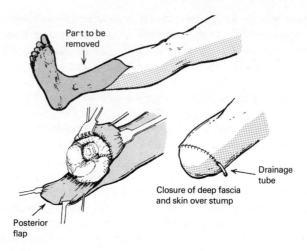

Fig. 25.4 Below-knee amputation.

has been removed. Physiotherapists have to use all their ingenuity in devising belts and pulleys and counterpressure against which the amputee can exercise his stump muscles.

In the British Isles most limbs are fitted at special centres. Patients are sent to these as early as possible after the amputation has been done in order that they may be prepared for successful limb fitting. In some patients, who have lost a hand, it may be possible to fit a cinéplastic limb which has powered joints and is operated by the patient's own tendons.

Two rather rare amputations which are occasionally performed for malignant disease require brief mention. In the *hind-quarter* amputation, the whole lower limb together with the bony wall of the pelvis is excised and the patient subsequently fitted with a limb attached to a form of tilting table which is held in place by a belt and sling over the opposite shoulder. This lower limb prosthesis is made up to size and requirements of the individual and will enable him to walk.

A *fore-quarter* amputation may be called for to remove malignant disease of the upper limb. In this case the whole arm together with the scapula and the clavicle is removed in one piece.

26
The Skin

The skin is the site of a great variety of diseases, being continually subjected to trauma, all manner of irritating substances and infection. Only a minority of these require surgical treatment; however, a number of them are considered here.

The skin provides a covering over the greater part of the body and is of supreme importance from the point of view of protection as well as for cosmetic reasons. The outer layer of the skin is constantly being worn away and this can be seen when removing clothes at the end of the day, for fine whitish scales can be shaken from them.

The deeper layers of the skin grow continuously and as these cells work their way to the surface they become keratinized (*'keratos'* is Greek for horny), thus making the skin waterproof and able to resist much of the wear and tear to which it is subjected.

Infections

Boils or furuncles

These have been mentioned already and are usually caused by staphylococcal infection of hair follicles. Treatment is to let out the pus, which can be done by applying fomentations or by incision. A good diet, healthy living, including plenty of fresh air, sunshine and the avoidance of chronic irritation which may come from the use of some soaps, detergents or other chemicals, are the best preventives against boils.

Carbuncle

This has been described already and is best considered as a group of boils which are partly confluent and which discharge pus through several openings; a large slough exists underneath the skin. This condition is seen in unhealthy patients and diabetics whose glycosuria is not adequately controlled. Treatment is the giving of penicillin or other antibiotic, applying local heat and removing dead tissue as it separates. There is no advantage in incising a carbuncle as this only adds to the subsequent scarring and in no way speeds resolution. If diabetes is present it must be treated.

Impetigo

This streptococcal infection of the skin is commonly seen in children, especially round the mouth and chin. It forms multiple pustules which are covered by a honey-coloured crust and the condition is readily spread because children naturally scratch the irritating lesion and then carry organisms, beneath their nails, to many other surfaces. Treatment is by one of the sulphonamides and the application of penicillin or a simple antiseptic locally.

Erysipelas

This is a streptococcal infection of the lymphatics which lie within the substance of and also just deep to the skin. The result is a brawny red raised area on the skin with an irregular edge which advances slowly and may spread widely. It is most often seen in aged and debilitated patients, but is much less common than formerly. Treatment is intramuscular penicillin and the local application of a soothing lotion such as one containing lead or ichthyol.

Tuberculosis

This used to be a common infection of the skin, it can appear in three different ways.

Lupus vulgaris. This is typically seen in the skin of the nose and around the ears. Tiny nodules appear which on pressure with a piece of glass give the appearance of apple jelly. As healing occurs in one part, spread occurs to another so that the disease, although painless, is difficult to cure and spreads for a long time. It may eventually clear up for no apparent reason. Treatment is mainly directed at improving the general health of the individual. At the same time streptomycin is given by injection and PAS and isoniazid by mouth.

Primary infection. Tuberculosis may occur as a primary infection in the skin of children. An ulcer with rather bluish edges appears and is very slow to heal. Suspicion that the ulcer is tuberculous is often first aroused by the massive enlargement of the regional lymph nodes.

Secondary inoculation. Occasionally someone who is working with meat, such as a butcher, develops a chronic ulcer in the hand or finger which is found to be tuberculous. Such ulcers are slow to heal and are due to *Mycobacterium tuberculosis* from the meat entering a small crack in the skin.

Syphilis

This can cause skin lesions in its primary, secondary and tertiary stages. They are described in the chapter on infection.

Diseases of sebaceous glands

The sebaceous glands are found in the skin of most parts of the body, but are especially concentrated in the face, the axilla and around the genitalia. These glands, which lie in the growing or Malpighian layer of the skin, have tiny tortuous ducts which open on the surface; the openings can readily be seen if the skin is examined through a magnifying glass.

Sebum, which is the substance excreted by the sebaceous glands, is the Latin word for suet. It well describes the greasy whitish material which the glands produce. The purpose of sebum is probably to protect and waterproof the skin. It is only when the glands produce sebum in too large amounts that a greasy appearance occurs.

Acne vulgaris

This common complaint usually affects the skin of the face at adolescence and is due to infection of enlarged sebaceous ducts by staphylococci. Many small boils or abscesses may occur and the condition can be quite disfiguring. Fortunately it usually clears up spontaneously as the period of adolescence passes, but occasionally much scarring remains as a permanent legacy from the secondary infection to which it is so susceptible. Treatment is with degreasing agents such as Cetrimide and astringent lotions applied to the affected skin, and expression of the pus and sebum from the large infected sebaceous glands. This should be carried out with strict aseptic technique. The use of ultraviolet light, which causes desquamation or peeling may assist resolution. Broad-spectrum antibiotics such as tetracycline control the infection, reduce scarring and may be given for long periods.

Sebaceous cysts

These are extremely common at all ages and are especially liable to arise in the scalp, in the skin behind the ears and on the back of the neck. Since a sebaceous cyst arises within the substance of the skin it can only be moved with it and is thus easily distinguished from a dermoid cyst, which lies deep to the skin. Sebaceous cysts can reach any size and if they become infected the contents are largely replaced by pus. Occasionally sebaceous cysts of the scalp ulcerate and give rise to a condition called Cock's peculiar tumour, which may be mistaken for an epithelioma. Sebaceous cysts are usually removed through a small incision made under local analgesia. The cysts shell out, the skin is sutured and a dry dressing applied.

Benign neoplasms

Many benign new growths or neoplasms occur in the skin and their incidence rises with increasing age. Most of them are of no significance and apart from the fact that they may be disfiguring, give little cause for anxiety.

Warts

Papillomas of the skin, or warts, may be single or multiple, can occur anywhere on the body and vary in appearance from a flat elevated area to a tumour on a stalk. They are often called veruccas and treatment is by excision. Occasionally warts are due to an infection, probably a virus, and then multiple outcrops may be seen on the hands and the face. They may occur as an epidemic among schoolchildren, especially in the summer if they use a swimming bath. Treatment of multiple warts is by curettage with a sharp spoon followed by touching the area with a silver nitrate stick. Alternatively diathermy may be used to get rid of them. When they occur on the sole of the foot, they are driven into the surface by the weight of the body and constitute plantar warts. They are then best treated by the application of 40 per cent salicylic plaster.

A special variety of wart or condyloma occurs around the anus in secondary syphilis and is highly infective.

Mole

Moles may be hairy, pigmented or both. A pigmented mole is a simple or benign melanoma ('*melanos*' is Greek for black), so called because of the dark pigment melanin which occurs in the cells. Pigmented moles are very common at all ages, but especially in old people. They seldom require excision except when they are particularly disfiguring, as on the face. Their importance lies in the fact that they be mistaken for malignant melanomas, which are extremely lethal.

Haemangioma

This is a tumour of blood vessels and not primarily of the skin, but since it occurs so commonly in the skin it is again mentioned here. In babies, haemangiomas often appear very soon after birth and grow rapidly during the first months of life. They are described as *cavernous* or *capillary* according to the size of the blood vessels of which they are composed. If left alone, they almost entirely disappear after a few years. Occasionally their size or position demands treatment; they may then be excised or frozen with the cryoprobe. Portwine lesions which are intradermal haemangiomas never disappear; they are treated by laser.

Molluscum sebaceum

This benign lesion on the face grows in a few weeks to resemble a rodent ulcer. It ulcerates centrally and heals with little scarring.

Malignant neoplasms

Basal cell carcinoma

A basal cell tumour or rodent ulcer is one which is locally malignant, but does not metastasize to distant parts of the body. It is typically seen in the skin of the face around the eyes, ears and nose and is more often found in those who are exposed to intense sunlight, although it is not usually seen in coloured patients. It is especially common in Australia and South Africa.

The ulcer takes the form of a tiny pit with heaped up edges and the skin has a rather gelatinous or translucent appearance. A little crusting often occurs over the centre of the ulcer, which spreads by its outer edge. The diagnosis is made by removing a small portion and examining it under the microscope. Treatment is by radiotherapy or radium, which gives excellent cosmetic results. Occasionally it is necessary to excise a rodent ulcer, when a generous surrounding area of healthy skin must also be removed if recurrence is to be prevented. Rodent ulcers are often multiple.

Squamous cell carcinoma

This malignant tumour of the skin occurs most commonly around the lips, in the mouth and over any part of the skin of the limbs. It starts as a small indurated area which breaks down centrally and the edge of the ulcer has a characteristic rolled over appearance. It spreads by the lymphatics to the nearby or regional lymph nodes; later it may be disseminated in the body by the bloodstream. Treatment is by wide excision or radiotherapy. Squamous cell tumours vary greatly in their malignancy and a biopsy often allows the pathologist to state how invasive any particular tumour is likely to be.

Some squamous lesions are produced by certain physical agents called carcinogens. They are commonly seen, for example, in men who work with tar or oil. Squamous cell cancer of the scrotum used to be frequently seen in chimney sweeps because their clothing was impregnated with soot, which contains many of the hydrocarbons of coal, and it was the first tumour to be the subject of industrial compensation in Great Britain. Mule spinners who worked in the cotton industry and whose overalls were saturated with oil developed similar lesions.

Melanoma

A malignant melanoma may occur in the skin on any part of the body, but shows a predilection for the sole of the foot, the skin just beneath the nails and the back. Unfortunately many melanomas occur in young adults, are extremely malignant and spread rapidly both by the bloodstream and the lymphatics.

Treatment is by a generous and wide excision followed by immediate skin grafting as soon as the diagnosis is made, but it is never possible to predict when a cure will be obtained. With rare exceptions the tumour is extremely resistant to radiotherapy of any kind. Chemotherapy by regional perfusion is sometimes helpful.

The nails

The nails are subject to many of those diseases which affect the skin, such as eczema and psoriasis, but only two conditions need concern us here.

Paronychia, perionychia

Either word describes inflammation of the tissues beside the edge of the nail, which is usually due to staphylococci and streptococci, especially where the skin tends to overhang the nail. There is swelling, tenderness and pain, often of a throbbing character. The suppuration destroys the tissue beside the nail and later, by undermining the nail, loosens it so that it may fall off (Fig. 26.1). Treatment consists of local heat, helping the pus to escape and removal of the unhealthy tissue so that a fresh nail may grow in its place. These conditions are treated in the day-surgery department, and any operation is performed under local analgesia introduced as a 'ring block' at the base of the finger.

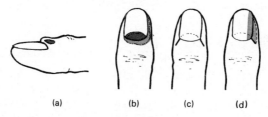

Fig. 26.1 Paronychia (a) pus in the nail fold, (b) lateral extension, (c) incisions in the nail fold, (d) unroofing the lateral extension.

Ingrowing nail

Typically seen in the great toe, this condition is due to an overgrowth of the tissues beside the nail, which then overhang it. The overgrowth is due to mechanical factors, such as the pressure of ill-fitting shoes, or to low-grade infection which causes hyperaemia and exuberant granulation tissue. In some families there appears to be a predisposition to ingrowing toe nails.

Prevention is better than cure, therefore the nails should be carefully cut so that infection is avoided. When the condition is established it is necessary to give the patient an anaesthetic and excise a strip of nail, nail bed and adjacent skin. This allows the boundary between the nail and skin to regrow normally.

Plastic surgery

Skin is more commonly injured than any other part of the body and because healthy skin serves such an important function in protecting the tissues, a great many operations are carried out to repair, replace or transplant it. Skin is one of the principal tissues with which plastic surgeons work, but they also use bone and cartilage to rebuild certain areas of the body.

Skin grafting is the method by which large denuded or scarred areas are replaced by healthy and supple epithelium. Grafts may be free, i.e. detached pieces of skin, or pedicled, i.e. the skin remains attached by one end until the blood supply has developed in the other. Alternatively, using microsurgical techniques, a flap of skin complete with blood vessels is anastomosed to the circulation in another part of the body.

Free grafts

These are of three main kinds:

Thiersch grafts. These are thin layers of the outer surface of the skin which are cut by means of a razor or dermatome, such as those devised by Blair-Humby or Padgett, or by an electric dermatome. Varying thicknesses of epithelium are removed and the donor site most frequently used is the upper and inner thigh. The skin is spread out and usually applied with a backing of tulle-gras or paraffin gauze, the thicker grafts being sutured in place.

Wolfe grafts. A Wolfe graft consists of the whole thickness of the skin and therefore the area from which it is taken has to be sewn up after its removal or covered with a Thiersch graft. If the graft is to 'take', every particle of fat has to be dissected from its deep surface before it is stitched into position. This method is most useful for areas where much wear is likely to take place, for example in the hands. Free flaps complete with vascular pedicle transplanted microsurgically are used in preference where possible.

Pinch, reverdin, or sieve grafts. These consist of tiny cones of skin which are obtained by picking up the skin with sharp forceps or the point of a needle and then slicing it across with a knife. The little circle of skin so obtained is thickest at its central part and thinnest at the periphery. Such grafts can be applied by scattering them over a wide area, where they subsequently grow together to form a complete layer of skin. They are rather unsightly and therefore not often used.

Pedicle or tubular grafts

These consist of flaps of skin with their attached subcutaneous tissue fashioned so that they keep their blood supply at one end while the free end is moved to the site where skin is required. When the graft has 'taken' the base of the pedicle is detached and the tube opened out and sewn into place. The ingenuity of plastic surgeons in employing tubed pedicles was only equalled by the fortitude of their patients, whose treatment might be spread over years, and micro-surgery is now outdating this technique.

Skin grafting

The essentials for successful skin grafting are that the donor skin should have been carefully cleaned with soap and water and all hairs shaved away. Antiseptics are not applied to the skin in case they injure it. There must be no infection either locally or in other parts of the body. The area which is to be grafted should be healthy and preferably covered by moist, red, healthy granulation tissue.

The graft must be held in position by means of firm pressure over its whole surface and should be left undisturbed until it has 'taken', which is usually after about 8 days. The first dressing is often done by the surgeon in the operating theatre and great care is always necessary when removing dressings from grafts in order not to damage them. Light plaster casts and various splints are called for to prevent movement of the graft during the critical days when it is growing its new blood supply. Dressings usually take the form of tulle-gras because it is possible to remove such an application without unduly disturbing the underlying skin. Patients should be warned not to interfere in any way with the dressings, but usually they are only too pleased to co-operate. The administration of antibiotics to patients who are undergoing skin grafting helps to control infection and are essential in this field of surgery.

Pressure sores

Pressure sores are commonly referred to as 'bed sores', 'decubitus ulcers' or 'ischaemic ulcers'. An increased understanding in the pathogenesis of pressure sores is reflected in the relatively new term 'distortion sores'. Prolonged pressure, however, is still accepted as the main cause, although few sores can be blamed on a single causative factor. Both nurses and doctors alike should be aware of the factors predisposing to sore formation, since their care should be aimed at reducing, if not eliminating, these causes.

Certain groups of patients fall into a high-risk category and these include the unconscious or comatose, obese, undernourished, wasted, elderly, incontinent and those suffering from systemic infections and circulatory, skin, neurological, metabolic or skeletal disorders. Additional to the above are imposed stresses applied by nursing and medical staff, albeit unwittingly, and it is to these factors that particular attention should be drawn. Bad lifting techniques, where patients are 'dragged' rather than raised to a seated position, cause friction on skin. Reduced activity is often a result of illness, but is also evident in patients who are capable of movement but feel restricted by their very admission to hospital. Excessive washing and massage, and unrelieved support of pressure points are also contributing factors. When a pressure sore has developed local treatment is required to prevent ulceration. Should ulceration of the area ensue, surgical intervention is often necessary to excise dead tissue, drain any pus and clean the wound. A dry occlusive dressing should be applied and occasionally it becomes necessary to aid healing by skin grafting, which is performed under general anaesthesia.

Recommended reading:

'A review of pressure sore pathogenesis' by P. Lowthian, *Nursing Times*, Jan 20, 1982, pages 117–121.

27
The Eye

The treatment of injuries and diseases of the eyes is extremely specialized, nursing skill of a high order being required. We are concerned here primarily with ophthalmic surgery, but much eye work is done by doctors who do not operate and are often called refractionists (because they measure the patient's refractive error and prescribe suitable spectacles). An oculist is a doctor who specialises in eye diseases, while an optician is someone who deals with optical instruments and an ophthalmic optician with spectacles.

A knowledge of the anatomy of the eye is essential for an understanding of the various diseases which may occur in this rather intricate part of human anatomy (Fig. 27.1).

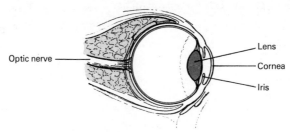

Fig. 27.1 Vertical section through the eye.

Cornea

This is the clear area in front of the eye which is kept moist by tears and is protected by the eyelids. The cornea is particularly susceptible to injury and this leads to *ulceration*. Occasionally a small foreign body, such as a splinter of metal, becomes imbedded in the cornea and requires removal by means of a mounted needle or spud. When the cornea is inflamed, the condition is called keratitis. Ulcers of the cornea often require cauterization in order to speed up healing.

Iris

The iris is the coloured circular area, blue or brown, which regulates the amount of light allowed to pass into the eye, and the aperture at its centre is called the pupil. A bright light causes the iris to close down and make the pupil tiny, whereas in the dark, the pupil is wide, due to dilatation. Inflammation of the iris is called *iritis* and if adhesions occur between the iris and the lens, which is immediately behind it, they fix the iris. These adhesions are called *synechiae*.

Lens

The lens is not a static structure, but can change its convexity and therefore its focal length through the agency of a muscle, the *ciliary muscle*, which by contraction relaxes the lens. When the lens becomes more spherical it allows one to focus on objects nearer to the eye. At rest, the eye is focused into the distance because of the tension of the ligaments which support the lens. When the lens is unable to focus properly the condition is called a *refractive error* and this calls for the use of spectacles. Opacity of the lens, which may be congenital and is seen in diabetes and the aged, is referred to as a *cataract*. A cataract can be removed and the patient then provided with specially powerful lenses in order to restore vision.

Retina

The posterior part of the eyeball is made up of a great number of sensory organs called rods and cones which are sensitive to light rays. Each is connected to a nerve fibre and all these fibres collect together and pass out of the posterior part of the eye as the *optic nerve*. The retina may become *detached* and if this happens a blind area or *scotoma*, corresponding to the amount of injury, is noticed by the patient. The retina is occasionally the site of tumours which are usually highly malignant, their pathological names being *glioma* and *retinoblastoma*.

Fundus

This term is applied to the posterior part of the eye and especially to what is seen with an ophthalmoscope. This instrument allows a view to be obtained of the *optic disc*, which is the area where the optic nerve leaves the retina, and also of many of the vessels supplying the retina. Elevation of the optic disc due to increased pressure within the skull is called *papilloedema* and is an important sign in brain tumour and other diseases of the central nervous system.

Anterior chamber

The cavity between the front of the lens and the cornea is referred to as the anterior chamber and is filled with a fluid called *aqueous humor*. This fluid circulates through the pupil and leaves the anterior chamber through the *canal of Schlem* at the perimeter of the iris. If this route becomes blocked, as it may do in old age and certain diseases of the eye, then the pressure rises in the anterior chamber causing great pain and hardness of the eyeball, a condition called *glaucoma*. If the pressure is not relieved, the eye will be destroyed and therefore eserine or pilocarpine is given in order to contract the pupil and open up the canal. If this is not successful the operation of iridectomy may be necessary in order to make an opening through the iris and allow the fluid to circulate.

Atropine causes dilatation of the pupil by paralysing the iris, which may then block the canal of Schlem and precipitate an acute attack of glaucoma. This is one of the risks of giving atropine drops to older patients or those with diseases of the iris.

Structures outside the eyeball

Attached to the outer surface of the eyeball are the extrinsic muscles which move the eye in all directions. If these muscles are not properly co-ordinated in the two eyes the imbalance causes double vision or *diplopia*. The result is a *squint* or *strabismus* in which the eyes may swing inwards and *converge*, or swing outwards and *diverge*. Squint is common in babies and childhood and is usually due to a lazy eye or lack of co-ordination, although the cause is not known.

The treatment of squint consists in the correction of any refractive error and the good eye is covered in order to re-educate the muscles on the faulty side. The imbalance may be corrected by advancing or recessing the muscles, that is by detaching them from the orbit and resuturing in the new position.

Orbital cellular tissue

The packing tissue between the eyeball and the bony orbit is made up largely of fat with a small amount of fibrous tissue, blood vessels and nerves. If this tissue becomes infected the resultant oedema forces the eye forwards and congests the eyelid, a condition referred to as *chemosis*. In hyperthyroidism or Graves' diseases there is lymphocytic infiltration and oedema of this fat and the eye muscles, and the pushing forward of the eye is called exophthalmos.

Eyelids

A foreign body such as a piece of grit or a tiny fly may get under one of the eyelids and cause great irritation until it is removed. If the lid is steadied by grasping the eyelashes it may be possible to see the foreign body and remove it. If this is not successful the lids may be everted or turned inside out by placing something firm such as a matchstick on the skin and pulling on the lashes.

A *stye* or *hordeolum* results from infection of a hair follicle of one of the lashes. Treatment is by hot bathing; sometimes removal of the affected hair allows the pus to discharge more readily.

A *Meibomian cyst* occurs when the duct of a tarsal gland in the lid becomes blocked. Subsequently it may become infected and produce an abscess. The cyst requires scraping out with a sharp spoon, followed by the application of something soothing. Inflammation of the lids as a whole is usually called *blepharitis*. Inflammation of the conjunctiva is called *conjunctivitis*, is common and produces a 'red eye'.

Ptosis. This means drooping of the eyelid and may be congenital or acquired. It is usually due to damage to the nerve supply to the muscle which raises the upper eyelid, and in extreme cases the patient has to tip the head backwards in order to see from under the lids. Treatment is by an operation in which a strip of fascia is threaded under the skin to hold up the lid.

Lachrymal apparatus

The lachrymal, or lacrimal, apparatus consists of a gland and sac for each eye, the gland lying to the outer side of the eye and just above the canthus, the sac lying at the inner canthus and having a duct, the nasolacrimal duct, which drains into the nose (Fig. 27.2). Lacrimal

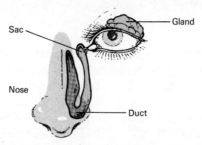

Fig. 27.2 Lacrimal gland at the outer border of the eye makes tears which collect in the lacrimal sac at the inner border and drain into the nose via the lacrimal duct.

fluid (or tears) is produced continuously and passes forward over the surface of the cornea lubricating and protecting it against injury and infection. The fluid is gathered up into a little pair of puncta or openings at the inner end of the two lids and drains continuously into the nose. If the tear duct is blocked, tears run down the cheeks all the time, a condition called *epiphora*. Treatment is by unblocking the duct with special probes or by an operation which provides a new lining with a skin graft at the site of the old one.

Congenital and hereditary eye diseases

Many eye conditions are congenital and they are often inherited in certain families. Occasionally congenital eye conditions result from disease or injury to the mother during pregnancy. The most important cause of this is rubella, or german measles, contracted by the mother during the first 3 months of pregnancy. As a result the baby may be born with congenital cataracts and may also have congenital heart disease.

At delivery, if there is serious infection of the birth canal, the baby's eyes may be infected and ophthalmia neonatorum results. Because of this it is usually routine practice to wipe the eyes with a sterile cotton wool swab as soon as the baby is born.

When the baby is born prematurely it may be necessary to give him oxygen to keep him alive. If the concentration of oxygen given is high and continuous, changes take place in the eye which lead to a layer of fibrosis behind the lens. This condition of *retrolental fibroplasia* led to many cases of blindness following the introduction of incubators supplied with oxygen for premature newborn babies.

Examination of the eyes

Acuity. Visual acuity or accuracy of vision is measured in a standard way so that the vision of different people can be compared. A set of *Snellen's types*, which is familiar to all, is hung on the wall, each line of letters has a number which represents the distance in metres at which a person with normal vision can read them. The patient stands 6 metres away and sees how many lines he can read. With normal vision the lowest line but one, numbered 6, can be read at this distance and eyesight is then expressed as 6/6. If he can only read the top line, numbered 60, the eyesight is said to be 6/60, and if less than this, resort is made to counting the surgeon's fingers when held in front of the patient.

Fields. The size of the visual fields can be measured by means of an apparatus which records the perimeter of vision. If there are any blind spots within this field they can be mapped out by means of a small object held on the end of a stick while the patient maintains the eyes looking in the same direction. Blind areas, or scotomas, are usually due to lesions in the retina or optic nerve.

Fundi. The fundi are usually examined with an ophthalmoscope, which has a battery in the handle but requires the patient to be out of direct light. Much can be learned from seeing the optic disc and the surrounding area of the back of the eye, since this allows inspection not only of the nerve elements and retina but also of the blood vessels. For example, in patients with severe hypertension the arteries often appear constricted like silver wires and may even nip the veins where they cross them. In diabetes and renal failure the changes are diagnostic.

Conjunctivae. The conjunctival sac may contain a foreign body, and a careful search has to be made for this. The presence of a small piece of grit in this area may abrade the cornea, and if there is any doubt as to injury of the latter a drop of fluorescin is put in the sac. This makes any irregularity of the surface of the cornea immediately visible.

Refraction. By means of this it is possible to determine refractive errors and the lenses necessary to correct them. The refractionist sits in a darkened room with a special mirror which has a tiny central hole through which he views the patient's fundus. By having a wide variety of lenses he can discover which is necessary to correct the patient's refractive error. A less accurate method is by using Snellens type and a spectacle frame in which different lenses can be interposed until one is found with which the patient sees clearly.

Slit lamp. This is a powerful light with a minute beam with which it is possible to examine all parts of the eye very accurately.

Nursing treatment

Drops or *guttae* are used for most of the drugs which are introduced into the eye. Typical antiseptic ones are silver proteinate and sulphacetamide. Analgesics are used to relieve pain in the eye and also to allow minor operations and investigations. The most commonly employed is 2 per cent cocaine.

It may be necessary to dilate the pupil and for this purpose 1 per cent atropine or 2 per cent homatropine is used. For constriction of the pupil 1 per cent eserine or 1 per cent pilocarpine is necessary.

Drops for the eye should be introduced by means of a special dropper. This is held so that it is just not touching the lids and, while the lower lid is steadied, the patient is asked to look up and the solution is allowed to flow into the inferior conjunctival fornix. The patient is warned before the drop is instilled and asked not to squeeze the eye shut. By using this technique there is no risk of touching or injuring the eye and the dropper is unlikely to be rendered unsterile so that it may be returned to the bottle for future use.

Other methods of introducing drugs into the eye are by means of a special tube containing ointment; from the nozzle of the tube a small ribbon of ointment is squeezed into the lower conjunctival fornix. Alternatively, the ointment may be applied on a glass rod which is gently laid into the lower conjunctival fornix, the lid being closed and the rod withdrawn. Lamellae, which consist of a drug impregnated in thin discs of gelatine, readily dissolve in the conjunctival sac and are also used.

Heat is applied to the eye in the following way. A wooden spoon is wrapped with cotton wool which is held in position with an open-wove bandage. The spoon is then placed in a basin of boiling water, lifted out, allowed to cool for a moment and held as near the eye as possible. The eye is kept closed and bathed in the steam. After ten minutes of this treatment the lids are carefully dried with cotton-wool swabs, working from within outwards and using each swab once only. Alternatively, electric pads may be used to provide the heat. It may be necessary to apply heat by these methods 3 or 4 times a day. Any prescribed ointment may then be applied. If the patient's eyesight is poor this procedure should be carefully supervised.

When it is necessary to irrigate the conjunctival sac, or an eye socket after enucleation, a small retort-shaped flask called an undine is used. This can be controlled by putting a finger over the filling aperture and releasing it gently so that the stream of fluid can be stopped or started at will. For irrigation of the eye, normal saline or bland alkaline lotion, e.g. $\frac{1}{2}$ per cent solution of sodium bicarbonate, may be ordered and should be used at blood heat; this may be tested by running the fluid over the hand. The patient is asked to co-operate by holding a receiver against the cheek to collect the lotion. First the fluid is allowed to flow on the cheek and then is slowly directed into the inner canthus of the eye. The patient is instructed to move the eyeball in all directions to ensure thorough irrigation, the undine being held 3 cm from the eye. At the completion of this treatment, the lids are carefully dried with cotton-wool swabs.

Postoperative care

When a patient has had a major operation on one of the eyes a special technique of nursing is necessary, both to maintain confidence and morale and to prevent any untoward injury. The patient is asked to avoid any sudden movement of the head and the nurse should explain the importance of this before operation. After operation sedatives are used freely and a comfortable sitting or semirecumbent position adopted. As pain begins to be felt because the local analgesic is wearing off, further sedation is given. Codeine may be all that is called for, but pethidine may be necessary by mouth or by injection. Morphia is generally avoided because of its pharmacological effect on the eye.

It is advisable for the ward to be kept as quiet as possible as any sudden noise might cause the patient to jump. The nurse should speak gently and give warning of anything she is going to do. Care must be taken to prevent the patient coughing, sneezing should be controlled by pressure on the upper lip and vomiting must be avoided at all costs.

When the patient is settled down for the night, it may be necessary in older patients or children to fix the arms and prevent plucking at the bandages while not fully conscious. If awake during the night the patient will need reassurance, and the nurse should be near at hand to give any explanation or help required.

The first dressing may be ordered for the day following operation, but in some cases is deferred until the fifth day. This is often done by the surgeon, usually in a special dressing room attached to the eye ward. Dark glasses may be worn when the bandages are finally removed. It is most important to avoid any pressure on an eye which has been operated upon, so that great care must be taken to ensure that the pad and bandage lie lightly in position.

The patient is discouraged from trying to strain at stool, and the bowels are either allowed to become constipated or very mild aperients are given. Enemata are not used.

After some eye operations the surgeon may recommend the patient to sit out of bed in a chair from the first or second day following operation, e.g. after cataract extraction. In other cases the patient may have to stay in bed longer, and after an operation for corneal graft or retinal detachment this may be 2 or even 3 weeks.

While helping these patients to move, the nurse must be careful to avoid any surprise and should give due warning of any change of position. The patient is ready for discharge from hospital after having learnt to walk about the ward; this may take from 10 to 14 days.

Special provision is made for blind and partially sighted people in Great Britain and patients are usually given full information about this by the medical social worker. Knowledge that the future does not have to be either difficult or lonely is of great help in strengthening morale and speeding convalescence.

28
Paediatric Surgery

Paediatric surgery, unlike any of the other specialities which have been described in this book, does not confine itself to one particular region of the body as does thoracic surgery, nor to one particular system as does orthopaedics, nor yet to any particular group of diseases, but deals with the surgical care of the whole child. This does not mean merely that smaller beds must be used in the wards and smaller instruments in the operating theatre, for there are many conditions which are only seen in this young age group. In addition the manner in which these patients respond to injury and disease is often quite different from that of adults.

It is convenient to consider the newborn or neonatal baby separately from the rest of this age group because special problems and conditions are encountered during the first 2 weeks of life. When a baby is born he suddenly changes from an environment where he is entirely dependent on his mother to one where he must breathe, adjust his water balance, use his gastro-intestinal tract, all within a matter of a few hours. The circulation also changes to accommodate itself to the new supply of oxygen, which now comes from the lungs instead of from the placenta.

A baby born before the thirty-sixth week is said to be *premature* and these babies present special problems in surgical management when they require operation. The majority are of low birth weight, i.e. under 2500 g and with a head circumference of 32 cm or less. Size is no contraindication to surgery, but tiny premature babies require to be nursed in a thermostatically controlled incubator with an oxygen supply so that they are in a constant environment.

Neonatal surgery

Atresia of the oesophagus

A newborn baby who has a blue attack and vomits when fed should be suspected of having atresia of the oesophagus until proved otherwise. This maxim has resulted in saving thousands of babies in recent years since, if treated early enough, this condition is usually capable of cure. In this condition the oesophagus fails to develop normally and terminates in a blind pouch in the upper part of the chest, while the lower part of the oesophagus usually communicates with the trachea near its bifurcation (Fig. 28.1). As a result when the baby is given milk, it spills over from the pouch into the trachea and causes a choking and cyanotic attack. It is then usually vomited and coughed up. It is recommended practice that a newborn baby be given sterile water as its first feed. Meanwhile with every deep breath a little air passes from the trachea into the lower part of the oesophagus, thus filling and distending the gut. The diagnosis is confirmed when a fine lubricated catheter, passed via the mouth or nose, is arrested within 10 or 12 centimetres. Visual proof is obtained by injecting not more than 1.0 ml of lipiodol down the catheter and taking a radiograph, when the blind upper pouch will be outlined.

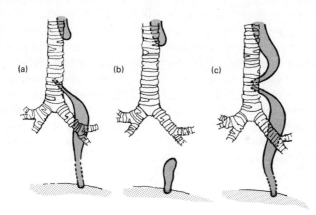

Fig. 28.1 Tracheo-oesophageal fistula: (a) Commonest type, (b) defect of oesphagus, (c) double fistula.

Nursing care. The baby is immediately transferred to hospital and nursed in the head down position, being turned from side to side every half hour so that the lungs expand well. Penicillin is given to combat infection in the chest and as soon as possible the patient is taken to the operating theatre, an intravenous infusion set up and the oesophagus reconstructed through a right-sided thoracotomy.

Since it is difficult for babies to regulate body temperature to their surroundings, it is particularly important to prevent undue chilling when they undergo surgery. One of the following methods can be used. The baby can be wrapped in ordinary domestic aluminium foil or several layers of gamgee. Where the facility of a 'baby therm' is available, this is ideal. This is a specially designed piece of apparatus with a heated mattress and overhead heating element on which the baby is placed for surgery. Raising the environmental temperature in theatre is helpful. The use of a humidifier to warm and moisten the gases breathed by the baby is also advisable. Atropine by hypodermic injection, 0.3 mg, may be ordered as premedication. The skin may be prepared in the normal way.

After operation the baby is nursed with the head of the cot a little raised. The temperature is recorded four hourly and the pulse and respiration more frequently at first. An incubator will be used. The postoperative care includes strict observation and recording of the amount of intravenous fluid given. The administration of parenteral fluid to infants is best recorded in terms of so many millilitres (ml) per hour.

Small feeds are given either by a fine indwelling polythene tube which passes down the oesophagus into the stomach, or through a gastrostomy tube. The pleural cavity is drained for 4 to 8 days and the tubing led to an underwater seal. The amount and type of drainage is observed and all precautions taken to ensure that the fluid level is 'swinging'. Care should be taken not to allow the entry of air into the pleural cavity through the drainage tube.

Usually the baby can swallow normally at the end of the first week and there is no disability so long as the anastomosis heals without narrowing. It should be remembered that atresia of the oesophagus may be associated with other congenital abnormalities, such as imperforate anus, and therefore a thorough examination should be made.

Intestinal obstruction

Any newborn baby who vomits bile or bile-stained material should be considered to have intestinal obstruction until it is proven otherwise. This second maxim has also saved innumerable babies by drawing attention to a condition which is not uncommon in the newborn and which is invariably fatal if not treated urgently. Vomiting should not be mistaken for the gentle regurgitation of a little fluid which many healthy babies produce after feeding. X-ray pictures of the abdomen are essential for diagnosis. Obstruction of the small bowel is caused by many conditions.

Malrotation. This is the commonest form of intestinal obstruction. During foetal life the small bowel passes out into the umbilical cord and later returns to the abdominal cavity in a regular order; if however it fails to do this in the correct way, the bowel lies twisted so that the caecum is usually found on the left side. The malrotation leads to obstruction of the small bowel, which may be intermittent. Treatment is by immediate operation through a generous incision which allows all the bowel to be lifted out of the wound and untwisted. It is returned in the correct order and if the duodenum is constricted by adhesions, Ladd's band, this is divided.

Duodenal stenosis. Narrowing may occur at any level of the small bowel, but is commonest in the duodenum, when it is called duodenal stenosis. In recent years it has been noticed that a high proportion of babies with duodenal stenosis are mentally deficient, many of them having Down's syndrome.

Atresia may occur where an area of bowel fails to develop; in the small bowel it is commonest in the ileum, but it is also frequently found in multiple sites.

Meconium ileus (cystic fibrosis of the pancreas) is a rare condition causing intestinal obstruction in the newborn and is due to pancreatic fibrosis with lack of adequate pancreatic secretion. Meconium is normally found in the bowel at birth. It is greenish black and composed of exfoliated intestinal epithelium, swallowed liquor and epithelial cells mixed with bile and the enzymes from the pancreas. The meconium in cystic fibrosis condition is abnormally viscid or sticky and obstructs the bowel. Treatment is by excision of the lower small bowel containing the viscid material and renewal of continuity of the bowel by anastomosing the two ends. The baby is given pancreatin by mouth.

Strangulated hernia. A hernia in the newborn may become strangulated, which means that the bowel in the hernial sac cannot be returned to the abdominal cavity and the blood supply to the bowel is obstructed. Immediate fluid replacement by the intravenous route, aspiration of the stomach followed by operation is necessary to relieve the obstruction. The commonest hernia to be affected is inguinal, but herniation through the diaphragm into the pleural cavity may also lead to intestinal obstruction. A baby may be born with a congenital diaphragmatic hernia, breathing is distressed and immediate operation is necessary.

Nursing care. A newborn baby with intestinal obstruction needs

care similar to that for oesophageal atresia. The stomach is aspirated
with a fine catheter passed nasally and the baby is turned regularly to
keep the lungs well expanded. Intravenous fluids are given sparingly
for fear of causing pulmonary oedema in the neonate. Fluids are
allowed by mouth as soon as bowel sounds return, and any urine or
faeces passed is charted. Expressed breast milk, obtained from the
mother, is used for feeding.

Exomphalos or omphalocele

In this condition there is a deficiency of the anterior abdominal wall
in the region of the umbilicus. The area is covered by a thin
transparent membrane and the sac may contain most of the bowel
and also the liver, spleen and other organs. Traditionally the
midwife should hand the baby to the surgeon if a cure is to result, a
saying which rightly stresses the importance of early operation in
this condition. Treatment is by excising the sac and repairing the
abdominal wall, although this may have to be done in two stages,
using merely the skin on the first occasion.

Imperforate anus

In this congenital abnormality the lower part of the alimentary canal
fails to develop. It is surprising how often a baby is brought to a
doctor with a history of vomiting and distension soon after birth
without the proper diagnosis having been made. There are three
degrees of this condition (Fig. 28.2). In the first, at the site of the
anus, there is a layer of skin between the rectum and the surface and
when the baby strains, coughs or cries a bulge is seen where the
opening should be. Simple incision and regular dilatation cures the
condition (Fig. 28.3).

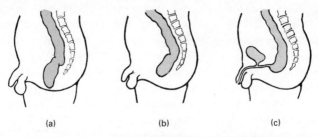

(a)   (b)   (c)

Fig. 28.2 Imperforate anus. From left to right, (a) Only skin covers the anus,
(b) More severe defect, (c) Long atretic area of the bowel. Bladder and urethral
fistula are also shown.

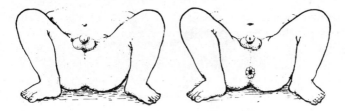

Fig. 28.3 Imperforate anus, before and after operation.

In the second degree, which is more severe, there is lack of development of the last 2 centimetres or more of the rectum and anal canal. This necessitates an operation carried out both by the abdominal and perineal route in order to mobilize the lower bowel sufficiently and bring it to the surface for anastomosis to the skin.

In the third and most severe degree, there is a long atretic area of lower bowel and it is necessary to perform a colostomy (transverse) to relieve the obstruction. Fistulas connecting bladder, urethra and vagina with the rectum often complicate the picture. Occasionally there is a small blind anal canal with an obstruction between it and the upper part of the alimentary tract.

Surgery of childhood

It is convenient here to consider the surgery of childhood, as opposed to the neonatal period, under two separate headings: in the first place there are conditions which require emergency surgery, and in the second there is a much larger group of conditions, usually congenital abnormalities, which can be treated at the time of choice.

Emergencies

Congenital hypertrophic pyloric stenosis. The baby, usually a male, starts to vomit at about 2 weeks of age. The vomiting becomes more and more forceful so that it is described as projectile. The baby seems to be always hungry, but loses weight and becomes dehydrated. The stools are scanty and green and the urine is concentrated.

This condition is due to hypertrophy of the muscle fibres constituting the inner circular layer at the pylorus and distal part of the stomach (Fig. 28.4). Careful examination of the baby's abdomen

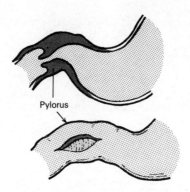

Fig. 28.4 Congenital pyloric stenosis. *Top*: section through the pylorus to show hypertrophied muscle. *Bottom*: Ramstedt's operation.

will often reveal visible peristalsis caused by the stomach trying to force its contents through the pylorus. It looks like a golf ball moving just below the surface from left to right across the upper abdomen. The diagnosis is confirmed by palpating the enlarged pylorus. To do this the nurse holds the baby on her lap and feeds him with a bottle. The surgeon, sitting on the baby's left, gently palpates the upper right abdomen just below the rib margin, the pylorus can be felt when it contracts, as an ovoid tumour.

Nursing care. Treatment consists of first correcting the dehydration and second relieving the pyloric obstruction. Dehydration is treated by intravenous infusion of fifth-normal saline. A rate of approximately 60 ml per kilogram body weight, twice in 24 hours is the usual amount. The stomach is washed out with a solution of normal saline; this is done twice daily and about an hour and a half before the baby is taken to the operating theatre. Great care is necessary to maintain body heat during operation and some surgeons ask for the baby to be bound to a 'crucifix' or padded wooden cross. When carrying the patient to and from the operating theatre the nurse must take great care that her movements are gentle. Premedication of atropine 0.3 mg by injection may be ordered.

The surgical correction of pyloric stenosis is known as Ramstedt's operation after the surgeon who introduced it, or pyloromyotomy. Either general or local anaesthesia is used and a small incision made in the upper right abdomen. The pyloric end of the stomach is lifted into the wound and a longitudinal incision made, followed by blunt dissection to split the thickened muscle coat right down to the mucosa, which is not opened. The abdominal wall is then closed and a dressing applied.

Postoperative nursing care. After operation the baby is nursed lying flat. Careful observations are important and it is usual to record the temperature at hourly intervals for 6 hours.

Feeding is started soon after operation, usually after about 2 hours, with a solution of glucose 5 per cent. Half-strength milk feeds follow and within 48 hours the baby should be back on a normal feeding régime. Some surgeons advocate that the baby should feed at the mother's breast soon after the operation.

The sutures, preferably subcuticular, are removed on the seventh or eighth day following operation. The baby, if well enough, goes home on the fourth day and is brought back to have the stitches removed. These patients are particularly prone to contract any infection present in the hospital, therefore they should be nursed in individual cubicles, preferably by mother. The sooner they can return home the safer they are.

Intussusception. In this condition, which is commonly seen in babies between the ages of 4 and 10 months, the bowel in the lower ileum telescopes on itself. A baby with intussusception is usually plump, healthy looking and often rather greedy. He suddenly draws up his legs and screams, goes pale due to the pain and often passes a motion which contains blood and mucus, giving it the appearance of red currant jelly, or blood may be seen on the finger cot after rectal examination.

The baby should be taken to hospital immediately. Dehydration is corrected by intravenous saline, as for pyloric stenosis, and a fine lubricated catheter is passed via the nose into the stomach so that its contents may be aspirated. It is noteworthy that these babies, being previously very fit and probably plump are often suffering more from shock than their appearance would suggest. At operation the telescoped bowel is gently milked back, but if the condition has been allowed to go on for more than 24 hours, the intussusception may be irreducible and the bowel requires excision and anastomosis, or short circuit.

The recovery rate is excellent provided the diagnosis is made in the first 24 hours and operation carried out forthwith. After this time the prognosis becomes progressively less good. In some hospitals an attempt is first made to reduce the intussusception by means of a barium enema.

Hirschsprung's disease. This is one of the causes of megacolon in infancy and childhood. The distal large bowel lacks a proper nerve plexus in its wall, is aganglionic and as a result cannot propel its contents. The normal colon proximal to this aganglionic segment becomes more and more dilated with faeces and the child has a swollen abdomen and becomes progressively constipated.

Treatment is by an operation called rectosigmoidectomy, in which the rectum and aganglionic segment of the colon is excised after pulling it through the anus. To do this it has first to be mobilized by an abdominal operation and the proximal colon is then sutured to the anal canal.

Congenital abnormalities requiring operation

Hernias in babies and children are common and present special problems.

Inguinal hernia. This is by far the commonest and when seen in the very small baby it is convenient to prescribe a rubber horse-shoe truss which can be worn the whole time. This keeps the hernia reduced and operation can then be carried out when the baby has been weaned; if the baby is bottle fed, then operation can be performed at any age which is convenient.

Umbilical hernia. In children this may be of two kinds. In the first year of life a direct bulge is seen at the site of the scar where the umbilical cord separated; it is particularly common in African and West Indian children. As time goes by, however, it corrects itself.

The other kind of umbilical hernia seen in children should really be called a *supra-umbilical hernia* since it occurs through a small triangular defect in the linea alba, just above the umbilicus. It is usually seen in girls at about 3 to 4 years of age. It is often made worse by coughing and constipation. A small surgical operation is necessary for its correction.

Cleft lip (hare lip). This condition results when the nasal and maxillary processes fail to unite properly. The cleft may be left, right or bilateral. It causes far more distress to the parents than to the baby, who can usually suck quite well. Treatment is by surgical operation, usually after 3 months of age. It is most desirable that the baby should be gaining weight, be fit and free from infection. These patients nowadays are often cared for in special plastic surgery units.

The baby is admitted to hospital a few days before operation and ideally the mother is admitted at the same time. It is important that the skin be in good condition with no spots or rashes. Before operation warmed clothing is put on and premedication given.

When the baby returns from the operating theatre it is most important that he have his own separate cubicle so as to avoid the risk of cross infection and preferably he shares it with his mother. He should be nursed lying flat with the head of the cot raised and the arms splinted for a few days following operation, while sedatives such as nepenthe and paraldehyde may be necessary. It is important that he should not cry, as this may damage the suture line, so he should be kept as contented as possible. There will be no dressing on the wound and it is important that this be kept clean and dry. Where there is much tension on the suture line, a Logan's bow is strapped to the cheeks to bring them together and relieve this tension.

It is usual to give the first feed on the morning of the day following operation and great care is needed to prevent infection of the suture line; the spoon and cup should be sterilized before each feed. The mouth must be carefully cleansed before and after feeding with a little sterile water.

The sutures are removed on the sixth to eighth day after operation. While this is being done, the baby should be on the nurse's lap, the head being firmly held, or a light anaesthetic may be given.

Cleft palate. This is a serious disability in which the child is born with a defect of the palate due to failure of the two halves to fuse in the midline. The baby cannot suck and the regurgitation of milk into the nasal cavity causes chronic infection so that there is usually a constant nasal discharge. Various degrees of severity are seen, the least serious being a cleft of the soft palate. In the more severe, both hard and soft palates are involved, while there may be the added complication of a unilateral or bilateral hare lip.

These babies are usually not subjected to operation for 2 or 3 years, and even then it may be necessary to remove the tonsils first, subsequently carrying out the treatment in stages. The baby is admitted to hospital some days before operation, and frequently anaemia is present and needs correction. Where facilities are available for the mother to be admitted with her child, this is advisable as mother will help to nurse the baby and there will be less crying and less general upset. The operation is a severe one and an intravenous infusion of saline or blood is necessary.

Postoperatively the child is nursed sitting up and the arms are splinted with cardboard so that the patient is unable to touch the wound. Drinks of one-fifth normal saline with 5 per cent glucose are given and the diet gradually increased until milk and finally solids are taken. Special care is needed to prevent infection of the wound. A sterile cup and spoon are used, and the spoon should be flattened at the end to avoid touching the roof of the mouth. After each feed 28 ml of sterile water is given, which helps to keep the mouth clean. A toddler's diet of soft food may be introduced about the seventh to eighth day following operation.

The hygiene of the mouth is important both before and after feeds. Cleansing is carried out very gently by irrigation, or a little cotton wool on an applicator with glycerine of thymol, or hydrogen peroxide may be used. The sutures may be of catgut, which will be absorbed, but if a non-absorbable substance is used a general anaesthetic is necessary in order to remove them. Finally, when the palate has healed, it is necessary for the child to receive speech therapy since the art of talking has to be learnt all over again in order to avoid the nasal twang which is so typical of this deformity.

Wry neck. Wry neck or torticollis has already been mentioned under deformities, but is referred to again here. It consists of shortening due to fibrosis of one sternomastoid muscle so that the head is pulled over to that side. If this condition is left uncorrected the baby develops asymmetry of the face, so that as time passes it will be noticed that the eyes are at different levels and one cheek much larger than the other. No amount of correction can give a good result after this has taken place. Treatment is therefore directed to stretching the muscle in the first weeks and months of life, and if this is not successful, carrying out a tenotomy or excision of the muscle at an early age before secondary changes occur.

Branchial cysts and fistulae. In early development the foetus passes through a stage when gill slits like those of fish are present. Part of these may survive in the adult and the remnants are referred to as branchial abnormalities. If part of such a slit becomes sequestrated, which means cut off from the rest of the tissues, a cyst is formed just behind the angle of the jaw, which contains fluid and cholesterin crystals. The cyst may produce no symptoms and may not even be noticed for many years. When the branchial cyst is infected, usually due to an attack of tonsillitis, an abscess forms. Typically a branchial cyst has many lymph nodes adherent to its wall. Treatment is by excision, but if infected, the abscess must first be drained.

A branchial cleft may remain patent on one side of the neck and take the form of a cervical sinus or branchial fistula. A tiny opening is seen in the skin at the level of the junction of the lower third and upper two-thirds of the sternomastoid muscle along its medial border and a little clear fluid oozes from the opening. The lesion may be bilateral. Infection eventually enters the fistula and causes recurring abscesses and scarring of the neck, therefore it is usual to excise the fistula in the first years of life. This is conveniently carried out through a series of step-ladder incisions which allow the track to be removed throughout most of its length. On the very rare occasions when the sinus is present throughout the entire length of the cleft, it opens immediately above the tonsil.

Cystic hygroma. This is a lymphangioma or tumour of lymphoid tissue which occurs in the neck in the newborn, or may develop in the first months of life. The swelling, which is often just behind the clavicles or in the nape of the neck, is brilliantly transilluminable and being multilocular cannot be aspirated with a needle. Excision is difficult since the tumour appears to infiltrate the tissues and plastic surgery may be necessary to produce a satisfactory result.

Thyroglossal cyst and fistula. The thyroid gland in development arises from the back of the tongue at the site of the foramen caecum. It descends into the neck to end up in front of the larynx and first rings of the trachea. In so doing it may leave behind it a track which opens in the neck as a thyroglossal fistula, or a small part of epithelium may develop into a cyst. This thyroglossal cyst is typically seen as a rounded midline swelling just above (or less often below) the hyoid bone (Fig. 28.5).

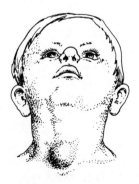

Fig. 28.5 Thyroglossal cyst in a baby.

Typically a thyroglossal cyst rises in the neck as the tongue is protruded, but, unlike the thyroid gland, does not move on swallowing. It may become infected so that it is preferable to remove it before this occurs. The operation is carried out through a transverse or crease incision and it is essential that the whole cyst together with the body of the hyoid bone be excised if recurrence is to be prevented.

A thyroglossal fistula discharges in the midline of the neck just above the manubrium sterni. If left, it soon becomes infected and scarred so that the opening becomes puckered. Treatment is by excision of the complete tract together with the hyoid bone to prevent recurrence.

Phimosis. This condition was referred to earlier, but it is convenient to recall it here. Phimosis means narrowing of the preputial opening and requires correction by the operation of circumcision. Phimosis is a rare condition in babies and is often erroneously thought to be present because the normal prepuce or foreskin cannot usually be retracted in the first year of life, so that at first glance it may appear to be constricted (see p. 230).

Hypospadias. This is a condition where the ventral surface of the penis is underdeveloped so that it is bowed. The urethra opens proximal to its normal site and there is an associated hooding of the prepuce. The bowing, or chordee, can be corrected in the first years of life, but surgical correction of the hypospadias is best postponed until 4 years of age (see p. 231).

Epispadias. This is a severe congenital abnormality in which the dorsal surface of the penis is underdeveloped. There may be incontinence with absence of the anterior bladder wall or *ectopia vesicae* (see p. 231).

Index

ether 86
ethmoidal sinus 125
ethmoidectomy 125
ethyl biscoumacetate 37
Ewing's tumour 282
exchange transfusion 41
exomphalos (omphalocele) 326
exophthalmos 315
exotoxins 18
external popliteal nerve damage 286
extradural haemorrhage 258
eye 313—21
  acuity 317
  anterior chamber 315
  examination 317—18
  fundus 314
    examination 318
  nursing treatment 318—20
  postoperative care 320—1
  visual fields 318
eyelids 316

Factor VIII (antihaemophiliac globulin) 37,
  44, 45
faecal fistula 102
Fallot's tetralogy 148
fat embolism 286
femoral arteriography 236
femoropopliteal bypass 236
fibrinogenemia 37
fibrocystic disease of bone 281
fibrocystic disease of pancreas 204
fibroma 70
fibrosis 4
fissure-in-ano (anal fissure) 191
fistula 27
fistula-in-ano (anal fistula) 27, 191
flat-foot (pes planus) 299—300
fluid(s)
  extracellular 49—50
  intracellular 49—50
  normal body 49—50
fluid balance 8, 49—51
  postoperative management 53—4, 96
fractures 284—92
  closed 284
  Colles' 288
  comminuted 284
  complicated 284—5
  complications: general 286
    local 285—6
  crush 284
  first-aid 287
  fissure 285
  greenstick 284
  healing of 286
  impacted 284
  instructions to patient 289 (fig)
  internal splinting 291
  maintenance of reduction 289
  open (compound) 284
  pathological 285
  rehabilitation 291—2
    occupational therapy 292
  skeletal traction 290

  nursing care 290—1
  skin traction 289—90
  symptoms and signs 285
  treatment 287—92
fragilitas ossium 285
frequency of micturition 210
fundoplication 145
furuncle (boil) 22, 303

galactocele 155
gall bladder 199
gall-stones (cholelithiasis) 200—3, 208
  operation 202—3
  postoperative care 203
  pre-operative treatment 202
  symptoms and signs 200—1
  tests 201—2
  types 200
ganglion 269
gangrene 15—16, 238
  diabetic 15
  post-fracture 285
  wet/dry 15—16
gas gangrene 23
gastrectomy
  Polya 174
  partial 174
gastric juice 167—8
gastric ulcer *see* peptic ulcer
gastrocnemius tear 266
gastroscopy 169—70
gastrostomy 176
gastrotomy 176
general paralysis of the insane 24
genito-urinary system 209—34
  blood tests 211—12
  cytoscopy 212
  frequency 210
  haematuria 45, 46, 210
  pain 209—10
  retention 210—11
  ultrasonography 213
  urine tests 211
  urography 212—13
    retrograde 213
genu recurvatum 298
genu valgum (knock-knee) 298
genu varum (bow-leg) 298
gibbus 264, 276
gingivitis 111
glioma 262
  of retina 314
goitre
  endemic 244—5
  malignant 246—7
  simple 244
  toxic 245
gold, radioactive 78
gonorrhoea 23, 229
Graves' disease *see* hyperthyroidism
gumma 24
gums 111
gynaecomastia 154

Haemaccel 42
haemangioma 70, 307